# ANNUAL REVIEW OF NURSING RESEARCH

VOLUME 37, 2019

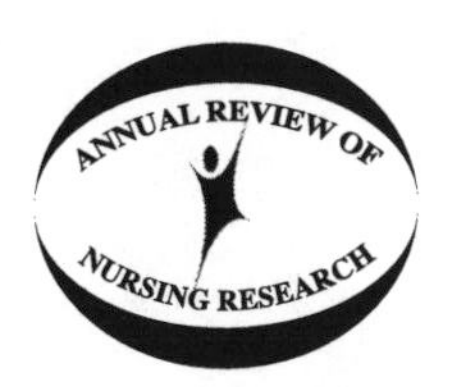

SERIES EDITOR

**Christine E. Kasper, PhD, RN, FAAN, FACSM**
Dean and Professor
Crenshaw Endowed Chair
University of New Mexico
College of Nursing
and
Professor, Daniel K. Inouye School of Nursing
Uniformed Services University of the Health Sciences,
Bethesda, MD

VOLUME EDITOR

**Rick Zoucha, PhD, PMHCNS-BC, CTN-A, FAAN**
Joseph A. Lauritis, C.S.Sp.
Endowed Chair for Teaching and Technology
Professor and Chair of Advanced Role and PhD Programs

# Annual Review of Nursing Research

## *Transcultural and Social Research*

VOLUME 37, 2019

*Series Editor*

CHRISTINE E. KASPER, PhD, RN, FAAN, FACSM

*Volume Editor*

RICK ZOUCHA, PhD, PMHCNS-BC, CTN-A, FAAN

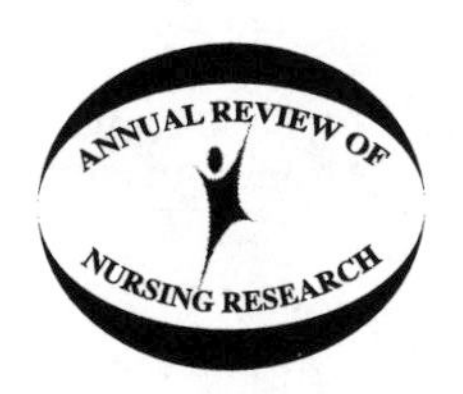


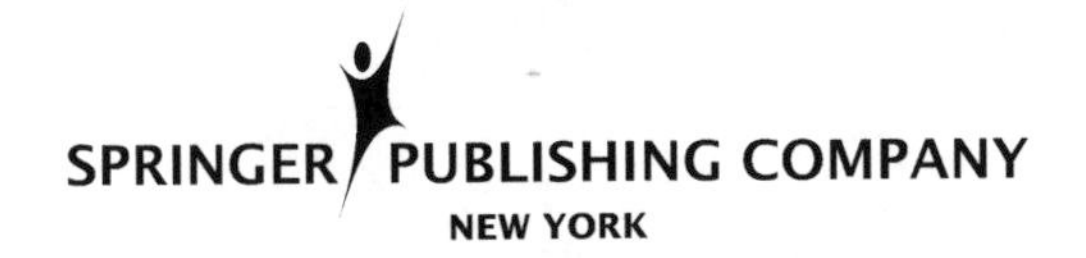

Springer Publishing Company, LLC
11 West 42nd Street
New York, NY 10036
www.springerpub.com

Composition: Exeter Premedia Services Private Ltd

ISBN: 978-0-8261-6205-2
e-book ISBN: 978-0-8261-6206-9
ISSN: 0739-6686
Online ISSN: 1944-4028

18 19 / 5 4 3 2 1

# Contents

# About the Volume Editor

**Rick Zoucha, PhD, PMHCNS-BC, CTN-A, FAAN,** is the Joseph A. Lauritis, C.S.Sp. Endowed Chair for Teaching and Technology, Professor and Chair of Advanced Role and PhD Programs at Duquesne University School of Nursing. He has a special interest in Transcultural and Global Nursing as well as Psychosocial Nursing. Dr. Zoucha has taught Transcultural Nursing in the BSN, Post-Master's, DNP, and PhD programs for the last 20 years. Dr. Zoucha teaches qualitative research methods in nursing in the PhD program. In addition, Dr. Zoucha is certified as an Advanced Practice Adult Psychiatric Mental Health Nurse, Clinical Nurse Specialist (Psychiatric Mental Health Clinical Nurse Specialist-Board Certified) by the American Nurses Credentialing Center. In addition, he is a Certified Transcultural Nurse-Advanced. Dr. Zoucha is a Fellow in the American Academy of Nursing.

His research interests include understanding various phenomena related to health and well-being in the Nicaraguan, Mexican American, African American, and African refugee and immigrant communities. Dr. Zoucha is a qualitative and mixed method researcher experienced in ethnography, ethnonursing, phenomenology, and participatory action research methods. He has served as PhD dissertation chair for studies seeking to understand cultural care phenomena related to people of the Puerto Rican, Taiwanese, Mexican American, African American, Peruvian, Dominican, Appalachian, and homeless cultures globally. He was inducted as a Transcultural Nursing Scholar in 2004. Dr. Zoucha was bestowed the Leininger Award in 1998. Dr. Zoucha has been invited to speak at national and international conferences as well as Visiting Professor/Scholar in Puerto Rico, Spain, New Jersey, Taiwan, Australia, and North Dakota regarding issues of cultural care.

# Contributors

**Michael J. Deem, PhD**
Assistant Professor
School of Nursing and Center for Healthcare Ethics
Duquesne University
Pittsburgh, PA

**Sr. Rosemary Donley, PhD, APRN-BC, FAAN**
Professor
Jacques Laval Chair for Social Justice
School of Nursing
Duquesne University
Pittsburgh, PA

**Yovanska Duarté-Vélez, PhD**
Assistant Professor
Department of Psychiatry and Human Behavior
Brown University
Providence, RI

**Griselle Batista Estrada, MSN, RN**
Clinical Assistant Professor
College of Nursing and Health Innovation
University of Texas at Arlington
Arlington, TX

**Abimbola Fapohunda, DrPH**
Faculty
Department of African Studies
University of Pittsburgh
Pittsburgh, PA

**Marianne R. Jeffreys, EdD, RN**
Professor, Nursing
The City University of New York (CUNY)
Graduate College, New York, NY and
CUNY College of Staten Island
Staten Island, NY

**Melissa A. Kalarchian, PhD**
Professor of Nursing and Psychology
Duquesne University
Pittsburgh, PA

**Carmen Kiraly, PhD(c), APRN**
Professor
School of Nursing
Suffolk County Community College
Brentwood, NY

**Chai Lo, DNP, PMHNP-BC**
Psychiatric Mental Health Nurse
Hennepin County Medical Center
Minneapolis, MN

**Joan Such Lockhart, PhD, RN, AOCN, CNE, ANEF, FAAN**
Professor and MSN Nursing Education Track Coordinator
Duquesne University School of Nursing
Pittsburgh, PA

**David A. Nolfi, MLS, AHIP**
Head, Research Engagement, Health Sciences/STEM Initiatives
Assessment Coordinator
Gumberg Library
Duquesne University
Pittsburgh, PA

**Melinda G. Oberleitner, DNS, RN**
Interim Dean, College of Nursing and Allied Health Professions
Professor, Department of Nursing
SLEMCO/BORSF Endowed Professor in Nursing
University of Louisiana at Lafayette
Lafayette, LA

**Drew Y. Sagar, MS, RN, ANP-C, PMHNP-C, PNP-BC**
Northeast Center for Brain Injury
Psychiatric Nurse Practitioner
Lake Katrine, NY

**Priscilla Limbo Sagar, EdD, RN, ACNS-BC, CTN-A**
Professor Emeritus of Nursing
Mount Saint Mary College
Newburgh, NY

**L. Kathleen Sekula, PhD, PMHCNS, FAAN**
Professor
School of Nursing
Duquesne University
Pittsburgh, PA

**Ashley Smith, RPN, BScPN, SANE-A, SANE-P**
Clinical Coordinator
SANE Clinic
Winnipeg, Manitoba, Canada

**Felicia Stokes, JD, MA, RN**
Director
American Nurses Association
Center for Ethics and Human Rights
Silver Spring, MD

**Melanie T. Turk, PhD, RN**
Associate Professor
School of Nursing
Duquesne University
Pittsburgh, PA

**Katelin N. Umland, MS, PMHNP-BC**
Psychiatric Mental Health Nurse Practitioner
Hennepin County Medical Center
Minneapolis, MN

**Hiba B. Wehbe-Alamah, PhD, RN, FNP-BC, CTN-A**
Professor, School of Nursing
University of Michigan
Flint, MI

**Kimberly M. Wolf, PhD, PMHCNS-BC**
Adjunct Faculty, Duquesne University
Pittsburgh, PA
Adult Psychiatric Mental Health Clinical Nurse Specialist
Hennepin County Medical Center
Minneapolis, MN

**Rick Zoucha, PhD, PMHCNS-BC, CTN-A, FAAN**
Professor and Chair of Advanced Role and PhD Programs
Duquesne University School of Nursing
Pittsburgh, PA

# Preface

Considering current and global events it is becoming more and more evident that the dissemination of Transcultural and Social research is imperative in addressing the growing health needs of a diverse population in the United States and globally. The purpose of this volume is to present to readers current and cutting-edge theoretical knowledge related to transcultural and social research in the context of nursing and health care. Volume 37 in the *Annual Review of Nursing Research* addresses the needs of those receiving care and care providers through the in-depth presentation of research and knowledge generation regarding transcultural nursing and health care.

The notion of culture and care is not a new phenomenon of interest in nursing and health care. Over 60 years ago nurse theorist and pioneer Madeleine Leininger considered and asserted that culture and nursing were linked and must be understood in the context of a relationship between culture and nursing care phenomena. She wisely asserted that there are "many cultures one world" and felt that caring in the context of culture can change the world. She considered that creating a caring environment in the family, then moving to local, regional, national and ultimately to a global view would have a lasting impact on nursing and health care. Culture and caring must always be considered and understood not only from the individual perspective but also the family and community. Leininger believed that culture influences human care beliefs and practices related to health, illness and well-being or to face death and disability (McFarland & Wehbe-Alamah, 2018).

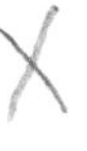

With the historical work of Leininger and those that followed, Volume 37 continues the journey of addressing the theoretical, educational, research and clinical work of scholars in promoting transcultural and social research. This work can serve as a guide for knowledge attainment, ideas regarding future research, informing practice and nursing and health care education.

In this volume readers will first be introduced to Leininger's Culture Care Diversity and Universality Theory as a foundation for the historical and theoretical work of Leininger. In addition, the chapter discusses the discipline of transcultural nursing and the continuing work of McFarland and Wehbe-Alamah. This is followed by the current state of Transcultural nursing theories, models and approaches by Sagar and Sagar. In addition, readers will be engaged in the most recent evidenced based updates regarding Jeffreys' cultural competence and confidence framework for nursing education. This set of works provides the reader with an introduction and foundation to the expanding scope of historical and current transcultural nursing theories models and approaches including application for nursing education. The presentation of transcultural theories, models and approaches is imperative in providing a grounding to understand and consider the remaining chapters in the volume.

In Volume 37, current issues related to culture have been added to provide a contemporary view of the needs of people of a variety of cultures, settings and specific health concerns. For this volume, the notion of culture includes racial and ethnic culture but has been expanded to cover sub cultures related to health, well-being and advocacy. In chapters 4 through 10, this volume tackles important issues such as Hispanic/Latino/Immigrant cancer survivor experiences, and cultural factors influencing suicide in Puerto Ricans. The volume addresses other important current issues such as transcultural mental health, forensic nursing practice, nursing ethics and a view of political and policy cultures affecting health.

The authors invited to publish in Volume 37 are considered experts in their areas of research, education, theory and clinical practice. They have provided cutting edge research and knowledge to inform the work of nurses and other health care professionals regardless of the culture and context of their work. The body of knowledge in nursing is always evolving and continues to provide a foundation and theoretical basis for the work of nurse scholars in research, education and practice. Volume 37 of the *Annual Review of Nursing Research* the transcultural and social research issue will provide a foundation and allow readers to move beyond their current view of culture and care to that of advocate and action taker in their context. To remind us of the words of Madeline Leininger, "Many cultures, one world" we do indeed have a say.

## REFERENCE

McFarland, M., & Wehbe-Alamah, H. (2018). *Transcultural nursing concepts, theories, Research, & practice* (4th ed.). New York, NY: McGraw-Hill.

*Rick Zoucha, PhD, PMHCNS-BC, CTN-A, FAAN*
*Volume Editor*

CHAPTER 1

# Leininger's Culture Care Diversity and Universality Theory

## *Classic and New Contributions*

Hiba B. Wehbe-Alamah

**ABSTRACT**

Introduction: Nurses and other healthcare providers need theoretical knowledge and practical skills to provide the people they care for with culturally congruent, competent, and sensitive care. Recognizing this need, Madeleine M. Leininger endeavored over six decades to establish the discipline of transcultural nursing. She developed a theory and research method designed to guide nurses to (a) understand cultural similarities and differences in how people care for themselves and others during health, illness, disability, dying, and death, and (b) provide culturally congruent, competent, and sensitive care. Purpose: The purpose of this article is to provide a brief overview of Leininger's theory of Culture Care Diversity and Universality, also known as the Culture Care Theory (CCT), and the related Ethnonursing Research Method (ERM). New developments to the CCT and ERM will be described. The CCT contributions to theory development, research, and scholarship will be highlighted. Conclusion: Findings from transcultural studies may help nurses provide culturally congruent care to diverse individuals, families, and populations.


http://dx.doi.org/10.1891/0739-6686.37.1

## INTRODUCTION

In a world characterized by increasing diversity and decreasing geographic boundaries, nurses and other healthcare providers need theoretical knowledge and practical skills to provide the people they care for with culturally congruent, competent, and sensitive care. Dr. Madeleine Leininger (1925–2012), an internationally renowned nurse theorist, researcher, educator, administrator, author, consultant, public speaker, scholar, human rights advocate, and leader in the field of Transcultural Nursing (Ray, 2013; Wehbe-Alamah, 2017) recognized this need in the early 1950s while working with children of diverse cultural backgrounds as a clinical mental health specialist in a child guidance center (McFarland & Wehbe-Alamah, 2015).

Over six decades, she proceeded to establish the discipline of transcultural nursing, developed and revised the Theory of Culture Care Diversity and Universality (also known as the Culture Care Theory, or CCT) and the Ethnonursing Research Method (ERM), founded the Transcultural Nursing Society in 1974, and established the *Journal of Transcultural Nursing* in 1989 (Wehbe-Alamah, 2017). She added to the body of transcultural nursing knowledge by contributing to more than 30 books, 300 articles, 60 book chapters, over 1,000 keynote addresses in the United States and around the world (Leininger's Info-Facts, 2008; McFarland, 2018b), and numerous audio and video recordings (Wayne, 2014). Leininger designed the CCT and ERM to help nurses (a) understand cultural similarities and differences in how people care for themselves and others during health, illness, disability, dying, and death, and (b) provide culturally congruent, competent, and sensitive care. The purpose of this manuscript is to provide an overview of the historical evolution and new developments to the CCT, and classic and new contributions to theory development, research, and scholarship. Applications of the CCT to theory development, research and scholarship will also be shared.

## HISTORICAL DEVELOPMENT

As a student pursuing a PhD in cultural and social anthropology in the mid-1960s, Leininger lived for 2 years with the indigenous Gadsup people of the Eastern Highlands of New Guinea (Leininger, 1966, 1995b, 1996; McFarland, 2018c). While observing and studying their cultural beliefs and practices, she noted striking differences and similarities in care and health practices between their non-Western culture and her own Western culture (Leininger, 1966; Leininger & McFarland, 2002, 2006). She began developing her CCT and ERM, which incurred numerous revisions and refinements over time (Leininger, 1978, 1985, 1991, 1995b; McFarland, 2018c). Many of these revisions were inspired by her students' research that she chaired or advised (Wehbe-Alamah, 2017).

Over the span of six decades, her theory, research method, and prolific intellectual contributions helped to establish the field of transcultural nursing and guided nurses and others in their scholarly pursuits toward understanding cultural diversities (differences) and universalities (commonalities) among people worldwide (Leininger & McFarland, 2002, 2006; McFarland, 2018c; Wehbe-Alamah, 2018d). A review of the literature completed in April 2017 identified 361documented studies conducted within the theoretical framework of the CCT (Wehbe-Alamah, 2018e). In 2012, Dr. Leininger charged Dr. Marilyn McFarland (first-generation mentee) and Dr. Hiba Wehbe-Alamah (second-generation mentee) with the continuation of her work with the CCT and the ERM. She continued to actively contribute to her work until her passing on August 10, 2012 and had two chapters (Leininger, 2015a, 2015b) published posthumously in the 2015 third edition of *Leininger's Culture Care Diversity and Universality: A Worldwide Nursing Theory* by McFarland and Wehbe-Alamah (McFarland, 2018b). During her lifetime, Dr. Leininger influenced and inspired many nurses to continue to explore new transcultural directions, theories, educational approaches, and areas of scholarship (McFarland, 2018c, p. 4).

## OVERVIEW OF THE CULTURE CARE THEORY

### Purpose and Goal

The purpose of the Theory of Culture Care Diversity and Universality is to discover, document, know, and explain the interdependence of care and culture phenomena with differences and similarities between and among cultures (McFarland & Wehbe-Alamah, 2015, pp. 5–6). The goal of the theory is to provide culturally congruent care that contributes to the health and wellbeing of people or to help them face disabilities, dying, or death using the three modes of culture care decisions and actions (McFarland, 2018b, p. 40).

### Major Tenets and Assumptive Premises

The CCT embodies four major tenets or positions developed and held by Dr Leininger. These are:

- Culture care expressions, meanings, patterns, and practices are diverse and yet there are shared commonalities and some universal attributes;
- Worldview, multiple social structure factors, ethnohistory, environmental context, language, and generic and professional care are critical influencers of culture care patterns to predict health, wellbeing, illness, healing, and ways people face disabilities and death;
- Generic emic (folk) and etic (professional) health factors in different environmental contexts greatly influence health and illness outcomes; and

- From an analysis of the above influencers, three major decision and action modes (culture care preservation and/or maintenance; culture care accommodation and/or negotiation; and culture care repatterning and/or restructuring) were predicted to provide ways to provide culturally congruent, safe, and meaningful health care to cultures (McFarland, 2018b, p. 41).

These major theoretical tenets led to the formulation of specific theoretical hunches or assumptive premises. These assumptions were derived from works with the theory and from subsequent evolving changes that were discovered and/or confirmed by Dr. Leininger and other researchers. The assumptive premises of the CCT include:

- Care is the essence and central dominant, distinct, and unifying focus of nursing;
- Humanistic and scientific care is essential for human growth, wellbeing, health, survival, and to face dying, death, and disabilities;
- Care (caring) is essential to curing or healing for there can be no curing without caring (this assumption was held to have profound relevance worldwide);
- Culture care is the synthesis of two major constructs [culture and care] that guide the researcher to discover, explain, and account for health, wellbeing, care expressions, and other human conditions;
- Culture care expressions, meanings, patterns, processes, and structural forms are diverse but some commonalities (universalities) exist among and between cultures;
- Culture care values, beliefs, and practices are influenced by and embedded in the worldview, social structure factors (e.g., [spirituality] religion, philosophy of life, kinship, politics, economics, education, technology, biological factors [new revision/addition], and cultural values) and the ethnohistorical and environmental contexts;
- Every culture has generic [lay, folk, naturalistic; mainly emic] and usually some professional [etic] care to be discovered and used for culturally congruent care practices;
- Culturally congruent and therapeutic care occurs when culture care values, beliefs, expressions, and patterns are explicitly known and used appropriately, sensitively, and meaningfully with people of diverse or similar cultures;
- Leininger's three theoretical modes of care offer new, creative, and different therapeutic ways to help people of diverse cultures;
- The Ethnonursing Research Method and other qualitative research paradigmatic methods offer important means to discover largely embedded, covert, epistemic, and ontological culture care knowledge and practices; and,

- Transcultural nursing is a discipline with a body of knowledge and practices to attain and maintain the goal of culturally congruent care for health and wellbeing (McFarland & Wehbe-Alamah, 2015, pp. 8–9).

## Central Constructs and Orientational Definitions of the Culture Care Theory

Leininger identified several central constructs used in the Culture Care Theory (Leininger, 1991, 1995b; Leininger & McFarland, 2002, 2006; McFarland & Wehbe-Alamah, 2015). These constructs have been described, adapted, and expanded in numerous ethnonursing studies by Leininger and other researchers (Leininger, 2015a; Mixer, 2015; Strang & Mixer, 2018). Leininger developed orientational definitions for the identified central constructs of her theory (Leininger, 1991, 1996, 2006). She maintained that orientational (not operational) definitions enable researchers to be open to the discovery of new theoretical construct dimensions and new qualitative knowledge from diverse cultural groups (McFarland, 2018b).

Following is a description of select central constructs definitions:

- *Care* refers to both an abstract and/or a concrete phenomenon. Leininger defined *care* as those assistive, supportive, and enabling experiences or ideas toward others (Leininger, 1995a, 2002a, 2006; McFarland, 2018b; McFarland & Wehbe-Alamah, 2015). *Caring* refers to actions, attitudes, and practices to assist or help others toward healing and wellbeing (Leininger, 1995a, 2002a, 2006; McFarland, 2018b; McFarland & Wehbe-Alamah, 2015). About 185 care/caring constructs have been discovered and supported in numerous studies conceptualized within the CCT between 1966 and 2016 (McFarland, 2018b). Some of the newest discovered care/caring constructs include collaborative care (McFarland & Leininger, via videotape, October 20, 2011); language as protective care (Wehbe-Alamah, 2015, 2018a); father protective care (Leininger, 2015a); mentoring and co-mentoring as care (Mixer, 2011); and herbs/community as care (Strang & Mixer, 2015).
- *Culture* refers to culture as the "learned, shared, and transmitted values, beliefs, norms, and lifeways of a particular culture that guide thinking, decisions, and actions in patterned ways… Culture can be viewed as the blueprint for guiding human actions and decisions and includes material and nonmaterial features of any group or individual… Culture is more than ethnicity or social relationships" (McFarland & Wehbe-Alamah, 2015, p. 10).

- *Generic (emic) care* refers to the "learned and transmitted lay, indigenous, traditional, or local folk (emic) knowledge and practices that are assistive, supportive, enabling, and facilitative acts for or toward others with evident or anticipated health needs in order to improve wellbeing or to help with dying or other human conditions" (McFarland & Wehbe-Alamah, 2015, p. 14).
- *Professional (etic) care* refers to "formal and explicit cognitively learned professional care knowledge and practices obtained generally through educational institutions" (McFarland & Wehbe-Alamah, 2015, p. 14).
- *Integrative care* refers to "safe, congruent, and creative ways of blending together holistic, generic, and professional care knowledge and practices so that the client experiences beneficial outcomes for wellbeing or to ameliorate a human condition or lifeway" (Leininger, 2002b, pp. 148–149). Leininger viewed integrative care as the preferred means to providing culturally congruent care (Wehbe-Alamah, 2018c). Through further development and evolution of Leininger's earlier work, Wehbe-Alamah & McFarland (2015a) recently added this construct to the CCT and the Sunrise Enabler. In the revised 2018 Sunrise Enabler (Figure 1.1), Integrative Care replaces Nursing Care Practices as the linking construct between Generic (folk) and Professional Care-Cure Practices in recognition of the integrative nature of culturally congruent care that transculturally prepared nurses and other healthcare providers could provide (McFarland, 2018b).
- *Culturally congruent care* refers to "culturally based care knowledge, decisions, and actions used in sensitive and knowledgeable ways to appropriately and meaningfully fit the cultural values, beliefs, and lifeways of clients for their health and wellbeing, or to prevent disabilities, illness, or death" (Leininger, 2006; McFarland & Wehbe-Alamah, 2015).
- *Culture care diversity* refers to "the differences or variabilities among human beings regarding culture care meanings, patterns, values, lifeways, symbols, or other features related to providing beneficial care to clients of a designated culture" (Leininger, 2002a, 2006; McFarland & Wehbe-Alamah, 2015, Wehbe-Alamah, 2018b).
- *Culture care universality* refers to "the commonly shared or similar culture care phenomena features of individuals or groups with recurrent meanings, patterns, values, lifeways, or symbols that serve as a guide for caregivers to provide assistive, supportive, facilitative, or enabling people care for healthy outcomes" (Leininger, 2006; McFarland & Wehbe-Alamah, 2015).

**Leininger's Sunrise Enabler to Discover Culture Care**

**CULTURE CARE**

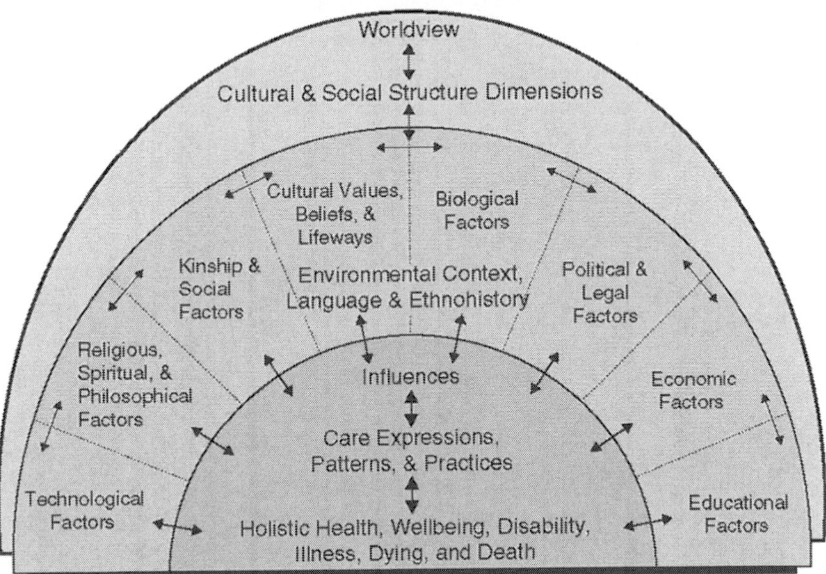


**Focus: Individuals, Families, Groups, Communities, or Institutions in Diverse Health Contexts of**

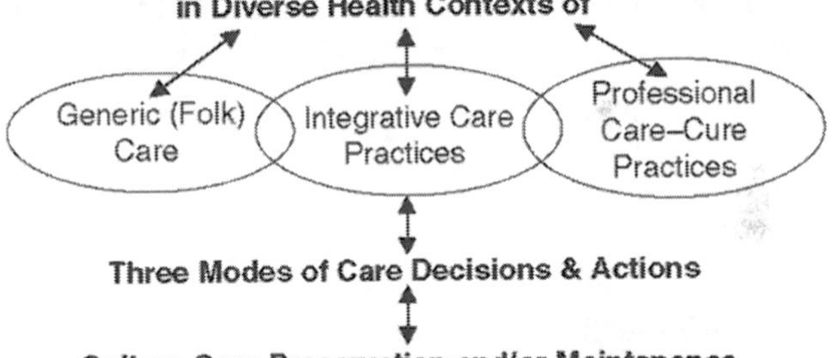


**Culture Care Preservation and/or Maintenance**
**Culture Care Accommodation and/or Negotiation**
**Culture Care Repatterning and/or Restructuring**

**Code:** ↔ (Influencers)



**Culturally Congruent Care for Holistic Health, Wellbeing, Disability, Illness, Dying, and Death**

FIGURE 1.1 Leininger's Sunrise Enabler to discover culture care. Used with permission by McFarland, M. & Wehbe-Alamah, H. (2018). *Transcultural Nursing Concepts, Theories, Research, & Practice* (4th ed., pp. 47). New York, NY: McGraw-Hill Education.

## THE ETHNONURSING RESEARCH METHOD

Dr. Leininger developed the ERM to facilitate the discovery of data focused on the CCT. While the CCT may be used with the ERM or other research methods, the ERM was designed for use specifically with the CCT. Ethnonursing is a qualitative nursing research method focused on naturalistic, open discovery and largely inductive (emic) modes and processes with diverse strategies, techniques, and enabling guides to document, describe, explain, and interpret people's worldview, meanings, symbols, life experiences, and other related aspects, as they bear on actual or potential nursing care phenomena (Leininger, 2002a; Wehbe-Alamah & McFarland, 2015b, p. 37). The central purpose of the ERM is "to establish a naturalistic and largely emic open inquiry discovery method to explicate and study nursing phenomena related to the Theory of Culture Care Diversity and Universality" (Wehbe-Alamah & McFarland, 2015b, p. 39). Inherent in ethnonursing research is an open inquiry approach that focuses on the discovery of insiders' (emic) as well as outsiders' (etic) knowledge related to holistic health care (Leininger, 2006; Wehbe-Alamah, 2018e).

Ethnonursing researchers focus on discovering healthcare beliefs, expressions, and practices related to worldview, cultural and social structure dimensions, environmental context, language, ethnohistory, generic (folk) care, integrative care, professional care practices, and other additional areas of the people's cultural lifeways (Leininger, 2006; Wehbe-Alamah, 2018e). They rely on a detailed guide to using the ERM and use criteria to evaluate qualitative research studies to evaluate their research findings (Wehbe-Alamah, 2018e, pp. 78–83). Their discovery is facilitated through the use of enablers or facilitators that serve to assist them as they examine the major tenets of the CCT and the domain of inquiry under study (Leininger, 2002a, 2006; Wehbe-Alamah, 2018e).

Ethnonursing researchers choose a combination of the following enablers as befitting the purpose, goal, and research questions of their study: The Sunrise Enabler to Discover Culture Care (Figure 1.1); Leininger's Stranger-to-Trusted-Friend Enabler; Observation-Participation-Reflection Enabler; Semi-Structured Inquiry Guide Enabler to Assess Culture Care and Health; Acculturation Health Care Assessment Enabler for Cultural Patterns in Traditional and Nontraditional Lifeways; Phases of Ethnonursing Data Analysis Enabler for Qualitative Data; The Leininger-Templin-Thompson (LTT) Ethnoscript Coding Enabler; and The Life History Health Care Enabler (Wehbe-Alamah, 2018e). Resulting qualitative data is abstracted into patterns and universal and/or diverse themes relevant to the population under study and are supported by descriptors provided by study informants as well as researchers' observations and/or reflections. Findings from ethnonursing research studies add to the body of transcultural nursing knowledge and guide nurses and others in providing culturally congruent and sensitive care to people of diverse cultural backgrounds through the use of the three culture care modes: Culture care preservation and/or maintenance, culture care accommodation and/or negotiation, and culture care repatterning and/or restructuring. However, study findings are not generalized to other similar or different cultural groups and do not negate the need for individualized cultural assessments.

## NEWEST REVISION TO THE CCT AND ERM

The CCT and ERM incurred numerous revisions over the course of six decades. Regional, national, and global care and health needs necessitate an ongoing evolution which is manifested by new revisions introduced in 2018 by McFarland & Wehbe-Alamah which include (Wehbe-Alamah, 2018d):

- Introduction of Biological Factors as a new construct to the CCT and a new addition to the Cultural and Social Structure dimension of the Sunrise Enabler to emphasize the importance of assessing hereditary and genetic illnesses and culture-bound syndromes that influence and are influenced by generic and professional care expressions, patterns, and practices (McFarland, 2018b; Wehbe-Alamah, 2018e).
- Revision of CCT and Sunrise Enabler to introduce construct of Integrative Care as previously discussed.
- Revision of Leininger's *Semi-Structured Inquiry Guide Enabler to Assess Culture Care and Health* involving major edits and updates to previous questions embedded under each inquiry mode; addition of a Biological Factors section with newly developed open-ended questions; and separation of the previous Professional and Generic Care Beliefs and Practices inquiry mode into two distinct sections: "Professional Care Beliefs and Practices" and "Generic (folk or lay) Care Beliefs and Practices" (Wehbe-Alamah, 2018e).
- Revision to the order and language content of Leininger's *Phases of Ethnonursing Data Analysis Enabler for Qualitative Data* (Wehbe-Alamah, 2018e).
- Introduction of minor edits to language used in all other enablers.

## CONTRIBUTIONS OF THE CCT

### Theory Development

Sagar (2018) described the influences of Leininger's Culture Care Theory on the development of subsequent transcultural theories, models, and guides. She confirmed her interpretation with relevant authors of respective guides and models that were inspired by the CCT. According to her, Leininger's Theory of Culture

Care, "Diversity and Universality has had a lasting effect not only in the provision of culturally congruent care for diverse individuals, groups, and communities but also by influencing new theories, models, and guides" (Sagar, 2018, p. 93). Select transcultural models and guides that have been influenced by Leininger's CCT are described below.

In 1991, Campinha-Bacote developed the first version of the *Process of Cultural Competence in the Delivery of Healthcare Services,* which was inspired by the earlier work of Leininger (1978), Cross et al. (1989), Pedersen (1988), Kleinman (1978), and Law (1993) (as cited by Campinha-Bacote, 2015; personal communication, March 27, 2018). This model was revised in 1998, 2002, and finally in 2010. In 2005, Campinha-Bacote (personal communication, March 27, 2018) developed the *Biblically Based Model of Cultural Competence in the Delivery of Healthcare Services* (Campinha-Bacote, 2005), which was also inspired by Leininger's CCT (Leininger & McFarland, 2006), as well as her own work (Campinha-Bacote, 2008), and that of others (Chapman, 2005; Cross et al., 1989; Kleinman, 1980; Law, 1993; Pederson, 1988; Wilkerson, 2002; Wood, 1998 as cited by Campinha-Bacote, 2015; Sagar, 2018, p. 88). Her Inventory for Assessing the Process of Cultural Competence Among Healthcare Professionals-Revised (IAPCC-R), Inventory for Assessing the Process of Cultural Competence Among Healthcare Professionals-Student Version (IAPCC-SV), Inventory for Assessing A Biblically Based Worldview of Cultural Competence Among Healthcare Professionals (IABWCC), and Inventory for Assessing the Process of Cultural Competence Among Healthcare Professionals in Mentoring (IAPCC-M) are also partially inspired by Leininger's work (personal communication, March 27, 2018). These instruments have been translated into several languages and used in the US and worldwide (Campinha-Bacote, 2015).

The *Andrews/Boyle Transcultural Nursing Assessment Guide for Individuals and Families (TCNGIF),* originally developed in 1986 (personal communication, March 28, 2018; Andrews, 1998; Andrews & Boyle, 2016), included 12 aspects of Leininger's social structure factors. Similarly, the *Andrews/Boyle Transcultural Nursing Assessment Guide for Groups and Communities* (TCNAGGC) incorporated eight major categories of Leininger's social structure factors (Sagar, 2018). Likewise, the *Andrews/Boyle Transcultural Nursing Assessment Guide for Health Care Organizations and Facilities* included nine areas from Leininger's social structure factors (Boyle, Andrews, & Ludwig-Beymer, 2012). These guides assist nurses and others with performing cultural and physical assessments that are imperative for the provision of culturally congruent care (Sagar, 2012, 2014, 2018).

Other transcultural models that were partially influenced by Leininger's Culture Care Theory include but are not limited to Giger and Davidhizar's (2004, 2008) Transcultural Assessment Model (TAM), Pacquaio's (2012) Model for

Culturally Competent Ethical Decision Making, Ray's (2010, 2016) Transcultural Caring Dynamics in Nursing and Health Care (TCDNHC) Model (Sagar, 2018), Jeffreys' Cultural Competence and Confidence Model (personal communication, March 28, 2018; Jeffreys, 2016), Lovering's (2012) Crescent of Care Model and the Model for Creating a Culturally Sensitive and Welcoming Academic Environment (Wehbe-Alamah & Fry, 2014).

In addition, the American Association of Colleges of Nursing (AACN, 2008) developed the *Tool Kit of Resources for Cultural Competent Education for Baccalaureate Nurses*. This document uses Leininger's Culture Care Theory (Leininger & McFarland, 2006), along with Campinha-Bacote's (2008) *Model of Cultural Competence* (most current version known as *Process of Cultural Competence in the Delivery of Healthcare Services*); Giger and Davidhizar's (2008) *Model of Transcultural Nursing*; Purnell's (2008) *Model of Transcultural Health Care;* and Spector's (2004) *Health Traditions Model.* Similarly, AACN's *Tool Kit for Cultural Competence in Master's and Doctoral Nursing Education* uses Leininger's Culture Care Theory, along with the four aforementioned nursing models, in addition to Jeffreys' (2016) *Cultural Competence and Confidence Model* (AACN, 2011). Both documents are vital in promoting cultural competence among baccalaureate and graduate nursing students (Sagar, 2018).

## Research

A review of the literature conducted in April 2017 using the search terms *Ethnonursing*, *Culture Care*, and *Leininger* resulted in the identification of 361 master's and doctoral studies (Wehbe-Alamah, 2018e, p. 79). This number does not include other studies that have been completed outside of academic requirements for graduate studies or studies that have been completed but not published. A review of journal and other publications of research conceptualized within the framework of the CCT and published between January 2013 and March 2018 confirmed that the CCT was used in numerous studies with different research designs including but not limited to ethnonursing, ethnography, phenomenology, and/or components of all of the above.

Studies using the CCT that have been published within the last 5 years are presented below according to year of publication:

- malaria care in the Maasailand (Strang & Mixer, 2018)
- linguistic conceptualizations of disease among the Luo of Kenya (Ojwang, 2018)
- culture expressions, meanings, beliefs, and practices of Mexican American women during the postpartum period (Hascup, 2018)

- social–cultural, religious, and health system barriers to hepatitis B screening among Hmong Americans (Fang, 2016; Fang & Stewart, 2018)
- community-informed health promotion to improve health behaviors in Honduras (Sullivan & Bettger, 2018, 2016)
- African American childbearing women in the Military Health System (Scott, 2017)
- unavoidable pressure ulcers (Clarey-Sanford, 2017)
- barriers to health care for Nigerian immigrants (Nwamu, 2017)
- Iranian–American older adults' attitudes and proactive actions toward planning ahead for end-of-life care (Rahemi, 2017)
- healing practices and medical plants use for riparian Brazilian mothers in early childhood care (Lima, Turrini, Silva, de Mero, & Augusto, 2017)
- African American children with autism (Burkett, Morris, Anthony, Shambley-Ebron, & Manning-Courtney, 2017; Burkett, Morris, Manning-Courtney, Anthony, & Shambley-Ebron, 2015)
- cultural influences of self-management of diabetes in coastal Kenya (Abdulrehman, Woith, Jenkins, Kossman, & Hunter, 2016)
- female genital mutilation (Jiménez-Ruiz & Almansa Martínez, 2017)
- exploring sexual history taking (Sowicz, 2016)
- nursing faculty's feelings of teaching cultural competence in the nursing education curriculum (Kalinowski, 2016)
- cultural care practices of pregnant teenagers in Barranquilla, Colombia (Muñoz-Henríquez, 2016)
- social support in family care of children with diabetes in Brazil (Pennafort, Queiroz, Nascimento, & Guedes, 2016)
- traditional practices in postnatal management among mothers in select Indian areas (Matere, 2016)
- needs of parents in caring for their children in a pediatric intensive care unit in Columbia (Sanabria & de Rodriguez, 2016)
- Somali immigrant new mothers' childbirth experiences (Missal, Clark, & Kovaleva, 2016)
- Somali immigrant perceptions of mental health and illness (Wolf et al, 2016)
- complexity of bipolar disorder (Stiles, 2016)
- sociocultural factors contributing to HIV risk among Ayoreo Bolivian sex workers (López Entrambasaguas, Granero-Molina, Hernández-Padilla, & Fernández-Sola, 2015)
- trust in qualitative research with culturally diverse participants (Burkett & Morris, 2015)
- studies of cancer survivors (Farren, 2015)
- Islamic values and nursing practice in Kuwait (Atkinson, 2015)

- health-related beliefs, practices, and experiences of migrant Dominicans in the northeastern United States (Sobon Sensor, 2015)
- application of the CCT in teaching cultural competence (Mixer, 2015)
- care provided to Arab Muslim clients with type 2 diabetes in Australia (Hussein, 2014)
- culture care experiences of Puerto Rican families with a child with special healthcare needs as perceived by the family caregiver (Rousseau, 2015)
- African American freshman students' experiences with stress and weight gain (Darden, 2015)
- Urban African American adolescent gang members (Morris, 2015)
- complementary and alternative medicine by Thai breast cancer survivors (Wanchai, Armer, & Stewart, 2012, 2015)
- end-of-life factors affecting nurse's ability to cope with culturally diverse patients and families (Popescu & Rosh, 2014)
- end-of-life care for rural Appalachian people and their families (Mixer, Fornehed, Varney, & Lindley, 2014)
- the applicability of the CCT on research published in the journals of Nursing in Brazil (Camargo et al., 2014)
- culture care beliefs and practices of Ethiopian immigrants (Chiatti, 2014)
- South Sudanese refugee women's healthcare access and use (Okegbile, 2014)
- nurses' ability to care within the culture of incarceration (Christensen, 2014)
- healthcare beliefs and practices of rural mestizo Ecuadorians (Moss, 2014)
- experience of fathers during the hospitalization of a preterm newborn in Bogota (Cañas-Lopera, 2014)
- lived experience of newly licensed registered nurses enrolled in a RN–BS completion program participating in a cultural and clinical immersion experience in Senegal (Patenaude, 2014)
- experiences of refugee women in a perinatal nutrition education program (Smith, 2014)
- practices and experiences of nurses working on a pediatric bone marrow transplant unit (Morrison & Morris, 2014)
- prenatal health behaviors of women from four cultural groups in Turkey (Taşçı-Duran & Sevil, 2013)
- adult inpatient falls (Rogers, 2013)
- use of culturally focused literature to enhance cultural competence of nursing students (Jenkins, 2013)
- culture care meanings and care expressions of men with a spinal cord injury from the Appalachian region of west Virginia (Imes, 2013)
- women's well-being and reproductive health in Indian mining community (D'Souza, Karkada, Somayaji, & Venkatesaperumal, 2013)

- faculty health and wellbeing (Mixer, McFarland, Andrews, & Strang, 2013)
- cultural meanings and practices of clinical nurse council leaders in shared governance (Allen, 2013)
- family homelessness and effect of substance abuse on social support systems (Clark & Lee, 2013)

An observed new and emerging trend is the use of the CCT by graduate students enrolled in Doctor of Nursing Practice programs in the conceptualization of translational scholarly projects focusing on clinical practice (McFarland, 2018a). Examples include:

- Using transcultural nursing education to increase staff cultural sensitivity and cultural assessment documentation in an in-home chronic disease self-management program (Neilly, Rader, Baker, Wehbe-Alamah, & Murray-Wright, 2018)
- Reducing 30-day emergency department visits and readmissions of bariatric surgical patients effectively through cultural competency training of nurses (Coleman, Garretson, Wehbe-Alamah, McFarland, & Wood, 2016)
- Implementation of hypertension and diabetes chronic disease management in an adult group in Les Bours, Haiti (Kelch, Wehbe-Alamah, & McFarland, 2015)
- Using Leininger's CCT as the building block for cultural competence and cultural assessment for a collaborative care team in a primary care setting (Courtney & Wolgamott, 2015)
- Advancing cultural assessments in palliative care using web-based transcultural education (Bhat, Wehbe-Alamah, McFarland, Filter, & Keiser, 2015)

### Other Scholarly Applications

Numerous other scholarly applications for the CCT have been noted. The CCT was used as the theoretical framework for the design and development in 2010 of the first prototype of a cultural simulation computer game, CultureCopia© (Wehbe-Alamah et al., 2015). In addition, the CCT has provided a conceptual framework for federal and other grants focused on or incorporating elements of cultural competence in academe and clinical practice (Andrews & Collins, 2015; Creech, Wehbe-Alamah, & Andrews, 2011–2015), and provided the groundwork for designing international service learning experiences and/or transcultural global courses (D'Appolonia & Kneckt Sabatine, 2015; Larson, 2015; Zoucha & Turk, 2015).

The Sunrise Enabler (Figure 1.1) is "a cognitive map of the Culture Care Theory and a visualization aid to see and to assess different holistic factors that tend to influence the care, health, wellbeing, disability, illness, death and dying of individuals, families, groups, communities, or institutions in their naturalistic settings" (Wehbe-Alamah, 2018e, p. 60). It has been used to assess, understand, and develop culturally congruent care approaches to diverse cultural groups. Accordingly, Lee (2018) shared the application of the CCT & Sunrise Enabler in understanding the culture care needs of Appalachian mothers experiencing homelessness and identified how the three modes of culture care decisions and actions can be used to provide them with culturally congruent and sensitive care. The same approach was used for highlighting the culture care needs of Haitians (Kelch & Wehbe-Alamah, 2018), Taiwanese (Chiang-Hanisko, 2018), Yupiit Alaska Natives (Embler, Weiss, & Mixer, 2018), and Lebanese and Syrian Muslims (Wehbe-Alamah, 2015). The CCT was also used to present cultural assessment findings and culturally congruent care approaches to select health-care issues such as childhood obesity (Wehbe-Alamah, Mixer, Collins, & Wright, 2010) and mental health (Vossos & Wehbe-Alamah, 2018).

## CONCLUSION

While Madeleine Leininger may have been the nursing theorist who provided a theoretical foundation for transcultural nursing, one must not forget the many others who built on her work and generated valuable transcultural models, guidelines, and instruments/tools. Researchers from all around the world have used the CCT alone or in conjunction with the ERM or other research methodologies to add to the vast body of transcultural nursing knowledge. Providing culturally congruent care that is respectful of diverse cultural beliefs, values, and practices is a moral and ethical responsibility for providers and a human right for recipients of professional care.

## REFERENCES

Abdulrehman, M. S., Woith, W., Jenkins, S., Kossman, S., & Hunter, G. L. (2016). Exploring cultural influences of self-management of diabetes in coastal Kenya: An ethnography. *Global Qualitative Nursing Research, 3*. http://dx.doi.org/10.1177/2333393616641825

Allen, S. R. (2013). An ethnonursing study of the cultural meanings and practices of clinical nurse council leaders in shared governance. ProQuest Dissertations Publishing.

American Association of Colleges of Nursing. (2008). *Tool kit of Resources for Cultural Competent Education for Baccalaureate Nurses*. Retrieved from http://www.aacnnursing.org/Portals/42/AcademicNursing/CurriculumGuidelines/Cultural-Competency-Bacc-Tool-Kit.pdf?ver=2017-05-18-143552-023

American Association of Colleges of Nursing. (2011). *Toolkit for cultural competence in master's and doctoral nursing education*. Retrieved from http://www.aacnnursing.org/Portals/42/AcademicNursing/CurriculumGuidelines/Cultural-Competency-Grad-Tool-Kit.pdf?ver=2017-05-18-143552-180

Andrews, M. (1998). A model for cultural change. *Nursing Management, 66*, 62–64.

Andrews, M. M., & Boyle, J. S. (2016). *Transcultural concepts in nursing care* (7th ed.). Philadelphia, PA: Wolters Kluwer/Lippincott Williams & Wilkins.

Andrews, M., & Collins, J. (2015). Using the Culture Care Theory as the organizing framework for a federal project on cultural competence. In M. McFarland & H. Wehbe-Alamah (Eds.), *Culture care diversity and universality: A worldwide nursing theory* (pp. 537–552). Burlington, MA: Jones and Bartlett Publishers, Inc.

Atkinson, C. (2015). Islamic values and nursing practice in Kuwait. *Journal of Holistic Nursing, 33*(3), 195–204. http://dx.doi.org/10.1177/0898010114564682

Bhat, A., Wehbe-Alamah, H., McFarland, M., Filter, M., & Keiser, M. (2015). Advancing cultural assessments in palliative care using web-based education. *Journal of Hospice and Palliative Care Nursing, 17*(4), 348–355.

Boyle, J. S., Andrews, M. M., & Ludwig-Beymer, P. (2012). Andrews/Boyle transcultural nursing assessment guide for health care organizations and facilities. In M. M. Andrews & J. S. Boyle (Eds.), *Transcultural concepts in nursing care* (6th ed., pp. 459–461). Philadelphia, PA: Wolters Kluwer|Lippincott Williams & Wilkins.

Burkett, K., & Morris, E. (2015). Enabling trust in qualitative research with culturally diverse participants. *Journal of Pediatric Health Care, 29*(1), 108–112. http://dx.doi.org/10.1016/j.pedhc.2014.06.002

Burkett, K., Morris, E., Anthony, J., Shambley-Ebron, D., & Manning-Courtney, P. (2017). Parenting African American children with autism: The influence of respect and faith in mother, father, single-, and two-parent care. *Journal of Transcultural Nursing, 28*(5), 496–504. http://dx.doi.org/10.1177/1043659616662316

Burkett, K., Morris, E., Manning-Courtney, P., Anthony, J., & Shambley-Ebron, D. (2015). African American families on autism diagnosis and treatment: The influence of culture. *Journal of Autism and Developmental Disorders, 45*(10), 3244–3254. http://dx.doi.org/10.1007/s10803-015-2482-x

Camargo, F., da Silva, R., Lima, A., dos Santos, L., da Silva, S., & dos Santos, I. (2014). The applicability of the theory of cultural care from nurses in periodics about health of Brazil (1992 – 2011). *Revista De Pesquisa, Cuidado é Fundamental Online, 6*(4), 1743.

Campinha-Bacote, J. (2005). *A biblically based model of cultural competence in the delivery of healthcare services*. Cincinnati, OH: Transcultural C.A.R.E. Associates.

Campinha-Bacote, J. (2008). The process of cultural competence in the delivery of healthcare services at. Retrieved from http://transculturalcare.net/the-process-of-cultural-competence-in-the-delivery-of-healthcare-services/

Campinha-Bacote, J. (2015). A biblically based model of cultural competence. Retrieved from http://transculturalcare.net/a-biblically-based-model-of-cultural-competence/

Cañas-Lopera, E. M. (2014). The experience of fathers during the hospitalization of a preterm newborn. La experiencia del padre durante la hospitalización de su hijo recién nacido pretérmino extremo. *Aquichan, 14*(3), 336–350.

Chiang-Hanisko, L. (2018). Transcultural nursing and health care in Taiwan. In M. McFarland & H. Wehbe-Alamah (Eds.), *Transcultural Nursing Concepts, Theories, Research, & Practice* (pp. 273–284). New York, NY: McGraw-Hill Education.

Chiatti, B. D. (2014). *Culture care beliefs and practices of an Ethiopian immigrant community: An ethnonursing study*. ProQuest Dissertations Publishing.

Christensen, S. (2014). Enhancing nurses' ability to care within the culture of incarceration. *Journal of Transcultural Nursing, 25*(3), 223–231. http://dx.doi.org/10.1177/1043659613515276

Clarey-Sanford, C. (2017). *Unavoidable pressure ulcers: An ethnonursing study*. ProQuest Dissertations Publishing.

Clark, A., & Lee, R. C. (2013). Transitioning through family homelessness and the effect of substance abuse on social support systems. *Western Journal of Nursing Research, 35*(9), 1230–1231. http://dx.doi.org/10.1177/0193945913487171

Coleman, S. K., Garretson, B. C., Wehbe-Alamah, H., McFarland, R., & Wood, M. (2016). RESPECT: Reducing 30-day emergency department visits and readmissions of bariatric surgical patients effectively through cultural competency training of nurses. *Online Journal of Cultural Competence in Nursing and Healthcare*, 6(1), 31–51. http://dx.doi.org/10.9730/ojccnh.org/v6n1a3

Courtney, R., & Wolgamott, S. (2015). Using Leininger's Theory as the building blocks for cultural competence and cultural assessment for a collaborative care team in a primary care setting. In M. McFarland, & H. Wehbe-Alamah (Eds.), *Culture Care Diversity and Universality: A Worldwide Nursing Theory* (pp. 345–368). Burlington, MA: Jones and Bartlett Publishers, Inc.

Creech, C., & Wehbe-Alamah, H., & Andrews, M. (2011–2015). *The University of Michigan-Flint Initiative to Strengthen Care to Underserved Populations (UM-FISCUP)*. Funded by U.S. Department of Health and Human Services, Health Resources and Services Administration, Advanced Education Nursing. Grant # D09HP22631.

D'Appolonia Knecht, L., & Knecht Sabatine, C. (2015). Application of Culture Care Theory to International Service- Learning Experiences in Kenya. In M. McFarland & H. Wehbe-Alamah (Eds.), *Culture care diversity and universality: A worldwide nursing theory* (pp. 475–501). Burlington, MA: Jones and Bartlett Publishers, Inc.

Darden, S. (2015). *How are the dimensions of technology, culture, kinship, and economics and the experience of stress described by African American students who gained weight during their freshman year in college?* ProQuest Dissertations Publishing.

D'Souza, M. S., Karkada, S. N., Somayaji, G., & Venkatesaperumal, R. (2013). Women's well-being and reproductive health in Indian mining community: Need for empowerment. *Reproductive Health, 10*(1), 24–24. http://dx.doi.org/10.1186/1742-4755-10-24

Embler, P., Weiss, M., & Mixer, S. (2018). Yuppit: Alaska Native People of Southwest Alaska. In McFarland, M. & Wehbe-Alamah, H. (Eds.), *Transcultural Nursing Concepts, Theories, Research, & Practice* (pp. 369–383). New York, NY: McGraw-Hill Education.

Fang, D. M. (2016). *Social-cultural, religious, and health system barriers to hepatitis B screening among Hmong: A case study*. ProQuest Dissertations Publishing.

Fang, D. M., & Stewart, S. L. (2018). Social–cultural, traditional beliefs, and health system barriers of hepatitis B screening among Hmong Americans: A case study. *Cancer, 124*, 1576–1582. http://dx.doi.org/10.1002/cncr.31096

Farren, A. T. (2015). Leininger's ethnonursing research methodology and studies of cancer survivors: A review. *Journal of Transcultural Nursing: Official Journal of the Transcultural Nursing Society / Transcultural Nursing Society, 26*(4), 418.

Giger, J. N., & Davidhizar, R. E. (2004). *Transcultural nursing: Assessment and intervention* (4th ed.). St. Louis, MO: Mosby Elsevier.

Giger, J. N., & Davidhizar, R. E. (2008). *Transcultural nursing: Assessment and intervention* (5th ed.). St. Louis, MO: Mosby Elsevier.

Hascup, V. (2018). Culture expressions, meanings, beliefs, and practices of Mexican American women during the postpartum period: An Ethnonursing Study. In M. McFarland & H. Wehbe-Alamah (Eds.), *Transcultural Nursing Concepts, Theories, Research, & Practice* (pp. 399–420). New York, NY: McGraw-Hill.

Hussein, A. (2014). An examination of the care provided to Arab Muslim clients with type 2 diabetes receiving health care in Australia in order to expand our understanding of culturally congruent care (Doctoral Dissertation). Retrieved from The Sydney eScholarship Repository. (http://hdl.handle.net/2123/13143)

Imes, H. S. B. (2013). *Discovering the culture care meanings and care expressions of men with a spinal cord injury from the Appalachian region of west Virginia: An ethnonursing study* (Order No. 3605252). ProQuest Dissertations & Theses Global (1477999542).

Jeffreys, M. R. (2016). *Teaching cultural competence in nursing and health care: Inquiry, action, and innovation*. New York, NY: Springer Publishing.

Jenkins, O. (2013). *Does use of culturally focused literature enhance cultural competence of nursing students?* ProQuest Dissertations Publishing.

Jiménez-Ruiz, I., & Almansa Martínez, P. (2017). Female genital mutilation and transcultural nursing: Adaptation of the rising sun model. *Contemporary Nurse, 53*(2), 196–197. http://dx.doi.org/10.1080/10376178.2016.1261000

Kalinowski, M. (2016). *Nursing faculty's feelings of teaching cultural competence in the nursing education curriculum.* ProQuest Dissertations Publishing.

Kelch, R., & Wehbe-Alamah, H. (2018). Providing culturally congruent care to Haitians using Leininger's Culture Care Theory. In M. McFarland & H. Wehbe-Alamah (Eds.), *Transcultural nursing concepts, theories, research, & practice* (pp. 232–250). New York, NY: McGraw-Hill.

Kelch, R., Wehbe-Alamah, H., & McFarland, M. (2015). Implementation of hypertension and diabetes chronic disease management in an adult group in Les Bours, Haiti. *Online Journal of Cultural Competence in Nursing and Healthcare, 5*(1), 50–63. http://dx.doi.org/10.9730/ojccnh.org/v5n1a4

Larson, M. (2015). The Greek connection: Discovering the cultural and social structure dimensions of the greek culture using Leininger's Theory of Culture Care: A model for a Baccalaureate Study-Abroad Experience. In M. McFarland & H. Wehbe-Alamah (Eds.), *Culture care diversity and universality: A worldwide nursing theory* (pp. 503–520). Burlington, MA: Jones and Bartlett Publishers, Inc.

Lee, R. (2018). Understanding the culture care needs of Appalachian mothers experiencing homelessness. In M. McFarland, & H. Wehbe-Alamah (Eds.), *Transcultural nursing concepts, theories, research, & practice* (pp. 385–398). New York, NY: McGraw-Hill.

Leininger, M. M. (1966). *Convergence and divergence of human behavior: An ethnopsychological comparative study of two Gadsup villages in the Eastern Highlands of New Guinea.* Doctoral dissertation. Seattle, WA: The University of Washington.

Leininger, M. M. (Ed.). (1978). *Transcultural nursing: Concepts, theories, and practice.* New York, NY: John Wiley & Sons.

Leininger, M. M. (1985). Transcultural care diversity and universality: A theory of nursing. *Nursing and Health Care, 6*(4), 202–212.

Leininger, M. M. (Ed.). (1991). *Culture care diversity and universality: A theory of nursing.* New York, NY: National League for Nursing Press.

Leininger, M. M. (1995a). Overview of Leininger's Culture Care Theory. In M. M. Leininger (Ed.), *Transcultural nursing: Concepts, theories, and practice* (2nd ed., pp. 93–114). Columbus, OH: McGraw-Hill College Custom Series.

Leininger, M. M. (1995b). *Transcultural nursing: Concepts, theories, and practice* (2nd ed.). Columbus, OH: McGraw-Hill College Custom Series.

Leininger, M. M. (1996). Culture care theory, research and practice. *Nursing Science Quarterly, 9*(2), 71–78.

Leininger, M. M. (2002a). Part I. The theory of culture care and the Ethnonursing Research Method. In M. M. Leininger & M. R. McFarland (Eds.), *Transcultural nursing: Concepts, theories, research, & practice* (3rd ed., pp. 71–98). New York, NY: McGraw-Hill Medical Publishing Division.

Leininger, M. M. (2002b). Part I. Toward integrative generic and professional health care. In M. M. Leininger & M. R. McFarland (Eds.), *Transcultural nursing: Concepts, theories, research, & practice* (3rd ed., pp. 145–154). New York, NY: McGraw-Hill Medical Publishing Division.

Leininger, M. M. (2006). Culture care diversity and universality theory and evolution of the Ethnonursing Method. In M. M. Leininger & M. R. McFarland (Eds.), *Culture care diversity and universality: A worldwide nursing theory* (2nd ed., pp. 1-41). Sudbury, MA: Jones & Bartlett Learning.

Leininger, M. M. (2015a). Leininger's Father Protective Care. In M. R. McFarland & H. B. Wehbe-Alamah (Eds.), *Leininger's culture care diversity and universality: A worldwide nursing theory* [Revised by H. B. Wehbe-Alamah] (3rd ed., pp. 119–136). Burlington, MA: Jones and Bartlett Learning.

Leininger, M. (2015b). The benefits of the Culture Care Theory and a look to the future for transcultural nursing. In M. McFarland & H. Wehbe-Alamah (Eds.), *Culture care diversity and universality: A worldwide nursing theory* (pp. 101–118). Burlington, MA: Jones and Bartlett Learning.

Leininger's Info-Facts. (2008). *Information and facts about Dr. Madeleine Leininger.* Retrieved from http://www.madeleine-leininger.com/cc/infofacts.pdf

Leininger, M., & McFarland, M. (2002). *Transcultural nursing concepts, theories, research, & practice* (3rd ed.). New York, NY: McGraw-Hill.

Leininger, M., & McFarland, M. (2006). *Culture care diversity and universality: A worldwide nursing theory* (2nd ed.). Burlington, MA: Jones and Bartlett Publishers, Inc.

Lima, R. F., Turrini, R. N., Silva, L. R., de Melo, L. D., & Augusto, S. I. (2017). Popular healing practices and medical plants use for riparian mothers in early childhood care. *Revista De Pesquisa, Cuidado é Fundamental Online, 9*(4), 1154–1163. http://dx.doi.org/10.9789/2175-5361.2017.v9i4.1154-1163

López Entrambasaguas, O. M., Granero-Molina, J., Hernández-Padilla, J., & Fernández-Sola, C. (2015). Understanding sociocultural factors contributing to HIV risk among Ayoreo Bolivian sex workers. *The Journal of the Association of Nurses in AIDS Care : JANAC, 26*(6), 781–793. http://dx.doi.org/10.1016/j.jana.2015.08.003

Lovering, S. (2012). The crescent of care: a nursing model to guide the care of Arab Muslim patients. *Diversity and Equality in Health and Care, 9*, 171–178.

Matere, K. V. (2016). Selected traditional practices among postnatal mothers. *Asian Journal of Nursing Education and Research, 6*(1), 11–16. http://dx.doi.org/10.5958/2349-2996.2016.00004.5

McFarland, M. R. (2018a). Culture care theory and translational science: A focus for Doctor of Nursing Practice scholarship. In M. R. McFarland & H. B. Wehbe-Alamah (Eds.), *Transcultural nursing: Concepts, theories, research, and practice* (pp.313–319). New York, NY: McGraw-Hill.

McFarland, M. R. (2018b). The theory of culture care diversity and universality. In M. R. McFarland & H. B. Wehbe-Alamah (Eds.), *Transcultural nursing: Concepts, theories, research, and practice* (pp.39–56). New York, NY: McGraw-Hill.

McFarland, M. R. (2018c). Transcultural nursing: History, focus, and future directions. In M. R. McFarland & H. B. Wehbe-Alamah (Eds.), *Transcultural nursing: Concepts, theories, research, and practice* (pp.3–11). New York, NY: McGraw-Hill.

McFarland, M. R. (with M. M. Leininger via videotape). (2011, October 20). *The Culture Care Theory and a look to the future for transcultural nursing.* Keynote Address presented at the 37th Annual International Conference of the Transcultural Nursing Society, Las Vegas, NV.

McFarland, M., & Wehbe-Alamah, H. (2015). The theory of culture care civersity and universality. In M. McFarland & H. Wehbe-Alamah (Eds.), *Culture care diversity and universality: A worldwide nursing theory* (pp. 1–34). Burlington, MA: Jones and Bartlett Publishers, Inc.

McFarland, M., & Wehbe-Alamah, H. (2018). *Transcultural nursing concepts, theories, research, & practice.* (4th ed.). New York, NY: McGraw-Hill

Missal, B., Clark, C., & Kovaleva, M. (2016). Somali immigrant new mothers' childbirth experiences in Minnesota. *Journal of Transcultural Nursing, 27*(4), 359–367. http://dx.doi.org/10.1177/1043659614565248

Mixer, S. J. (2011). Use of the Culture Care Theory to discover nursing faculty care expressions, patterns, and practices related to teaching culture care. *The Online Journal of Cultural Competence in Nursing and Healthcare, 1*(1), 3–14.

Mixer, S. J. (2015). Application of Culture Care Theory in teaching cultural competence and culturally congruent care. In M. McFarland & H. Wehbe-Alamah (Eds.), *Culture care diversity and universality: A worldwide nursing theory* (pp. 369–387). Burlington, MA: Jones and Bartlett Publishers, Inc.

Mixer, S. J., Fornehed, M. L., Varney, J., & Lindley, L. C. (2014). Culturally congruent end-of-life care for rural Appalachian people and their families. *Journal of Hospice & Palliative Nursing, 16*(8), 526–535. http://dx.doi.org/10.1097/NJH.0000000000000114

Mixer, S. J., McFarland, M. R., Andrews, M. M., & Strang, C. W. (2013). Exploring faculty health and wellbeing: Creating a caring scholarly community. *Nurse Education Today, 33*(12), 1471–1476. http://dx.doi.org/10.1016/j.nedt.2013.05.019

Morris, E. (2015). An examination of subculture as a theoretical social construct through an ethnonursing study of Urban African American Adolescent gang members. In M. McFarland & H. Wehbe-Alamah (Eds.), *Culture care diversity and universality: A worldwide nursing theory* (pp. 255–285). Burlington, MA: Jones and Bartlett Publishers, Inc.

Morrison, C., & Morris, E. (2014). Practices and experiences of nurses working on a pediatric bone marrow transplant unit. *Biology of Blood and Marrow Transplantation, 20*(2), S101. http://dx.doi.org/10.1016/j.bbmt.2013.12.136

Moss, J. A. (2014). Discovering the healthcare beliefs and practices of rural mestizo Ecuadorians. an ethnonursing study. *Investigación y Educación En Enfermería, 32*(2), 326–336.

Muñoz-Henríquez, M. (2016). What cultural care practices mean to pregnant teenagers in Barranquilla (Colombia). *Aquichan, 16*(1), 43–55.

Neilly, C., Baker, S., Rader, A., Wehbe-Alamah, H., & Murray-Wright, M. (2018, March). *Using transcultural nursing education to increase cultural sensitivity and cultural assessment documentation by staff of an in-home chronic disease self-management program.* Poster presented at the 17th Annual Michigan Council of Nurse Practitioner Conference, Detroit, MI.

Nwamu, A. (2017). *Barriers to healthcare: A phenomenological study of Nigerian immigrants.* ProQuest Dissertations Publishing.

Ojwang, B. O. (2018). Linguistic conceptualizations of disease among the Luo of Kenya. *Qualitative Health Research, 28*(3), 433–445. http://dx.doi.org/10.1177/1049732317747875

Okegbile, E. O. (2014). *South Sudanese refugee women's healthcare access and use.* ProQuest Dissertations Publishing.

Pacquaio, D. F. (2012). Cultural competence in ethical decision making. In M. M. Andrews & J. S. Boyle (Eds.), *Transcultural concepts in nursing care* (6th ed., pp. 403–420). Philadelphia, PA: Wolters Kluwer|Lippincott Williams & Wilkins.

Patenaude, K. J. (2014). Exploring the lived experience of newly licensed registered nurses enrolled in a RN-BS completion program participating in a cultural and clinical immersion experience in Senegal, west Africa. ProQuest Dissertations Publishing.

Pennafort, V. P., Queiroz, M. V., Nascimento, L. C., & Guedes, M. V. (2016). Network and social support in family care of children with diabetes. *Revista Brasileira De Enfermagem, 69*(5), 856. http://dx.doi.org/10.1590/0034-7167-2015-0085

Popescu, L., & Rosh, E. A. (2014). Transcultural nursing in the end-of-life: Factors affecting nurse's ability to cope with culturally diverse patients and families. *Revista De Asistenţă Socială*, (2), 89–101.

Purnell, L. D. (2008). The Purnell model for cultural competence. In L. D. Purnell & B. J. Paulanka (Eds.), *Transcultural health care: A culturally competent approach* (3rd ed., pp. 15–44). Philadelphia, PA: FA Davis.

Rahemi, Z. (2017). Iranian-American older adults' attitudes and proactive actions toward planning ahead for end-of-life care. ProQuest Dissertations Publishing.

Ray, M. A. (2010). *Transcultural caring dynamics in nursing and health care*. Philadelphia, PA: FA Davis.

Ray, M. A. (2013). Madeleine M. Leininger, 1925–2012. *Qualitative Health Research, 23*(1), 142–144. http://dx.doi.org/10.1177/1049732312464578

Ray, M. A. (2016). *Transcultural caring dynamics in nursing and health care* (2nd ed.). Philadelphia, PA: FA Davis.

Rogers, L. M. (2013). *Opening the black box: Understanding adult inpatient falls*. ProQuest Dissertations Publishing.

Rousseau, K. (2015). *An exploration of the culture care experiences of Puerto Rican families with a child with special health care needs as perceived by the family caregiver*. ProQuest Dissertations Publishing.

Sagar, P. L. (2012). *Transcultural nursing theory and models: Application in nursing education, practice, and administration*. New York, NY: Springer Publishing.

Sagar, P. L. (2014). *Transcultural nursing education strategies*. New York, NY: Springer Publishing.

Sagar, P. (2018). Culture Care Theory: A trailblazing theory. In McFarland, M. & Wehbe-Alamah, H. (Eds.), *Transcultural nursing concepts, theories, research, & practice* (pp. 85–96). New York, NY: McGraw-Hill.

Sanabria, M. L., & de Rodríguez, L. D. (2016). Needs of parents in caring for their children in a pediatric intensive care unit/Necesidades de los padres para cuidar a sus hijos en una unidad de cuidados intensivos Pediátrica/Necessidades dos padres para cuidar aos seus filhos numa unidade de tratamento intensivos pediátrica. *Investigación y Educación En Enfermería, 34*(1), 29. http://dx.doi.org/10.17533/udea.iee.v34n1a04

Scott, T. H. (2017). *Perceptions of care during the prenatal period: An ethnonursing study of African American childbearing women in the Military Health System*. ProQuest Dissertations Publishing.

Smith, M. (2014). *The experience of refugee women in a perinatal nutrition education program*. ProQuest Dissertations Publishing.

Sobon Sensor, C. (2015). *Health-related beliefs, practices and experiences of migrant Dominicans in the northeastern United States*. ProQuest Dissertations Publishing.

Sowicz, T. J. (2016). *Exploring sexual history taking in one health center: A focused ethnography*. ProQuest Dissertations Publishing.

Spector, R. E. (2004). *Cultural diversity in health and illness* (6th ed.). Upper Saddle River, NJ: Pearson Education.

Stiles, B. M. (2016). *Identifying the complexity of bipolar disorder: A focused ethnography*. ProQuest Dissertations Publishing.

Strang, C. W., & Mixer, S. J. (2015). Discovery of the meanings, expressions, and practices related to malaria care among the Maasai. *Journal of Transcultural Nursing, 27*(4), 333–341. Advance online publication. http://dx.doi.org/10.1177/1043659615573841

Strang, C., & Mixer, S. (2018). Culturally competent research using the Culture Care Theory: Malaria Care in Maasailand. In M. McFarland & H. Wehbe-Alamah (Eds.), *Transcultural nursing concepts, theories, research, & practice* (pp. 339–358). New York, NY: McGraw-Hill.

Sullivan, B. J., & Bettger, J. P. (2018, 2016). Community-informed health promotion to improve health behaviors in Honduras. *Journal of Transcultural Nursing, 29*(1), 14–20. http://dx.doi.org/10.1177/1043659616670214

Taşçı-Duran, E., & Sevil, U. (2013). A comparison of the prenatal health behaviors of women from four cultural groups in Turkey: An ethnonursing study. *Nursing Science Quarterly, 26*(3), 257–266. http://dx.doi.org/10.1177/0894318413489180

Vossos, H., & Wehbe-Alamah, H. (2018). Using a culturally congruent approach in mental health care. In M. McFarland & H. Wehbe-Alamah (Eds.), *Transcultural nursing concepts, theories, research, & practice* (pp. 199–213). New York, NY: McGraw-Hill.

Wanchai, A., Armer, J. M., & Stewart, B. R. (2012). Performance care practices in complementary and alternative medicine by Thai breast cancer survivors: An ethnonursing study. *Nursing & Health Sciences, 14*(3), 339–344. http://dx.doi.org/10.1111/j.1442-2018.2012.00730.x

Wanchai, A., Armer, J. M., & Stewart, B. R. (2015). Thai nurses' perspectives on the use of complementary and alternative medicine among Thai breast cancer survivors in northern Thailand. *International Journal of Nursing Practice, 21*(2), 118–124. http://dx.doi.org/10.1111/ijn.12231

Wayne, G. (2014). *Madeleine M. Leininger: The founder of transcultural nursing*. Retrieved from https://nurseslabs.com/madeleine-leininger

Wehbe-Alamah, H. (2015). Folk care beliefs and practices of traditional Lebanese and Syrian Muslims in the Midwestern United States. In M. McFarland & H. Wehbe-Alamah (Eds.), *Culture care diversity and universality: A worldwide nursing theory* (pp. 137–182). Burlington, MA: Jones and Bartlett Publishers, Learning.

Wehbe-Alamah, H. (2017). *Historical development and worldwide contributions of the Transcultural Nursing Society, in memory and honor of founder, Dr. Madeleine Leininger*. Video presented at the 42nd Annual Conference of the Transcultural Nursing Society in New Orleans, LA.

Wehbe-Alamah, H. (2018a). Culture care of Syrian Muslims in the Midwestern United States: An ethnonursing research study. In M. McFarland & H. Wehbe-Alamah (Eds.), *Transcultural nursing concepts, theories, research, & practice* (pp. 421–432). New York, NY: McGraw-Hill.

Wehbe-Alamah, H. (2018b). Essential transcultural nursing care concepts, principles, guidelines, and policy statements for culturally congruent and competent health care practice, education, and research. In M. McFarland & H. Wehbe-Alamah (Eds.), *Transcultural nursing concepts, theories, research, & practice*. New York, NY: McGraw-Hill.

Wehbe-Alamah, H. (2018c). Integrating generic and professional health care practices. In M. McFarland & H. Wehbe-Alamah (Eds.), *Transcultural nursing concepts, theories, research, & practice* (pp. 131–141). New York, NY: McGraw-Hill.

Wehbe-Alamah, H. (2018d). Madeleine Leininger's Theory of Culture Care Diversity and Universality. In M. Smith (Ed.), *Nursing theories and nursing practice*. Philadelphia: PA: F. A. Davis Company.

Wehbe-Alamah, H. (2018e). The Ethnonursing Research Method: Major features and enablers. In M. McFarland & H. Wehbe-Alamah (Eds.), *Transcultural nursing concepts, theories, research, & practice* (pp. 57–84). New York, NY: McGraw-Hill.

Wehbe-Alamah, H., Farmer, M. E., McFarland, M., Tower, A., Jones, M., Shah, V., et al. (2015). Development of an extensible game architecture for teaching transcultural nursing. *Online Journal of Cultural Competence in Nursing and Healthcare, 5*(1), 64–74. http://dx.doi.org/10.9730/ojccnh.org/v5n1a5

Wehbe-Alamah, H., & Fry, D. (2014). Creating a culturally sensitive and welcoming academic environment for diverse health care students: A model exemplified with muslim physical therapist students. *Journal of Physical Therapy Education*, *28*(1), 5-15.

Wehbe-Alamah, H., & McFarland, M. (2015a). *Leininger's Culture Care Theory and Ethnonursing Research Method: The classic and the new.* Paper presented at the 41st Annual Conference of the Transcultural Nursing Society in Portland, Oregon.

Wehbe-Alamah, H., & McFarland, M. (2015b). Transcultural nursing course outline, educational activities, and syllabi using the Culture Care Theory. In M. McFarland & H. Wehbe-Alamah

(Eds.), *Culture care diversity and universality: A worldwide nursing theory* (pp. 553–578). Burlington, MA: Jones and Bartlett Publishers, Inc.

Wehbe-Alamah, H., Mixer, S., Collins, J., & Wright, K. (October 2010). "*Eating Our Health Away: Addressing the Obesity Pandemic using an Evidence-Based and a Culturally Congruent Approach.*" Presented at the 36th Annual Conference of the Transcultural Nursing Society, Atlanta, GA.

Wolf, K. M., Zoucha, R., McFarland, M., Salman, K., Dagne, A., & Hashi, N. (2016). Somali immigrant perceptions of mental health and illness: An ethnonursing study. *Journal of Transcultural Nursing, 27*(4), 349–358. http://dx.doi.org/10.1177/1043659614550487

Zoucha, R., & Turk, M. (2015). Using the Culture Care Theory as a guide to develop and implement a transcultural global health course for Doctor of Nursing Practice students for study in Italy. In M. McFarland & H. Wehbe-Alamah (Eds.), *Culture care diversity and universality: A worldwide nursing theory* (pp. 521–535). Burlington, MA: Jones and Bartlett Publishers, Inc.

CHAPTER 2

# Current State of Transcultural Nursing Theories, Models, and Approaches

Priscilla Limbo Sagar and Drew Y. Sagar


## ABSTRACT

Dr. Madeleine Leininger—founder and mother of transcultural nursing (TCN)—worked tirelessly with nurses from around the world to expand its body of knowledge. Leininger's Sunrise Model is based on culture care bridging generic folk care and professional care and uses three action modes to provide culturally congruent care. Other proponents of TCN and followers of Dr. Leininger developed theories and models and further added to the body of expanding knowledge in TCN. This article includes some exemplars of theories and models developed by Andrews and Boyle, Campinha-Bacote, Choi, Giger and Davidhizar, Jeffreys, Purnell, and Spector to further integrate TCN in nursing education, practice, administration, and research. The authors gathered some application of these theories and models in nursing education, practice, administration, and research. Research agenda for the future and gaps in knowledge focusing on increasing diversity of nursing workforce, preventing health disparities, and adding to TCN body of knowledge are likewise included.



http://dx.doi.org/10.1891/0739-6686.37.25

## INTRODUCTION

Conceptual models guide research and practice and provide the structure to view human beings and their health (Andrews & Boyle, 2016). Reciprocally, models give structure to practice; outcomes of nursing practice provide evidence of the model's credibility (Butts, 2016). The various definitions of nursing theory, models, and conceptual frameworks are beyond the scope of this article. The goal of this chapter is to provide a current state of TCN theories, models and approaches and its further integration in nursing education, practice, administration, and research. To achieve this goal, the authors provided some exemplars of TCN theory and models and approaches, current research in nursing education and practice, and agenda for future research.

Leininger laid the foundation for TCN; her followers and other proponents of TCN are continually adding to the growing body of TCN knowledge and best practices. Whether explicitly acknowledged or implied, many areas converge and are similar among TCN theories and models (Sagar, 2018). Accrediting agencies such as The Joint Commission in healthcare practice and those in academic setting namely the American Association of Colleges of Nursing (AACN) Commission on Collegiate Nursing Education (CCNE, 2013) and the National League for Nursing (NLN, 2016) Commission for Nursing Accreditation (CNEA) have standards inclusive of diversity and cultural competence. Both AACN (2008) and the NLN have faculty toolkits to facilitate teaching culturally and linguistically congruent care. AACN's (2008) *Cultural Competency in Baccalaureate Nursing Education: End-of-Program Competencies for Graduates and Faculty Toolkit* uses theories and models of Leininger, Campinha-Bacote, Giger and Davidhizar, Purnell, and Spector. In its *Toolkit for Cultural Competence in Master's and Doctoral Education,* the AACN (2011) added the Jeffreys model along with these theories and models.

To eliminate disparate quality and access to care, the U.S. Department of Health and Human Services (USDHHS) Office of Minority Health (OMH) (2013) worked with various sectors of society to refine the culturally and linguistically appropriate services (CLAS) standards that it initially published in 2000. There were 14 original standards during its publication in 2000; the enhanced CLAS has 15 standards (USDHHS, OMH, 2013).

The CLAS standards contain mandates for language access services (LAS) among institutions receiving federal funding (USDHHS, OMH, 2013). Indeed, language is vital when navigating the healthcare system. Effective and respectful provider–patient communication is central to culturally congruent care. The rest of the standards are guidelines to facilitate the elimination of health inequities (USDHHS, OMH, 2013). The Agency for Healthcare Research and Quality's (2016) *2015 National Healthcare Quality and Disparities Report and 5th Anniversary*

*Update on The National Quality Strategy* exhorted the use of CLAS standards as a framework to aid organizations offer services that are "responsive to patients' diverse cultural health beliefs and practices, preferred languages, health literacy, and other communication needs" (p. 16).

## EXEMPLARS OF TRANSCULTURAL NURSING THEORIES AND MODELS

### Andrews and Boyle: Transcultural Interprofessional Practice Model

Aimed at clarifying TCN clinical practice application, the initial publication of *Transcultural Concepts in Nursing Care* evolved from a collaboration with faculty and doctoral students at the University of Utah (Andrews & Boyle, 2012). Successive editions of their books provided comprehensive history of TCN, supported a lifespan approach, and offered guidelines in assessment for planning culturally congruent care. In the seventh edition of their book, Andrews and Boyle (2016) published their own theory of *Transcultural Interprofessional Practice (TIP) Model*. Four interconnected and interrelated components make up the TIP Model: cultural context, interprofessional healthcare team, communication, and problem-solving process (Andrews & Boyle, 2016). The interprofessional focus of this model may be applied to undergraduate and graduate programs in nursing and allied health.

The *Transcultural Nursing Assessment for Individuals and Families* makes up a guide with 12 categories for cultural assessment and development of culturally congruent care: biocultural variations; communication; cultural affiliations; cultural sanctions and restrictions; developmental considerations; economics; educational background; health-related beliefs and practices; kinship and social networks; nutrition; religion and spirituality; and values orientation (Boyle & Andrews, 2016a, pp. A1–A6).

Boyle and Andrews (2016b) also developed *Transcultural Nursing Assessment for Groups and Communities*. Included in this guide are eight categories namely: family and kinship systems; social and life networks; political or government systems; language and traditions; worldview, value orientations, and cultural norms; religious beliefs and practices; health beliefs and practices; and healthcare systems (Boyle & Andrews, 2016b, pp. B1–D3). This guide lends itself very well to community assessments in undergraduate and graduate nursing and allied healthcare courses.

To aid in assessing organizational cultural competence, Boyle, Andrews, and Ludwig-Beymer (2012) developed the *Andrews/Boyle Assessment Guide for Healthcare Organizations and Facilities*. Comprising the nine categories in this guide are: environmental context; language and ethnohistory; technology;

religious/philosophical; social factors; cultural values; political/legal; economic; and education (Boyle et al., 2012, pp. 459–461). The quest for organizational competence is a lifetime journey and must involve policy making, administrative, management, and provider levels as the organization partners with the community it serves (Ludwig-Beymer, 2016).

### Campinha-Bacote: The Process of Cultural Competence in the Delivery of Healthcare Services

Campinha-Bacote (2007) developed the original version of *A Culturally Competent Model of Care* in 1991 citing the blending of concepts from Leininger (1978), Pedersen (1988), and Law (1993). Representing the model were four interrelated constructs: cultural awareness, cultural knowledge, cultural skill, and cultural encounters (Campinha-Bacote, 2007, 2011). She added *cultural desire* in 1998, renaming her model *the Process of Cultural Competence in the Delivery of Healthcare* Services. Campinha-Bacote (2015) further revised her model in 2002, depicting the kindling of an individual's desire for cultural competence with an erupting volcano. To assess cultural competence, Campinha-Bacote (2007) developed two assessment tools: *The Inventory for Assessing the Process of Cultural Competence Among Healthcare Professionals-Revised* (IAPCC-R) and its version for student nurses, the *IAPCC-Student Version* (IAPCC-SV). These tools have been used extensively in nursing education, practice, administration, and research to measure perceived cultural competence among student nurses and practitioners (Sagar, 2018). The research studies utilizing her model and the IAPCC-R pointed out cultural encounters as the pivot and key to the process of becoming competent; with this realization in 2010, Campinha-Bacote (2015) accordingly modified her representation of the model with cultural encounters as the central construct.

Campinha-Bacote's *Biblically Based Model of Cultural Competence in the Delivery of Healthcare Services* flows from her work and those of Leininger and McFarland (2006) and others (Chapman, 2005; Cross et al., 1989; Kleinman, 1980; Law, 1993; Pederson, 1988; Wilkerson, 2002; Wood, 1998, all authors as cited by Campinha-Bacote (2015). This model urged healthcare professionals to see the image of God or "Imago Dei" in their patients and to integrate love, caring, and humility, among other virtues. The graphic representation shows "Imago Dei" as the key and sixth construct of the model, continually infusing the five original constructs of cultural awareness, cultural knowledge, cultural skill, and cultural encounters (Campinha-Bacote, 2015).

### Choi: Theory of Cultural Marginality

As an immigrant living and working in the United States, Hesseung Choi (2008, 2013) noted situations among immigrant adolescents and the impact of such process on their mental health development. This led Choi to develop the Theory of Cultural Marginality (TCM) to foster understanding of the unique experiences of immigrants "straddling" two cultures.

TCM has three major concepts: marginal living, across culture conflict recognition, and easing cultural tension. In marginal living, the individual is passive and feels in between two cultures. According to Choi (2008, 2013), one of the qualities of marginal living is forming new relationship amid old relationships. Across culture conflict recognition indicates the initial understanding of two divergent cultural beliefs, values, behaviors, and norms. Two distinct value systems and expectations confront the individual, requiring difficult choices that lead to conflict. Easing cultural tension naturally occurs as an adjustment response for resolution of across-culture conflict through four response patterns modified from the works of Weisberger among German Jews: assimilation, reconstructed return, poise, and integration (Choi, 2013).

Assimilation signifies the response pattern when individuals become absorbed into the new or dominant culture. As a strategy for survival in the new culture, immigrants endeavor to learn new customs, mingle with people, and acquire proficiency in the new language (Choi, 2008). Whether it is due to obstacles and conflicts from the new culture or due to longing for their old culture, an individual may exhibit the response pattern of reconstructed return. The response pattern of poise may render the individual free from cultural attachment to the old or new culture, with a sense of being "neither belonging to the old culture nor the new culture." Individuals may still yet continue to experience emotional conflicts even while responding in poise (Choi, 2008). During the response pattern of integration, the individual merges and integrates the old and new culture to form a third culture (Choi, 2008, 2013). Individuals at the integration response pattern are likely to respond successfully when confronted with cultural tension.

### Giger and Davidhizar: Transcultural Assessment Model

In an attempt to assist students in providing care to culturally diverse clients, Giger and Davidhizar (2008); Giger (2013) developed the Transcultural Assessment Model (TAM) in 1988. They based the TAM on the work of Leininger; Spector; Orque and Bloch; and Hall. The TAM is formulated on a theoretical construct or metaparadigm of integral requisites transcultural nursing and cultural diversity, culturally competent care, recognizing that each individual is unique despite cultural similarities with others of the same background or ethnicity, culturally sensitive environment, and health and wellness based on behaviors specific to cultural background (Giger & Davidhizar, 2008, Sagar, 2012).

TAM has six cultural phenomena: biological variations, environmental control, time, social orientation, space and communication (Giger, 2013; Giger &

Davidhizar, 2008). Each one of the six cultural phenomenon occurs in cultures and relates to each other, overlaps with one another, and with varying degrees of utility and application (Giger, 2013).

Giger and Davidhizar's TAM has been extensively used in nursing practice, education, and research for over 20 years. Giger (2013) cited other notable instances of TAM's applicability such as its incorporation by Spector in 1993 into her Health Traditions Model (HTM) and its integration by the USDHHS Office of Minority Health as an overarching model for culturally congruent care in 2004. The TAM is the only TCN model to be recognized by the American Academy of Nursing with its prestigious Edge Runner award (Giger, 2013).

### Jeffreys: Cultural Competence and Confidence Model

The Cultural Competence and Confidence (CCC) Model interrelates concepts that influence or predict cultural competence, integrating the construct of transcultural self-efficacy *(TSE* or *confidence)* as the key factor (Jeffreys, 2010, 2016). On a global scale, educators, researchers, and learners in allied health professions use this evidence-based, decidedly applicable theoretical framework (Sagar, 2018). Jeffreys (2010) defines TSE as the perceived confidence to perform or learn transcultural skills when caring for diverse clients. In the CCC model, cultural competence is directed towards culturally congruent care; has three dimensions: cognitive, practical, and affective; and could be positively influenced by formal education and learning experiences (Jeffreys, 2010, 2016).

According to Jeffreys (2010, 2016), the cognitive learning dimension covers cultural knowledge and comprehension that impact professional care for diverse clients across the life span. Jeffreys observed similarities between the psychomotor domain of learning and the practical learning dimension of the CCC. In TCN context, this involves verbal and nonverbal communication skills during cultural assessment. The affective learning dimension vital for "professional value and attitude development consists of attitudes, values, and beliefs" (Jeffreys, (2010, p. 52).

Based on the CCC, Jeffreys (2010, 2016) developed the Transcultural Self-Efficacy Tool (TSET) in 1994, an 83-item questionnaire that measures and evaluates transcultural nursing skills among diverse client populations. The TSET

### Purnell: Model for Cultural Competence

Originally intended for a framework for clinical assessment, Purnell (2013, 2014, 2016) developed his Model for Cultural Competence in 1991. Depicted in his organizing framework for cultural competence in nursing is a series of four concentric circles or spheres of cultural influence. From the outermost toward the center signifies the global sphere, followed by the third representing the community, the second which denotes family, and the innermost representing the self. The center of the model is a dark circle, representing unknown phenomenon about culture (Purnell, 2013, 2014).

Radiating from the dark center of the PMCC are 12 wedge-shaped sections signifying cultural domains. The 12 cultural domains are cultural heritage; healthcare practice; healthcare practitioners; family roles and organizations; communication; workforce issues; biocultural ecology; high risk behaviors; spirituality and religious practices; nutrition; pregnancy; and death rituals (Purnell, 2013, 2014). The 12 domains could be used in their entirety or applicable domains could be selected. A jagged line at the bottom represents nonlinear aspects of cultural consciousness (Purnell, 2005, 2014).

The MCC has been adapted for use in multiple settings and is among the most widely used models in nursing education; its 12 domains could be threaded in the curriculum both in theoretical courses and in clinical assessments (Sagar, 2014). Notably, this model is not only frequently used in nursing practice, administration, and research but also applied in health-related fields and in international projects. Additional applications are incorporated in employee orientation, continuing staff education, and institutional practice guidelines. Marrone (2013) demonstrated how the MCC could be applied to organizational educational, healthcare, and professional organization cultural competence.

### Spector: Health Traditions Model

Currently in its ninth edition, Spector's (2013, 2017) textbook *Cultural Diversity in Health and Illness* was originally published in 1977 as a fulfillment of a promise to her students. When Spector (2009, 2013) developed the Health Traditions Model (HTM) in 1993, she incorporated Giger and Davidhizar's six cultural phenomena of biocultural variations, communication, environmental control, social orientation, space, and time (Giger, 2013; Giger & Davidhizar, 2008). Spector (2017) emphasized that tradition is the vital element of and its role is fundamental in HTM. Many individuals use ethnocultural, traditional methods instead of or in conjunction with modern healthcare regimen.

According to Spector (2013, 2017), the HTM centers on holistic health, exploring traditional individual approaches to maintain, to protect health, and to restore health. Furthermore, she regarded health as the internal balance of an individual with the outside world in the physical, mental, and spiritual aspects. Holistically, the nine interrelated facets of health for an individual comprise personal maintenance of health, protection of health, and restoration of health physically, mentally, and spiritually. As an illustration, to restore health, an individual may use coining (physical), traditional healer (mental), and exorcism (spiritual).

Spector coined the word *CulturalCare* to encompass the development of healthcare delivery that meets the mandates and guidelines of CLAS standards and other mandates for culturally competent care (Spector, 2013, 2017). In addition, Spector (2013, 2017) developed a Heritage Assessment Tool for assessing an individual's depth of self-identification with one's personal heritage. She further added family and community assessment tools in the 2017 edition of her book and referred to the three tools as the Heritage Chain for Cultural Assessments (Spector, 2017).

## APPLICATION IN NURSING EDUCATION

Kolade (2016) conducted a phenomenological study of minority nursing faculty using LaFromboise, Coleman and Gerton (1993) model of bicultural competence and Campinha-Bacote's (2015) Process of Cultural Competence in the Delivery of Healthcare Services. Kolade used face to face interviews with five female assistant professors ranging from 8 to 13 years as faculty in three nursing programs in Tennessee. The data yielded six themes: "missing mentorship, lack of collegial support, harnessing external support, I feel more like a minority here, acculturation, and feeling isolated" (Kolade, 2016, p. 110). Feeling like a minority had two subthemes of relating to faculty and relating to students.

Using a pre-and post-survey after a 2-week summer pipeline program, Katz, Barbosa-Leiker, and Benavides-Vaello (2016) explored changes in knowledge and opinions of underserved American Indians and Hispanic high school students. The term 'pipeline' denotes programs at any level of education targeting, enrolling, and supporting graduation among minority, low-income, and women aimed at increasing their representation in various fields (Katz et al., 2016).

Hudiburg, Mascher, Sagehorn, and Stidham (2015) conducted a study aiming to promote awareness of cultural heritage and value in diverse populations of school aged children. The goal of this intervention is to improve educational outcomes by removing the stigma of cultural diversity. The Pittsburgh State University launched a program to teach Culturally Responsive Teaching (CRT) among student teachers. The CRT aimed to transform the curriculum to make it culturally relevant to students. Using Purnell's MCC, the curriculum was modified using 16 of the 19 of its major assumptions. The curriculum was developed with an on library technologies. A group of 25 student teacher were trained to meet the needs of American Indian (AI) children in Northeast Oklahoma (Hudiburg et al., 2015). Criteria for qualification of participants included teaching in schools with a predominantly AI enrollment or that the participants were AI themselves. Because this project was ongoing at the time of publishing, long term benefits are anticipated. Many of the teachers have expressed positive outcomes and an increased awareness of the individuality of their students rather than viewing them as a collective group (Hudiburg et al., 2015).

With expanded TCN body of knowledge, it is vital to integrate TCN concepts into all levels of nursing and healthcare curricula. Sagar (2014) suggested educational strategies such as threading into curricula; creating separate course or courses; guiding students in independent studies; using case scenarios in clinical; assigning self-learning modules; and incorporating into simulations. Weaving into curricula and creating separate courses prevent hit or miss situation of integration. In an already packed curriculum, every faculty in nursing and healthcare are passionate about diverse areas in healthcare. The next generation of healthcare professionals need awareness, knowledge, and skills in culturally appropriate services to collaborate with each other in caring for patients, families, and communities whose cultures are different from their own.

Faculty and academia are also urged to be creative in facilitating reflection and journaling; developing unfolding case scenarios; teaching with literary works; and using online resources (Sagar, 2014). The arts and humanities provide powerful tools in teaching compassion and caring. Stories such as *Victoria and Abdul* (Basu, 2017), *The Spirit Catches You and You Fall Down* (Fadiman, 1997), *News of the World* (Jiles, 2016), *Pachinko* (Lee, 2017), and *the Immortal Life of Henrietta Lacks* (Skloot, 2010) all vividly portray bias, cultural imposition, cultural shock, ethnocentrism, prejudice, racism, among other reactions when cultures collide. The vividness of portrayal through stories is more powerful and alive than plain textbook descriptions. These narration and novels or part thereof could be assigned for individual or group projects in nursing and allied health courses.

Sagar (2014) illustrated the use of modules in teaching the CLAS standards among nurses and healthcare professionals in academic and staff development settings. Other modules included are theory of heat and cold, asthma in an orthodox Jewish child, and posttraumatic stress disorder (PTSD) in women. Modules are all inclusive, stand-alone educational tool that learners can complete at their own time independently without an instructor (Sagar, 2014). While modules have been used for many years, they have evolved from hard copies in binders to intranet and web-based formats that enhance self-learning and accessibility.

## APPLICATION IN NURSING PRACTICE

Biological variation (Giger, 2013; Giger & Davidhizar, 2008), biocultural variations and cultural aspects of incidence of a disease (Boyle & Andrews, 2016a, 2016b), or biocultural ecology (Purnell, 2013) are quite vital in assessment, diagnosing, planning, implementing, and evaluating care of individuals, families, and groups. For example, women carrier of the hemophilia gene have 50% chance of transmitting the gene to their sons who will be hemophiliac; their daughters have 50% chance of being carriers of hemophilia (Beery, Workman, & Eggert 2018). Genomic care ensures that an individual's genetic history about health and disease becomes part of general assessment for individuals and families. This is not to advocate that each person needs some kind of genetic testing; it reminds all healthcare professionals to be mindful of genetic issues when assessing individual health or risk factors for diseases (Beery et al., 2018).

In a cross-sectional correlation study of 61 Korean American (KA) families, Choi, Kim, Park, and Dancy (2012) explored parental knowledge, parental/ filial self-efficacy, parent–child communication, and parent–child conflicts through a questionnaire. A total of 33 boys and 30 girls aged 11 to 14 participated in the study, along with 54 fathers and 61 mothers. Findings suggested a necessity of education programs or counseling services for KA parents of adolescents, especially fathers with ineffective parental skills and limited communication with their children (Choi & Kim, 2013).

Booker (2015) explored African Americans' (AA) use of biomedicine and spiritual medicine to moderate experience of pain. In this study, Booker noted that AAs may be deeply spiritual in general and deeply devoted to Christian tradition in particular. Furthermore, there is often a blending of African traditions with Christianity among AAs in order mitigate the difficulties in life (Cherry & Giger, 2012, as cited by Booker, 2015). Furthermore, chronic pain may be modulated by a series of interrelated systems including but not necessarily limited to biophysiologic, psychological, and spiritual responses. This possibly accounts for a tendency among AAs to present with a combination of spiritual, psychological and somatic complaints. While there may be a strong spiritual component interwoven with the somatic, there may also be a sense of retribution by the divine. Cherry and Giger (as cited by Booker, 2015) noted that if illness is perceived as punitive than there likely will be doubt in treatment efficacy.

Merritt (2013) illustrated an application of the Giger and Davidhizar TAM with regards to the dynamics of communication with the Chinese parents of an infant in a neonatal intensive care unit (NICU). Merritt reported that there has been a great deal of attention in current literature on Spanish speaking populations. However, Mandarin is spoken by nearly as many people and there is a paucity of information dealing with this population. It bears repetition that although people may belong to a particular ethnicity, they are still quite unique individuals. In this respect, much of how individuals understand language, nuance, and context will be influenced by the degree of their acculturation (Merritt, 2013).

There is an intense emotional response under any circumstance in which an infant requires NICU care. There may be a feeling of blame among Chinese parents or fault associated with a medically compromised infant thus the likelihood of a great deal of concern for the future implications of this illness for the infant (Merritt, 2013). This situation is made more complex wherein a parent is from a different culture, may have limited understanding of the language, and may feel driven to affirm complete understanding while there is in fact limited understanding (Merritt, 2013). It is common in a situation such as this for a family to consider health providers as deserving of respect and may be hesitant to express concerns or ask questions. It is recommended to promptly assess the degree of understanding of the patient and or family, to provide communication in a nonthreatening manner, and to validate understanding. To ensure culturally and linguistically appropriate care, healthcare professionals must utilize language access services (LAS) when communicating and provide written materials in the appropriate language (Merritt, 2013).

Guangzhou, China's population is increasingly becoming more diverse. The team of Li, He, Luo, and Zhang (2016) employed cross sectional survey of 1,156 multicultural nurses in three general hospitals to evaluate three areas: perceived transcultural self-efficacy (TSE) of nurses; demographic characteristics of nurses and self-efficacy; and reliability of the Chinese version of Jeffreys' TSET (TSET-CV). In this research, the Cronbach alpha was .99 for the total TSET scores, with reliability ranging from .97 to .98 and subscales of cognitive (87.9%), Practical (87%), and affective (89.2%). According to Li et al., older nurses from minority background with more years of experience along with higher professional titles and income scored higher in the TSE. The Li et al. study indicates the importance of in-service education to improve transcultural self-efficacy of nurses.

In a span of a few decades attributed to mass immigrations, the once homogenous population of Greece has become multicultural and multiethnic. Sarafis and Michael (2014) utilized the TSET Greek Version (TSET-GR) among 136 nursing students and 202 nurses in two general hospitals in Athens, Greece. The participants completed the questionnaire either in the classroom or at the workplace. Cronbach alpha coefficient ranged from .92 to .98 for the cognitive, practical, and affective subscales. This study confirms the construct validity and internal consistency of the TSET-GR and its applicability to assess cultural competence among Greek nurses (Sarafis & Michael, 2014).

While the cultural domains of the MCC (Purnell, 2014) are viewed as a complex whole, individual domains may be applied to specific needs and settings (Sagar, 2012, 2014). Debiasi and Selleck (2017) conducted a study to explore improvement in the ability of nurse practitioners (NPs) to provide culturally appropriate care in two NP-run clinics. Their study involved 13 NPs and 50 patient volunteers of various ethnicities. The NPs performed a self-assessment of their proficiency while at the same time patients completed a modified Cultural Sensitivity Survey. A self-learning module using the MCC was then emailed to NPs for completion. This was followed by patients' reevaluation of the care provided by NPs post intervention (Debiasi & Selleck, 2017). The results of the intervention showed that the majority of patients felt the NP competency had improved in 20 of 21 of survey questions.

## APPLICATION: NURSING RESEARCH

Qualitative methods such as the ethnonursing method, grounded theory, and phenomenology are suited to explore lived experiences; acculturation; cultural values; beliefs about health and illness among cultural groups. Quantitative methods could tap the research gap and healthcare Disparities in access and quality of care among African Americans, Native Americans, Hispanic Americans and Asian Americans. The Institute of Medicine (IOM) report, *Unequal Treatment: Confronting Racial and Ethnic Disparities in Health Care* (Smedley, Stith, & Nelson, 2003) urged diverse stakeholders to tackle this problem. The IOM report not only highlighted the need for research to identify reasons for racial and ethnic disparities but also called for development of strategies for interventions to prevent them (Smedley et al., 2003).

Conducting research among the underserved frequently poses a challenge of access and congruency of method. Digital story telling has recently shown promise in health promotion and research to access vulnerable and underrepresented populations. Briant, Halter, Marchello, Escareno, and Thompson (2016) implemented the transportation theory in a pilot project to explore whether digital story telling is a culturally congruent tool to promote health among Hispanics and Latinos in the lower Yakima Valley in Washington State. Briant et al. collaborated with *Creative Narrations*, a national organization expert for developing digital stories. Nine bilingual *promotores* (health educators) participated and created digital stories in the train-the-trainer digital story telling workshops. The promotores later conducted three community workshops for 5 weeks each consisting of 2 hours; mostly women aged 30 years or older attended the small workshops and created nine digital stories. Semistructured, follow-up interviews were conducted for community participants to assess their experiences (Briant et al., 2016). Although small, this pilot study evidenced a strong support for digital storytelling, an emergent health promotion tool combining digital technology and the globally pervasive storytelling that requires minimum literacy.

Applying Campinha-Bacote's model, Ingram (2011) reviewed literature from the 1990s to 2011 to explore how nurses can address cultural issues related to individual's low health literacy. In the US, one of every five adult reads at or below the fifth grade level (Doak et al. 1996 as cited by Ingram, 2011) well below the eighth or ninth grade levels to function adequately in this century. Ingram further stated difficulties encountered by clients with low literacy in completing forms; in understanding instructions; in following-up with appointments; and in taking medications as directed. When caring for clients with low literacy, Ingram urged nurses to improve their own cultural competence and to use resources targeting low literacy. This suggestion regarding resources is consistent with current literature citing culturally congruent use of photonovels, soap operas, cartoons, videos, and digital storytelling for health promotion. When constructing surveys and questionnaires, researchers need to be mindful of literacy levels.

While some models and theories may not be proposed for research, they are value in guiding education, practice, and administration (Purnell, 2016). Some attention to the practice theory gap is in order. Is TCN research being translated to practice? Or is it what Dahnke and Dreher (2016) pointed to us as the second theory to practice gap namely conducting research for knowledge's sake and not for applicability to nursing practice? Application of translation of research into practice (TRIP) is a comprehensive process of fostering adoption of evidence-based practices in healthcare settings (Titler, 2016). The AACN (2018), in its *Defining Scholarship for Academic Nursing Task Force Consensus Position Statement,* urged academic faculty commitment to the pursuit of inquiry to generate knowledge connecting practice with education and the improvement of health and healthcare.

## CONCLUSIONS

When planning to use TCN theory, model, or approaches, there is the challenge to reflect on the applicability or fit of a theory or model to the mission, goals, and philosophy of a particular setting. Douglas (2002)—a decade and a half ago—urged the testing of theory or model as applied in education, practice, administration, and research to identify gaps and agenda for future research hence allowing them to grow, evolve, and be tested in order to survive. Thus, theory and models add to the body of knowledge in evidence-based practice (EBP); reveal further gaps in knowledge; guide clinical practice; and provide guidelines in education and preparation of future practitioners (Sagar, 2012).

In addition to Leininger's groundbreaking work for over a decade, TCN theory and models have emerged from Andrews and Boyle, Campinha-Bacote,

Choi, Giger and Davidhizar, Jeffreys, Purnell, and Spector, to name a few. In the future, more TCN theories and models will be developed and tested to further add to the TCN body of scientific knowledge and best practices for culturally and linguistically congruent care for an increasingly diverse population.

## Questions for Reflection

1. Does your practice setting use a theory or model? If it does, is it a TCN theory or model?
2. Name one theory or model. How would you facilitate the integration of this theory or model in educational institution? Do you see congruency between this theory or model with the mission, goals, and objectives of your institution?
3. Name one theory or model. How would you facilitate the integration of this theory or model in your practice? Do you see congruency between this theory or model with the mission, goals, and objectives of your particular setting?
4. How would you explain the two kinds of theory gap between nursing research and practice? Enumerate three approaches whereby you can help narrow these theory gaps.

## REFERENCES

Agency for Healthcare Research and Quality. (2016). 2015 National healthcare quality and disparities report and 5th anniversary update on the national quality strategy. Retrieved from https://www.ahrq.gov/sites/default/files/wysiwyg/research/findings/nhqrdr/nhqdr15/2015nhqdr.pdf

American Association of Colleges of Nursing. (2008). *Cultural competency in baccalaureate nursing education: End-of-program competencies for graduates and faculty toolkit.* Washington, DC: Author.

American Association of Colleges of Nursing. (2011). *Toolkit for cultural competency in master's and doctoral nursing education.* Washington, DC: Author.

American Association of Colleges of Nursing. (2018). *Defining scholarship for academic nursing task force consensus position statement.* Retrieved from http://www.aacnnursing.org/Portals/42/News/Position-Statements/Defining-Scholarship.pdf

Andrews, M. M., & J. K. Boyle. (2012). *Transcultural concepts in nursing care.* Philadelphia, PA: Wolters Kluwer/Lippincott, Williams, & Wilkins.

Andrews, M. M., & J. K. Boyle. (2016). *Transcultural concepts in nursing care.* Philadelphia, PA: Wolters Kluwer/Lippincott, Williams, & Wilkins.

Basu, S. (2017). *Victoria and Abdul.* New York, NY: Knopf Doubleday.

Beery, T. A., Workman, L. M. & Eggert, J. A. (2018). *Genetics and genomics in nursing and healthcare.* Philadelphia, PA: F.A. Davis.

Booker, S. J. (2015). Older African Americans' beliefs about pain, biomedicine and spiritual medicine. *Journal of Christian Nursing, 32*(3), 148–155. Retrieved from http://www.nursingcenter.com/cearticle?an=00005217-201507000-00009&Journal_ID=642167&Issue_ID=3133855

Boyle, J. S. & Andrews, M. M. (2016a). Andrews/Boyle transcultural assessment guide for individuals and families. In M. M. Andrews & J. K. Boyle (Eds.), *Transcultural concepts in nursing care* (7th ed.; pp. A1–A6). Philadelphia, PA: Wolters Kluwer/Lippincott, Williams, & Wilkins.

Boyle, J. S., & Andrews, M. M. (2016b). Andrews/Boyle transcultural assessment guide for groups and communities. In M. M. Andrews & J. K. Boyle (Eds.), *Transcultural concepts in nursing care* (7th ed., pp. B1–D3). Philadelphia, PA: Wolters Kluwer/Lippincott, Williams, & Wilkins.

Boyle, J. S., Andrews, M. M., & Ludwig-Beymer, P. (2012). Andrews/Boyle transcultural assessment guide for health care organizations. In M. M. Andrews & J. S. Boyle, *Transcultural concepts in nursing care* (6th ed., pp. 459–461). Philadelphia, PA: Wolters Kluwer/Lippincott, Williams, & Wilkins.

Briant, K. J., Halter, A., Marchello, N., Escareno, M., & Thompson, B. (2016). The power of digital storytelling as a culturally relevant health promotion tool. Retrieved from https://www.ncbi.nlm.nih.gov/pmc/articles/PMC5065376/pdf/nihms803404.pdf

Butts, J. B. (2016). Components and levels of abstractions in nursing knowledge. In J. B. Butts & K. L. Rich (Eds.), *Philosophies and theories for advanced nursing practice* (pp. 87–108). Burlington, MA: Jones & Bartlett Learning.

Campinha-Bacote, J. (2007). *The process of cultural competence in the delivery of healthcare services.* Cincinnati, OH: Transcultural C.A.R.E. Resources.

Campinha-Bacote, J. (2011). Coming to know cultural competence: An evolutionary process. *International Journal for Human Caring, 15*(3), 42–48.

Campinha-Bacote, J. (2015). The process of cultural competence in the delivery of healthcare services. Retrieved from http://transculturalcare.net/the-process-of-cultural-competence-in-the-delivery-of-healthcare-services

Choi, H. (2008). Theory of cultural marginality. In M. J. Smith & P. R. Liehr, *Middle range theory for nursing* (2nd ed., pp. 243–259). New York, NY: Springer Publishing.

Choi, H. (2013). Theory of cultural marginality. In M. J. Smith & P. R. Liehr (Eds.), *Middle range theory for nursing* (3rd ed., pp. 289–307). New York, NY: Springer Publishing.

Choi, H., & Kim, S. (2013). Parenting experiences and the need for parent education programs among parents of adolescents in Korea. *Journal of Nursing and Care, 4*, 233. http://dx.doi.org/10.4172/2167-1168.1000233.

Choi, H., Kim, M., Park, C. J., & Dancy, B. L. (2012). Parent child relationships between Korean American adolescents and their parents. *Journal of Psychosocial Nursing, 50*(9), 21–27.

Commission on Collegiate Nursing Education. (2013). Standards for accreditation of baccalaureate and graduate nursing programs. Retrieved from http://www.aacnnursing.org/Portals/42/CCNE/PDF/Standards-Amended-2013.pdf?ver=2017-06-28-141019-360

Dahnke, M. D., & Dreher, H. M. (2016). *Philosophy of science for nursing practice: Concepts and applications* (2nd ed.). New York, NY: Springer Publishing.

Debiasi, L., & Selleck, C. (2017). Cultural competence training for primary care nurse Practitioners: An intervention to improve culturally competent care. *Journal of Cultural Diversity, 24*(2), 39–45. Retrieved from https://0-search-proquest-com.opac.msmc.edu/central/docview/1974490916/fulltextPDF/6968681CC3D24056PQ/1?accountid=28089

Douglas, M. (2002). Developing frameworks for providing culturally competent health care (Editorial). *Journal of Transcultural Nursing, 13*(3), 177.

Fadiman, A. (1997), *The spirit catches you and you fall down*. New York, NY: Farrar, Straus, & Giroux.

Giger, J. N. (2013). *Transcultural nursing: Assessment and intervention* (6th ed.). St. Louis, MO: Elsevier/Mosby.

Giger, J. N., & Davidhizar, R. E. (2008). *Transcultural nursing: Assessment and intervention* (5th ed.). St. Louis, MO: Elsevier/Mosby.

Hudiburg, M., Mascher, E., Sagehorn, A. S., & Stidham J. (2015). Moving toward a culturally competent model of education: Preliminary results of a study of culturally responsive teaching in an American Indian community. *School Libraries Worldwide, 21*(1), 137–148. Retrieved from https://0-search-proquest-com.opac.msmc.edu/healthcomplete/advanced?accountid=28089

Ingram, R. R. (2011). Using Campinha-Bacote's process of cultural competence model to examine relationship between health literacy and cultural competence. *Journal of Advanced Nursing, 68*(3), 695–704.

Jeffreys, M. R. (2010). A model to guide cultural competence education. In M. R. Jeffreys (Ed), *Teaching cultural in nursing and health care* (2nd ed., pp. 45–59). New York, NY: Springer Publishing.

Jeffreys, M. R. (2016). *Teaching cultural in nursing and health care* (3rd ed.). New York, NY: Springer Publishing.

Jiles, P. (2016). *News of the world.* New York, NY: Harper Collins.

Katz, J. R., Barbosa-Leiker, C. & Benavides-Vaello, S. (2016). Measuring the success of a pipeline program to increase nursing workforce diversity. *Journal of Professional Nursing, 32*(1), 6–14.

Kolade, F. M. (2016). The lived experience of minority faculty: A phenomenological study. *Journal of Professional Nursing, 32*(2), 107–114.

LaFromboise, T., Coleman, H. L., & Gerton, J. (1993). Psychological impact of biculturalism: Evidence and theory. *Psychological Bulletin*, 114, 395–412.

Lee, M. J. (2017). *Pachinko.* New York, NY: Grand Central.

Li, J., He, Z., Luo, Y., & Zhang, R. (2016). Perceived transcultural self-efficacy of nurses in general hospitals on Guangzhou, China. *Nursing Research, 65*(5), 371–379.

Leininger, M. M. & McFarland, M. M. (2006). *Culture care diversity and universality: A worldwide nursing theory*. Sudbury, MA: Jones & Bartlett.

Ludwig-Beymer, P. (2016). Creating culturally competent organizations. In M. M. Andrews & J. K. Boyle (Eds.), *Transcultural concepts in nursing care* (7th ed., pp. 242–271). Philadelphia, PA: Wolters Kluwer/Lippincott, Williams, & Wilkins.

Marrone, S. R. (2013). Organizational cultural competence. In L. D. Purnell (Eds.), *Transcultural health care: A culturally competent approach* (4th ed., pp. 60–73). Philadelphia, PA: F.A. Davis.

Merritt, L. (2013). Communicating with Chinese American families in the NICU using the Giger and Davidhizar Transcultural Model. *Neonatal Network, 32*(5) 335–341. Retrieved from https://0-search-proquest-om.opac.msmc.edu/healthcomplete/docview/1439534841/fulltextPDF/69684CEE3A914B22PQ/1?accountid=28089

National League for Nursing. (2016). Commission for Nursing Accreditation. *Accreditation standards for nursing education programs*. Retrieved from http://www.nln.org/docs/default-source/accreditation-services/cnea-standards-final-february-201613f2bf5c78366c709642ff00005f0421.pdf?sfvrsn=12

Purnell, L. D. (2013). *Transcultural health care: A culturally competent approach* (4th ed.). Philadelphia, PA: F.A. Davis.

Purnell, L. D. (2014). *Guide to culturally competent health care* (3rd ed.). Philadelphia, PA: F.A. Davis.

Purnell, L. D. (2016). Models and theories focused on culture. In J. B. Butts & K. L. Rich, *Philosophies and theories for advanced nursing practice* (pp. 517–557). Burlington, MA: Jones & Bartlett Learning.

Sagar, P. L. (2012). *Transcultural nursing theory and models: Application in nursing education, practice, and administration.* New York, NY: Springer Publishing.

Sagar, P. L. (2014). *Transcultural nursing education strategies.* New York, NY: Springer Publishing.

Sagar, P. L. (2018). Culture Care Theory: A trailblazing theory. In M. R. McFarland & H. B. Wehbe-Alamah (Eds.), *Leininger's Transcultural nursing: Concepts, theories, research, and practice.* (4th ed., pp. 85–96) New York, NY: McGraw Hill Education.

Sarafis, P., & Michael, I. (2014). Reliability and validity of the transcultural self-efficacy tool questionnaire (Greek version). *Journal of Nursing Measurement, 22*(2), E41–E51.

Skloot, R. (2010). *The immortal life of Henrietta Lacks.* New York, NY: Broadway Books.

Smedley, B. D., Stith, A. Y., & Nelson, A. R. (2003). *Unequal treatment: Confronting racial and ethnic disparities in health care* (Committee on Understanding and Eliminating Racial and Ethnic Disparities in Health Care, Institute of Medicine. Washington, DC: National Academies Press.

Spector, R. E. (2009). *Cultural diversity in health and illness* (7th ed.). Boston, MA: Pearson Education.

Spector, R. E. (2013). *Cultural diversity in health and illness* (8th ed.). Boston, MA: Pearson Education.

Spector, R. E. (2017). *Cultural diversity in health and illness* (9th ed.). Boston, MA: Pearson Education.

Titler, M. (2016). Developing an evidence-based practice. In G. LoBiondo-Wood & J. Haber (Eds.), *Nursing research: Methods and critical appraisal for evidence-based practice* (8th ed., pp. 418–441). St. Louis, MO: Elsevier.

U.S. Department of Health and Human Services, Office of Minority Health. (2013). *Enhanced national CLAS standards.* Retrieved from https://www.thinkculturalhealth.hhs.gov/assets/pdfs/EnhancedNationalCLASStandards.pdf

CHAPTER 3

# Evidence-Based Updates and Universal Utility of Jeffreys' Cultural Competence and Confidence Framework for Nursing Education (and Beyond) Through TIME

Marianne R. Jeffreys


## ABSTRACT

Nurses and other health care professionals are challenged to engage in the ongoing process of cultural competence development of self and others with a desired outcome goal of achieving cultural congruence in clinical, research, education, and workplace (CREW) settings. Jeffreys' Cultural Competence and Confidence (CCC) model provides an evidence-based, easily applicable theoretical framework that has been a valuable cognitive map guiding educators, researchers, and learners worldwide. Gleaned from 25 years and over 70 studies incorporating the CCC model and/or one of its psychometrically validated questionnaires, this chapter traces the research steps underlying theory and instrument development, presents evidence-based updates, and shows the universal utility of the CCC framework for nursing education (and beyond) through TIME (**t**heory, **i**nnovations, **m**easurement, and **e**valuation). The chapter begins by introducing the



http://dx.doi.org/10.1891/0739-6686.37.43

CCC theory, its underlying assumptions, and an updated CCC visual diagram. A time-sequenced appendix traces initial questions, conceptualization, series of studies, and other scholarly work in theory development and evaluation that lead up to the present and future. Universal utility applications are highlighted through two approaches: a) aggregated studies grouped by study design, topic, and/or populations; and b) innovation spotlight exemplars featuring course and curricular enhancements, service-learning, cultural immersion, employee education, workshops, complementing and scaffolding activities, program evaluation, train-the-trainer, partnerships, and utility to new and/or prioritized topics, pedagogy, and technology. Appendices, figures, tables, and exhibit boxes provide easy to apply practical ideas and research recommendations as well as psychometric and other statistical details related to the CCC model, Transcultural Self-Efficacy Tool (TSET) and Cultural Competence Clinical Evaluation Tool (CCCET).

## INTRODUCTION

Cultural competence and the achievement of cultural congruent care are imperative for nurses, other healthcare professionals, and society everywhere, especially amidst a rapidly changing world, shifting demographics, and cultural conflicts. Although "cultural competence and cultural congruence in nursing care are not new ideas" (Marion et al., 2016) the article "Implementing the New ANA Standard 8: Culturally Congruent Practice" introduces a new focus challenging nurses and other healthcare professionals to topple the status quo, raise the bar, and take action. Within a professional discipline, taking action means implementing evidence-based and theoretically supported actions. It requires commitment, connectedness, curiosity, depth and breadth of knowledge. It requires comprehensive understanding why theories, methodologies, and strategies worked or didn't work at a depth and connectedness beyond superficial perusal of literature limited to the last few years. Process and details over time matter (Jeffreys, 2017).

Notably the new ANA standard distinguishes between cultural competence and cultural congruence (Marion et al., 2016, ANA), an important detail that is frequently missed but one that was evident, prevalent, and visionary in Leininger's seminal and lifetime work (Leininger, 1991; Leininger & McFarland, 2006; McFarland & Wehbe-Alamah, 2015, 2018). Simply stated, cultural competence is an ongoing process with the expected goal of achieving culturally congruent care. Cultural congruence is a tailored "fit" between an individual's cultural values, beliefs, health practices, and care decisions and actions. Care and caring extend beyond clinical settings to research, education, and workplace arenas. Creating culturally safe environments where the diversity of diversity is embraced fits within this inclusive caring framework.

Consequently, nurses and other healthcare professionals are challenged to engage in the ongoing process of cultural competence development of self and others with a desired outcome goal of achieving cultural congruence in clinical, research, education, and workplace (CREW) settings. Comprehensively understanding the multidimensional process, developing strategies for ongoing, optimal cultural competence development for diverse learners and settings, and achieving optimal outcomes can seem like a daunting and overwhelming task without an organizing framework and a valid way to measure and evaluate innovations and outcomes (Jeffreys, 2016a). The Cultural Competence and Confidence (CCC) model provides an evidence-based, easily applicable theoretical framework that has been a valuable cognitive map guiding educators, researchers, and learners worldwide (Douglas & Pacquiao, 2010; Jeffreys, 2016a; Loftin, Hartin, Branson, & Reyes, 2013; McFarland & Wehbe-Alamah, 2015, 2018; Sagar, 2014; Shen, 2015). The model's most frequently requested corresponding questionnaire, the Transcultural Self-Efficacy Tool (TSET), has been psychometrically validated, translated, and incorporated within over 70 studies in a variety of settings. More recently, the Cultural Competence Clinical Evaluation Tool (CCCET) and the Clinical Setting Assessment Tool-Diversity and Disparity (CSAT-DD) expand and offer options aimed to measure providers' cultural behaviors (care provision, assessment, sensitivity) and clientele characteristics and healthcare needs (Jeffreys, 2016a, 2016b).

The purpose of this chapter is to trace the research steps underlying theory and instrument development, present evidence-based updates, and show the universal utility of the CCC theoretical framework for nursing education (and beyond) through TIME. The acronym TIME (*t*heory, *i*nnovations, *m*easurement, and *e*valuation) serves as a reminder that in a scholarly practice discipline: (a) evidence-based theory should guide innovations; (b) the development of innovations should incorporate valid measurement of outcomes (formative and summative) at the onset of innovation design; and (c) thorough evaluation of outcomes guides future decision and action. The chapter begins by introducing the CCC theoretical framework, its underlying assumptions, and an updated CCC visual diagram. A time-sequenced appendix traces the author's initial questions, conceptualization, series of studies, and other scholarly work in theory development and evaluation that lead up to the present and future. Universal utility applications for clinical, research, education, and the workplace (CREW) settings are highlighted through two approaches: a) aggregated studies grouped by study design, topic, and/or populations; and b) innovation spotlight exemplars. Appendices, figures, tables, and exhibit boxes provide easy to apply practical ideas as well as psychometric and other statistical details for researchers and educators who want to know more. Ideas for future expansion conclude the chapter.

## OVERVIEW OF THE CCC THEORY AND MODEL

Preparing nurses and other health professionals to provide quality health care in the increasingly multicultural and global society of the 21st century requires a comprehensive approach that emphasizes cultural competence education throughout professional education and professional life. Although several models have been proposed to describe the process of cultural competence (Campinha-Bacote, 2003; Purnell, 2013) or the process of achieving culturally congruent care through the assessment of cultural diversity and universality (Leininger, 2002; McFarland & Wehbe-Alamah, 2015, 2018), Jeffreys' CCC model focuses specifically on interrelating concepts that explain, describe, influence, and/or predict the phenomenon of learning (developing) cultural competence and incorporates the construct of transcultural self-efficacy (confidence) as a major influencing factor. Within the CCC theory, cultural competence is defined as a multidimensional learning process that integrates transcultural skills in all three dimensions (cognitive, practical, and affective) and involves transcultural self-efficacy. TSE is the perceived confidence for learning or performing transcultural skills needed for culturally congruent care.

The term *learning process* emphasizes that the cognitive, practical, and affective dimensions of TSE and transcultural skill development can change over time as a result of formalized education and other learning experiences. The main goal of the model is to promote culturally congruent care through the development of cultural competence. TSE was proposed in 1994 as a new construct vital to the process of cultural competence and cultural congruence (Jeffreys, 1994) (Appendix A). A new, expanded focus advocates that cultural congruence extends beyond care directed towards healthcare consumers to include cultural congruence in clinical/community, research, education, and workplace (CREW) settings.

The CCC model recognizes that despite the learning opportunities presented to students, nurses, and other healthcare professionals, some individuals persist at cultural competence development while others do not. According to Bandura (1986), self-efficacy perceptions and self-efficacy appraisal influence learning, motivation, persistence, and commitment to situation-specific tasks. Self-efficacy appraisal is an individualized process influenced by four information sources: actual performances (most powerful), vicarious experiences (observing role models), forms of persuasion (encouragement by others), and emotional arousal (Bandura, 1986). Inefficacious individuals may avoid tasks, lack

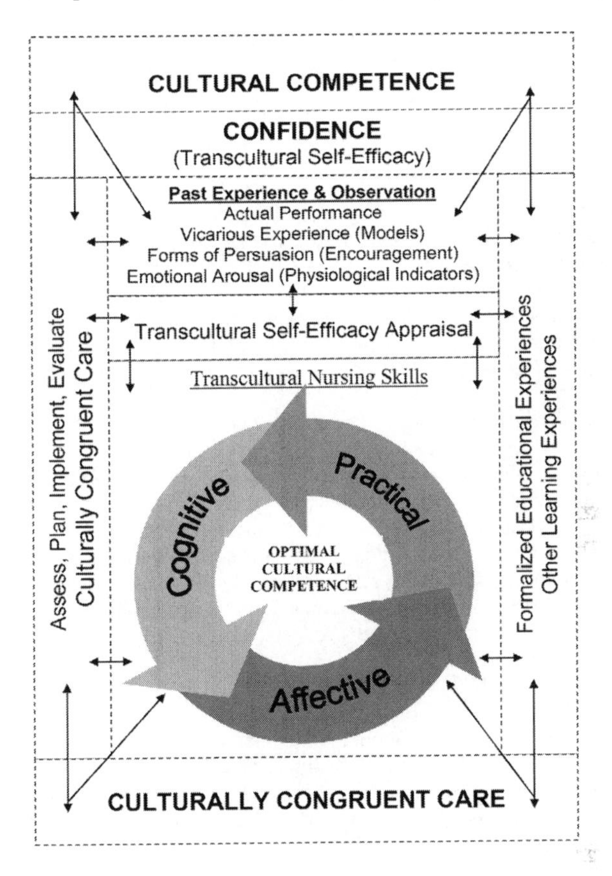


**FIGURE 3.1** Jeffreys' Cultural Competence and Confidence (CCC) Model - (2016)
Reprinted from *Teaching Cultural Competence in Nursing and Health Care: Inquiry, Action, and Innovation* (3rd ed., p. 69), by M. R. Jeffreys, 2016, New York, NY: Springer Publishing.

motivation and commitment, and give up easily. Supremely efficacious (overly confident individuals) view tasks as unimportant, see no need to prepare, and may not see a need to perform the task. In contrast, individuals with resilient TSE view obstacles as challenges, actively seek out additional resources, and expend extra energy aimed at cultural congruence and optimal cultural competence in all settings.

*Optimal cultural competence* is at the core (core value or goal) and had been added to the 2016 model illustration as a visible reminder of its significance.

(Figure 3.1). Optimal cultural competence: (a) goes beyond competence (a minimum expectation) toward the pinnacle or peak performance goal; (b) embraces the diversity of diversity; (c) fosters multicultural harmony; (d) facilitates cultural safety; (e) promotes the delivery of the highest level of culturally congruent

1. Cultural competence is an ongoing, multidimensional learning process that integrates transcultural skills in all three dimensions (cognitive, practical, and affective), involves TSE (confidence) as a major influencing factor, and aims to achieve culturally congruent care.
2. TSE is a dynamic construct that changes over time and is influenced by formalized exposure to culture care concepts (transcultural nursing). *
3. The learning of transcultural nursing skills is influenced by self-efficacy perceptions (confidence). *
4. The performance of transcultural nursing skill competencies is directly influenced by the adequate learning of such skills and by TSE perceptions. *
5. The performance of culturally congruent nursing skills is influenced by self-efficacy perceptions and by formalized educational exposure to transcultural nursing care concepts and skills throughout the educational experience. *
6. All students and nurses (regardless of age, ethnicity, gender, sexual orientation, lifestyle, religion, socioeconomic status, geographic location, or race) require formalized educational experiences to meet culture care needs of diverse individuals. *
7. The most comprehensive learning involves the integration of cognitive, practical, and affective dimensions. *
8. Learning in the cognitive, practical, and affective dimensions is paradoxically distinct yet interrelated. *
9. Learners are most confident about their attitudes (affective dimension) and least confident about their transcultural nursing knowledge (cognitive dimension). *
10. Novice learners will have lower self-efficacy perceptions than advanced learners. *
11. Inefficacious individuals are at risk for decreased motivation, lack of commitment, and/or avoidance of cultural considerations when planning and implementing nursing care.
12. Supremely efficacious (overly confident) individuals are at risk for inadequate preparation in learning the transcultural nursing skills necessary to provide culturally congruent care.
13. Early intervention with at-risk individuals will better prepare nurses to meet cultural competency. *
14. The greatest change in TSE perceptions will be detected in individuals with low self-efficacy (low confidence) initially, who have then been exposed to formalized transcultural nursing concepts and experiences. *

**FIGURE 3.2** Assumptions of Jeffreys' Cultural Competence and Confidence (CCC) model.
*Note.* All conceptual models and theories have underlying assumptions; however, validation of proposed underlying assumptions via valid quantitative and qualitative evidence is often missing. Some assumptions cannot be validated; they are merely "assumptions" or "tenets" that one holds true. Other proposed assumptions can be measured empirically. Many of CCC model's underlying assumptions have been validated via numerous studies in practice and academic settings worldwide using the model's corresponding TSET questionnaire. Assumptions tested and supported empirically are indicated by an asterisk (*).
*Source:* Reprinted from *Teaching Cultural Competence in Nursing and Health Care: Inquiry, Action, and Innovation* (3rd ed., pp. 75–76), by M. R. Jeffreys, 2016, New York, NY: Springer Publishing.

patient care for individuals, families, and communities; and (f) requires ongoing active learning. Within the model, "*diversity of diversity*" acknowledges that culture is more than just "labels" and requires individualized assessment. Diversity may exist based on birthplace, citizenship status, reason for migration, migration history, food, religion, ethnicity, race, language, kinship and family networks, educational background and opportunities, employment skills and opportunities, lifestyle, gender, sexual orientation, socioeconomic status (class), politics, past discrimination and bias experiences, health status and health risk, age, insurance coverage, and other variables.

As a result of formalized education and other types of learning, the cognitive, practical, and affective dimensions of TSE and transcultural skill development can change over time. Cognitive skills include knowledge and comprehension about ways in which cultural factors may influence (care among) individuals of different cultural backgrounds and throughout various phases of the life cycle; practical refers to verbal and nonverbal communication skills; and affective pertains to attitudes, values, and beliefs including self-awareness, awareness of cultural gap (differences), acceptance, appreciation, recognition, and advocacy. While individually distinct, the three dimensions are all interrelated and influence optimal cultural competence. *Optimal* cultural competence in self and in others involves seven essential steps: self-assessment; active promotion; systematic inquiry; decisive action; innovation; measurement; and evaluation however it is not a linear process and does not result in an end or final product labeled "I am culturally competent." Envisioning and experiencing continual movement, development, and interaction between all steps offers infinite possibilities for further development through ongoing inquiry, action, and innovation.

A unique feature of the model is that its major concepts, propositions, and constructs are supported by quantitative studies using the Transcultural Self-Efficacy Tool (TSET), a questionnaire with consistently high psychometric properties (validity and reliability). Notably, over 70 studies utilizing the CCC model and/or its associated TSET, support underlying assumptions of the model. (Figure 3.2). Findings from the CCCET, multimethod, and qualitative studies also substantiate the CCC model.

## THEORETICAL APPLICATION AND EMPIRICAL SUPPORT: LITERATURE OVERVIEW

The Cumulative Index to Nursing and Allied Health Literature (CINAHL), Academic Search Complete, Medline, Google, Google Scholar, and Virginia Henderson Library Repository databases were searched for studies that incorporated the CCC model and/or one of its associated questionnaires, revealing a variety of sources including peer-reviewed journal articles in English and other languages, doctoral dissertations, DNP capstone projects, conference brochures and abstracts, posters, PowerPoint presentations, and reports. An added strength for this chapter in the *Annual Review of Nursing Research* is that it is prepared by the theorist and researcher who is privy to knowledge that may not be accessible to others and who can share insights and practical do's and don'ts for others to build upon and expand the work begun over the last 25 years. (Appendices A and B). Between 1999 through to the present, the author received numerous requests from educators and researchers to review and/or administer the TSET. Prior to each book edition (Jeffreys, 2006, 2010, 2016a) the author attempted to reach requesters via e-mail, letter, and/or phone and to send a TSET-User Questionnaire. Prior to her first book and TSET copyright transfer to Springer Publishing Company (2006), author had requested researchers to send a copy

**TABLE 3.1**
*Summary of Study Locations, Settings, and Purposes*

| Location and setting | | | |
|---|---|---|---|
| **Countries** | **United States (U.S.)** | | **59** |
| | **Outside U.S.** | | **14** |
| (*n* = 9) | | Australia | 2 |
| | | Canada | 2 |
| | | China | 2 |
| | | Greece | 3 |
| | | Norway | 1 |
| | | Philippines | 1 |
| | | South Korea | 2 |
| | | Turkey | 1 |
| **Studies in academia** | **Nursing students** | | **56** |
| (*n* = 62) | | Practical nurse | 1 |
| | | Associate degree nursing (ADN) | 14 |
| | | Baccalaureate | 34 |
| | | Masters | 5 |
| | | Doctoral (DNP) | 3 |
| | **Healthcare science students** | | **1** |
| | **Nursing faculty** | | **5** |
| | **Administrators** | | **1** |
| **Studies in the clinical workplace** | Staff RNs | | **12** |
| | Nurse practitioners | | **3** |
| | Multidisciplinary health professionals | | **1** |
| (*n* = 17) | Healthcare personnel | | **1** |

(*Continued*)

TABLE 3.1

*Summary of Study Locations, Settings, and Purposes (Continued)*

| Purpose | | |
|---|---|---|
| **Educational intervention (EI)— Academia** (*n* = 16) | <u>**Educational intervention**</u> | **16** |
| | Immersion-Domestic | 2 |
| | Immersion-International | 6 |
| | Faculty development program | 1 |
| | Service-learning | 6 |
| | Simulation | 1 |
| | Standardized patient | 1 |
| **Educational intervention (EI)— Employees** (*n* = 6) | <u>**Educational Intervention**</u> | |
| | Modules | 1 |
| | Professional development program | 3 |
| | Self-instruction learning packet | 1 |
| | Train-the-trainer | 1 |
| **Course or program evaluation** (*n* = 21) | **Course evaluation** | **10** |
| | **Program evaluation** | **12** |
| **Instrumentation** (Main purpose(s) design, translation, or other validation) (*n* = 11) | <u>TSET</u> | |
| | Initial design study series | 4 |
| | Translation | 3 |
| | Factor analysis | 5 |
| | **Cultural Competence Clinical Evaluation Tool (CCCET)** | **2** |
| **Perceptions or relationship studies** (*n* = 20) | Perceptions (TSE) | **12** |
| | Relationship (of TSE to other variables) | **8** |

of TSET psychometric properties and research results. Address changes and/or lack of response, and/or researchers who had not followed through with their research and/or who had not completed their study occurred. Several completed TSET-User Questionnaires were accompanied by a more detailed study report, master's thesis, or dissertation. Hand searches of books and references cited in other published and unpublished materials also uncovered some studies. Serendipitous discoveries yielded some results, such as conference abstracts or handouts.

There were several anticipated limitations in this review method. First, depending on type of source reviewed, more-or-less detail could be expected. For example, dissertations contained (or should have contained) the most details while articles and other sources, were more restricted due to space requirements, target audience, and/or purpose. Second, it remains unknown how many researchers requesting the TSET conducted and completed studies; however, the author did make a systematic attempt to follow up with researchers. Third, the author can only read English, therefore materials written exclusively in other languages could not be reviewed. Several journal articles contained abstracts and tables written in English but not the narrative, therefore the English sections were included. Lastly, the author relied on written reports and/or personal correspondence concerning the methodology and back-translations of TSET-translated versions.

Several unexpected discoveries or challenges will be mentioned to alert others who may conduct similar searches. Misspelling of the author's last name occurred several times, even in same article, with her name spelled several different ways so indexing and future citation errors could/did occur. Similarly, other misspellings or typographical errors in the full name of the model, TSET, and/or subscale names were discovered.

Using the described method, a total of 73 studies used the CCC model as a framework and/or administered all 3 subscales of the TSET and/or Cultural Competence Clinical Evaluation Tool (CCCET). (See Appendix C). (A few studies administered only 1 TSET subscale and were excluded). Most studies were conducted in the United States (*n* = 59) with fourteen studies conducted in Australia, Canada, China, Greece, Norway, the Philippines, South Korea, and Turkey. (Table 3.1). Several studies targeted more than one setting or sample, therefore they were included in more than one table subcategory. For example, Andrews and colleagues' collaborative train-the-trainer multiphase study provided 37 webinars and face-to-face training sessions to 1,024 RNs, 113 NPs, 149 nursing faculty, and 1,830 nursing students from 45 states over 5 years of grant-funding (Andrews et al, 2011; Andrews & Collins, 2015; Collins & Andrews, 2016). Most studies were conducted in academia (*n* = 62) primarily with undergraduate nursing students (*n* = 48). Over half (*n* = 34) targeted baccalaureate nursing students, followed by associate degree nursing students (*n* = 14) although nursing students in practical, associate degree, masters, and Doctor of Nursing Practice (DNP) programs as well as health science students were also studied. Five studies surveyed nursing faculty and one study also included academic administrators. Of the seventeen studies conducted with healthcare providers or workers in the clinical workplace (including clinics, hospitals, community health), most involved staff RNs (*n* = 12), three with nurse practitioners, and two with multidisciplinary healthcare providers and/or workers.

Studies were further categorized according to the predominant or primary purpose of the study as stated in the document reviewed; however, many studies listed several purposes in overlapping areas. Appendix C is organized by the following categories that emerged related to the primary study purpose: (a) instrumentation; (b) educational intervention (academia); (c) educational intervention (clinical workplace); (d) course evaluation; (e) program evaluation; (f) perceptions; and (g) relationship of TSE to other variables. Regardless of study purpose, to obtain valid quantitative research results, researchers must use a valid measurement tool and follow the recommended procedures for data collection, analysis, and interpretation, therefore instrumentation is discussed first. Appendix A provides additional details for researchers.

## INSTRUMENTATION: TSET DEVELOPMENT, VALIDITY, AND RELIABILITY

The TSET was developed using general and specific conceptual and psychometric guidelines concerning the questionnaire design process. Based on the literature in transcultural nursing, education, psychology (self-efficacy), and psychometrics, the TSET is a comprehensive tool reviewed by 6 doctoral prepared experts in transcultural nursing and education to determine content validity. The TSET has been rigorously tested since 1994, with high reports of validity and reliability; thereby lending ongoing support for the CCC model. In addition, several published reviews by external multidisciplinary evaluators noted the strong psychometric properties (validity and reliability) and comprehensiveness of the TSET and CCC model as providing a strong conceptual and psychometric framework relevant to multiple disciplines (Capell, Veenstra, & Dean, 2007; Gozu et al., 2007; Harper, 2008; Krentzman & Townsend, 2008; Lin, Lee, & Huang, 2017; Loftin et al., 2013; Shen, 2015). Details concerning TSET initial design are provided in Appendix A (#1-21), with ongoing evaluation listed throughout the appendix.

### Internal Consistency

Internal consistency is concerned with the degree to which questionnaire items correlate with each other and reflect the same concept. Cronbach $\alpha$ (coefficient $\alpha$) is commonly calculated to determine internal consistency. Cronbach $\alpha$ scores, collected over time, contribute to the growing psychometric history of a questionnaire and its usability for a variety of samples, purposes, and settings. Using all available Cronbach $\alpha$ scores, 3 groupings of analyses were conducted: (a) studies by TSET author including instrument design testing and psychometrics as well as subsequent studies; (b) studies by researchers other than TSET author including TSET-translated versions and TSET-Multidisciplinary Heal thcare Provider (MHP) version; and (c) studies by researchers other than TSET author excluding TSET-translated versions and TSET-MHP.

**TABLE 3.2**

*Transcultural Self-Efficacy Tool (TSET) Cronbach α Scores: Overview and Synthesis*

| | # of studies | # of Cronbach scores | Total | Cognitive | Practical | Affective | Post-test total | Post-test cognitive | Post-test practical | Post-test affective | Sample size range |
|---|---|---|---|---|---|---|---|---|---|---|---|
| **Studies by TSET author (Jeffreys)** | | | | | | | | | | | |
| | 9 | | .98 | .97 | .97 | .96 | .98 | .97 | .97 | .97 | 9 to 1260 |
| ***Combined*** (Pretest and post-test TSET total and subscale Cronbach α calculations within study) | | 16 | .98 | .97 | .97 | .96 | | | | | |
| Range of Cronbach α scores including original series of studies (.91 to .99) total and all subscales | | | .97–.99 | .94–.99 | .96–.99 | .91–.99 | | | | | |
| **Studies by other researchers (7 TSET-translated and 1 TSET-MHP included)** | | | | | | | | | | | |
| | 26 | 24 | .97 | | | | | | | | 16 to |
| | | 10 | | | | | .98 | | | | 1156 |
| | | 7 | | .96 | .97 | .93 | | .98 | .97 | .97 | |

*(Continued)*

| | | | | | | | | | | | |
|---|---|---|---|---|---|---|---|---|---|---|---|
| ***Combined*** | | 31 | .97 | | | | | | | | |
| (All times TSET total and TSET subscales Cronbach $\alpha$ calculations as part of study) 1–4 times, such as pretest and 1 or more administrations in a longitudinal study) | | 26 | | .96 | .97 | .93 | | | | | |
| Range of Cronbach $\alpha$ scores | | | .81–.99 | 82–.99 | .80–.99 | .4–.99[a] .87–.99[b] | | | | | |
| **Studies by other researchers (TSET translated and TSET-MHP excluded)** | | | | | | | | | | | |
| Other researchers | 18 | 18 | .96 | | | | | | | | 16 to 749 |
| (TSET translated and TSET-MHP excluded) | | 16 | | .96 | .97 | .92 | | | | | |
| | | 9 | | | | | .98 | | | | |
| | | 7 | | | | | | .98 | .98 | .97 | |
| ***Combined*** | | 28 | .97 | | | | | | | | |
| (All times TSET total and TSET subscales Cronbach $\alpha$ calculations as part of study) 1–4 times, such as pretest and 1 or more administrations in a longitudinal study) | | 24 | | .97 | .97 | .94 | | | | | |
| Range of Cronbach $\alpha$ scores | | | .81–.99 | 82–.99 | .80–.99 | .4–.99a .87–.99[b] | | | | | |

[a].4 only obtained 1 time.

[b].87 to .99 if outlier of .4 removed. Average then equals .96.

Table 3.2 presents number of studies and number of Cronbach scores reported and included in the calculation of the average for the total TSET and its subscales. Because sample size can influence internal consistency and Cronbach $\alpha$, sample size range is also included. Although not all pretest-post-test designs evaluated Cronbach $\alpha$ for each TSET administration, for the purposes of this review, post-test scores were also appraised separately from one-time appraisal. When multiple administrations of a survey occur, one concern could be the influence of completing the survey previously on follow-up (repeat administration of surveys). Among researchers who administered pretest and post-tests (intervention study or program study with integrated educational intervention throughout course or curriculum), and conducted $\alpha$ testing with both pretest and post-test, $\alpha$ coefficient results were close (largest difference was .02 [Schmidt, 2012]), aggregate difference was .01), specifically aggregated pretest .99 to mean aggregated post-test .97), individual range from .81 to .99. Notably, all but 1 alpha total TSET score was below .9; the coefficient was .81, an acceptable value. Therefore, it was concluded that multiple administrations of the TSET in these studies did not influence internal consistency as measured by Cronbach $\alpha$. During the TSET design phase, test–retest reliability was adequate and as expected with a 2-week interval from prior to the start of any nursing "content" to 2 weeks for beginning nursing students (Appendix A, #17). Post-test scores are also provided separately and are aggregated into the overall calculation of Cronbach $\alpha$ scores.

Grouping 1. The analyses encompassed all studies by TSET author. Because an intended purpose would be to obtain baseline information, guide educational interventions within and between courses and program levels, and evaluate outcomes, preliminary testing was done with entry-into-practice students. Cultural competence at entry into practice has the potential to make the furthermost positive difference in meeting healthcare needs of diverse patient populations. Additionally, preliminary testing was done with associate degree nursing (ADN) students in an urban, northeast public university setting in a city known for diverse cultures. Consequently, diverse students would be caring for patients and communities who were culturally different and who represented a broad spectrum of diversity ("diversity of diversity" concept). Another advantage of piloting with ADN students was that in the United States (in 1994 and currently), the greatest number of nurses graduate from ADN programs and ADN programs have highest number of nontraditional and culturally diverse students. Moreover, the author had research, teaching, and curricular expertise with nontraditional associate degree nursing students and convenient access to the desired population and setting with institutional review board approval.

Meticulous detail to questionnaire design was time consuming but necessary (Appendix A, #1-21). The initial instrument development study of ADN students provided key data for evidence-based decision-making (Jeffreys & Smodlaka, 1996). Study two, a multi-site study ($n$ = 1,260), included nursing students from 2 traditional baccalaureate programs and 5 ADN programs and broadened knowledge and psychometric history of TSET beyond one setting and included a more diverse student population (Jeffreys & Smodlaka, 1998). In addition to high Cronbach $\alpha$ scores for the total TSET and all subscales, the exploratory factor analysis study yielded factors that made sense conceptually and was consistent with the underlying framework and related scholarly literature; Cronbach $\alpha$ scores of all factors ranged from .88 to .95. Two contrasting group (cross-sectional and longitudinal) studies with ADN students provided additional evidence that the TSET could detect within groups (over time pre and post educational intervention longitudinally) and between groups (novice and advance learners – cross-sectionally), yielding consistently high Cronbach $\alpha$ scores (.91 to .99) (Jeffreys & Smodlaka, 1999a, 1999b). Three subsequent studies with associate degree nursing students and 2 small samples of graduate nursing students yielded consistent results ranging from .97 to .99 (average .98) for the total TSET with subscale Cronbach $\alpha$ averages .97 (Cognitive and Practical) and .96 (Affective) (Jeffreys, 2011; Jeffreys & Dogan, 2010, 2012).

Grouping 2. The analyses comprised 26 studies by researchers other than the author, including 7 administering TSET-translated versions and 1 TSET-MHP version with sample size ranging from 16 to 1156. The TSET was administered to nursing students (ADN, BS, MS, DNP) and non-nursing health science students, faculty, administrators, and nurses in clinical practice settings. Using twenty-four Cronbach $\alpha$ scores reported for the total instrument, aggregated results demonstrated high internal consistency of .97. Post-test total instrument Cronbach $\alpha$ yielded a similarly high score of .98. Aggregated score average of seven studies reporting Cronbach subscale calculations yielded the following: Cognitive Pretest .96 and Post-test .98; Practical Pretest and Post-test .97; and Affective Pretest .93 and Post-test .97. When combining all times Cronbach $\alpha$ was calculated for the total instrument as part of a study (1-4 times, such as pretest and 1 or more administrations in a longitudinal study), Cronbach $\alpha$ scores were high at .97 (total), .96 (Cognitive), .97 (Practical) and .93 (Affective).

Grouping 3. The analyses contained 18 studies by researchers other than the author but excluded the 7 studies administering TSET-translated versions and 1 TSET-MHP version. Sample size ranged from 16 to 749 and excluded health science students and nurses and nursing students outside the United States. Aggregated, average scores using all previously mentioned combinations (Table 3.2) remained high and ranged from .92 to .98.

Section Summary Statement. The consistently high Cronbach $\alpha$ scores generated from 35 studies conducted by TSET author ($n$ = 9) and other researchers reporting $\alpha$ coefficients of the TSET, TSET-MHP version, or TSET-translated version provides strong support for the questionnaire's internal consistency overall (total questionnaire) and each subscale, thereby contributing to the growing psychometric history of the TSET and further advancing the body of knowledge, applicability, and utility of the CCC model and TSE construct across settings and sample populations globally. Despite varied sample size and whether single or repeated TSET administration, and regardless of study groupings analyses, Cronbach $\alpha$ is consistently high for the total instrument and its subscales.

## THEORY, INNOVATION, MEASUREMENT, AND EVALUATION (TIME): UTILITY

As with most theoretical models that strive to make abstractions immediately relevant, useful, and purposeful in a practice discipline, the CCC model (Figure 3.1) was proposed as tentative and requiring modification when new data became available. Subsequently, researchers around the world who applied the theory, model. and its corresponding questionnaire (TSET and/or CCCET) according to the recommended specifications have continued to confirm many of the testable underlying assumptions originally proposed (Figure 3.2). In addition, more sophisticated statistical techniques previously not available have expanded the possibilities to substantiate the theory and support the excellent psychometric properties of the TSET (Jeffreys, 2016a; Jeffreys & Dogan, 2010). Feedback from researchers and educators using the model indicates that they selected and implemented the model for one, several, or all proposed purposes, goal, and uses of the model, noting its ease and benefits in providing a comprehensive framework.

A theory's utility can be demonstrated by the innovations it inspires and the easily measurable desirable outcomes it produces. Innovations can take many forms. One purpose of the theory and TSET is to provide baseline information before designing cultural competence educational intervention strategies. Several researchers administered the TSET and/or CCCET as an exploratory strategy for obtaining baseline self-efficacy in each domain (cognitive, practical, affective), so that items or areas of higher or lower ratings could assist in determining prioritized educational target areas. Several descriptive studies aimed to assess TSE perceptions ($n$ = 12) or examine TSE in relation to other variables ($n$ = 8). Researcher-recommended results include developing diagnostic-prescriptive cultural competence education programs or strategies for various groups of learners (healthcare professionals and students), settings (academia, clinical, workplace), and/or topics.

An innovative example of this was Hoyer's study designed to "explore transcultural self-efficacy in nursing education administrators/faculty and to gain

TABLE 3.3
*Educational Strategies Specifically Mentioned Within Resources Reviewed*

| | **Educational Strategies Specifically Mentioned within Resources Reviewed**[a] Presented in rank order (most frequent to least frequent) |
|---|---|
| 1 | Cultural assessment |
| 2 | Case study |
| 3 | Immersion-international, Lecture, Reflection |
| 4 | Clinical, Discussion |
| 5 | Articles, Films/videos/videoclips, Self-heritage, Test questions |
| 6 | Service-learning |
| 7 | Cultural interview, Journaling, Physical assessment, Group work, Project |
| 8 | Guest presenter, Story-telling |
| 9 | Book, Care plans, Immersion-domestic, Modules/tutorials, Paper component, Professional development program, Simulation |
| 10 | Brainstorming, Computer-based education, Concept-mapping, Cultural food buffet, Debate, Documentation, Gaming/games, Online vs. f2f, Paper/essay/book review, Poster, PowerPoint, Reflexive photography, Role play, Standardized patient, Technical skills V-Sim, Web links or LMS resources |

[a]Excludes resources by Jeffreys.

understanding of confidence related to [lesbian, gay, bisexual, transgender] LGBT issues" (Hoyer, 2016, p. 222). In her study, 4,374 nursing education administrators and faculty employed at Collegiate Nursing Education (CCNE) nursing programs in Michigan, Indiana, Ohio, Illinois and Wisconsin were surveyed online over a 3-week period with the TSET and additional LGBT questions. Three areas, receiving continuing education in transcultural nursing, LGBT education, and confidence discussing LGBT issues with the management team contributed to an increase in TSET scores within all three subscales. There was a positive relationship between TSET results and confidence with providing nursing education related to LGBT issues. Consequently, Hoyer proposed,

> Findings from this study may inform this issue in two ways: first, to encourage leadership to include LGBT content within the nursing student's formal education to positively impact practice for LGBT patients; and second, to provide data to nursing academic institutions for the need to expand LGBT

**BOX 3.1**

*Transcultural Nursing Course*

Innovation: "Throughout the semester the following methods of instruction were implemented: Lecture, discussions, brainstorming, videos and DVD (*The Multicultural Health Series, Part I and Part II* and *Cultural Issues in the Clinical Setting* (Kaiser Permanente, 2002, 2003, 2004) and *Hold Your Breath* (Grainger-Monsen & Haslett, 2005), PowerPoint presentations by faculty and students, book review of *The Spirit Catches You and You Fall down* (Fadiman, 1997), cultural meal and guest speakers. Eshleman and Davihizar (2006) suggest integrating a cultural meal and guest speakers into the curriculum to promote cultural competency. Therefore, students were required to complete a variety of assignments including: Self-heritage assessment, group cultural assessment, cultural film review, cultural educational pamphlet, and an interview of a client from another culture. In addition, the nursing students, course faculty and the university's multicultural coordinator planned a cultural meal for junior and senior level nursing students, nursing faculty, and university administrators. Using media, 20 multicultural case studies were shown to the students throughout the semester to simulate real life scenarios the students may experience during their nursing careers. Moreover, *The Spirit Catches You and You Fall Down* was assigned to the students to assist them to recognize some barriers patients from diverse populations may face while implementing our health care system." (Adams & Nevel, 2016, pp. 248–252).

Measurement: A convenience sample of 55 generic baccalaureate and RN-BSN students completed the TSET at the beginning (pretest) and at the end (post-test) of the course.

Evaluation: A significant increase from pretest to post-test was found in all three subscales (cognitive, practical, and affective) following the transcultural nursing educational strategies implemented throughout the course.

**REFERENCES**

Eshleman, J., & Davidhizar, R. E. (2006). Strategies for developing cultural competency in an RN-BSN program. *Journal of Transcultural Nursing, 17*(2), 179–183.

Fadiman, A. (1997). *The spirit catches you and you fall* down. New York, NY: Farrar, Straus and Giroux.

Grainger-Mosen, & Haslett, J. (Producers). (2005). *Hold your Breath [DVD]*. (Available from Fanlight Productions, 4196 Washington Street, Boston, MA 02131.)

Kaiser Permanente. (2002). *Cultural issues in the clinical setting (Series A and B)* [videocassette]. Available from Kaiser Permanente National Video Communications and Media Services, 825 Colorado Blvd., Suite 301, Los Angeles, CA, 90041.

Kaiser Permanente. (2003). *The multicultural health series (Part 1)* [videocassette]. Available from Kaiser Permanente National Video Communications and Media Services, 825 Colorado Blvd., Suite 301, Los Angeles, CA, 90041.

Kaiser Permanente. (2004). *The multicultural health series (Part 2)* [videocassette]. Available from Kaiser Permanente National Video Communications and Media Services, 825 Colorado Blvd., Suite 301, Los Angeles, CA, 90041.

educational opportunities to nursing education faculty and administrators. (Hoyer, 2016, p. 222)

Immediate post-study local interventions included committee formation and monthly meetings for cultural competence enhancements visibly inclusive of LGBT issues that targeted faculty, administrators, and students.

Another type of innovation is instrumentation studies involving TSET translations following the recommended permission procedures and methodology for translation, back-translation, pilot testing, and expanded studies examining psychometric properties of translated versions. Three studies involved TSET translations with three additional factor analysis studies for translated versions of the TSET-Chinese, TSET-Greek, and TSET-Turkish (Appendix C – Instrumentation). Recent requests to translate into additional languages suggest that instrumentation research may currently be in progress.

Of the 73 studies, most encompassed innovations targeting individual, multiple, multidimensional, and/or integrated educational interventions. Researchers utilized the CCC model as a guide and the TSET as a pretest and post-test following educational interventions with a select focus on a type of intervention or on interventions integrated in a complementary, scaffolded fashion throughout a course and/or program. Although space limitations may have been a concern in some of the sources reviewed, educational strategies specifically mentioned within resources reviewed are presented in Table 3.3. Major ones are mentioned; however, they should not be construed as producing greatest results (educational outcomes) but simply informational.

## INNOVATION SPOTLIGHTS

The next sections present a brief synopsis of select innovations, measurement, and evaluation. Together with innovation exemplar boxes, these resources aim to provide readers, researchers, and educators with a springboard of evidence-based and theoretically linked teaching-learning strategies (congruent with the CCC model) to spark new ideas, innovations, and adapt into their clinical, research, education, and/or workplace setting. Appendix C and the reference list provide additional resources for readers who seek more information concerning each innovation.

### Transcultural Nursing Course

Adams and Nevel (2007, 2016) evaluated the effectiveness of a transcultural nursing course on baccalaureate nursing students' transcultural self-efficacy. (Box 3.1) Innovation details demonstrate how the course incorporated comprehensively

**BOX 3.2**

*Service-Learning in an Associate Degree Nursing Course*

Innovation: A community health nursing course

> required all students to complete 23 service-learning hours, 10 reflection hours, and 7 mandatory lecture hours. Students completed service-learning activities in diverse community settings. Students were permitted to complete their service-learning hours at a variety of agencies and activities, ranging from community health fairs and health screenings to health promotion and education in the communities with a focus on women and children. All activities were overseen by nursing faculty. Students were also required to write reflection journal entries for every activity and lecture they attended, which were provided to the nursing faculty for evaluation. (Rogers-Walker, 2016, pp. 307–310).

Measurement: A convenience sample of 55 culturally diverse third-semester students enrolled in a community health nursing course completed the TSET during the first 3 weeks of the course (pretest) and during the last 2 weeks of the course (post-test).

Evaluation: TSE perceptions significantly increased from pretest to post-test on all four measures (cognitive, practical, affective, and total score) following completion of a community health course with a service-learning component.

planned and scaffolded teaching-learning activities purposely designed to tap into all learning domains. The visible interconnectedness creatively taps into all learning domains, utilizes all senses, and provides ongoing feedback to learners. Strategies are purposely crafted to continually engage diverse learners to develop the attitudes, knowledge, skills, and confidence within a culturally safe academic environment that values diverse learners and embraces diversity, including diverse ways of learning. The results of this study supported the CCC theoretical assumption that transcultural self-efficacy is dynamic and changes following effective transcultural nursing educational strategies.

The researchers recommended future administrations of the TSET to evaluate new teaching-learning strategies introduced within the course. Subsequently, Adams (2012) conducted a non-equivalent, multiple year, quasi-experimental study to evaluate service-learning as an innovative teaching-learning strategy, demonstrating significant changes in TSE on all TSET subscales following the strategy. She proposed that the results of her study should

> inspire servant leaders in higher education and communities to work collaboratively to develop service-learning cultural immersions for nursing

**BOX 3.3**

*Cultural Immersion Abroad*

Innovation: Following completion of a community health nursing course,

> The 14 students participating in an immersion completed a one credit cultural selective class to prepare for the immersion experience. These students then either spent 2 weeks in El Paso, Texas/Juarez, Mexico or 2 and ½ weeks in South Africa. Both groups of students experienced the culture by living in the communities and providing health care to the population (Larsen & Reif, 2016, p. 300).

Measurement: Study abroad participants completed the TSET online 1 week before and immediately following their immersion experience. Nursing students not participating in a study abroad experience ($n = 25$) acted as a control group and completed the TSET at the same times.

Evaluation: TSE scores increased significantly on all subscales for pretest to post-test for both immersion group and control group. Additionally, cultural immersion participants had significantly greater positive change scores on each subscale when compared with student non-participants (Larsen & Reif, 2011, 2016).

> students to address health disparities, render culturally competent nursing care to diverse populations, demonstrate health education and promotion skills, and become engaged citizens in their communities. (Adams, 2012, p. iv)

### Service-Learning in an Associate Degree Nursing Course

Although justification of resources and adequate preparation of faculty to lead service-learning and/or immersion experiences are concerns for all programs, time and financial constraints of associate degree nursing (ADN) programs present additional challenges. Using a quasi-experimental, one group pretest post-test survey research design, Rogers-Walker (2014, 2016) evaluated the effectiveness of service-learning among associate degree nursing students by determining if there was significant increase in students' TSE perceptions prior to and after participating in required service-learning activities. (Box 3.2). TSE perceptions significantly increased from pretest to post-test on all 3 TSET subscales and total score following course completion. She recommended early introduction of cultural competence education within ADN

**BOX 3.4**

*Complementing, Connecting, and Scaffolding Courses and Domestic and International Immersion Experiences*

Innovation:

"Nursing Seminar – Fall semester: Course content addressed cultural awareness, cultural knowledge, and cultural skills. Discussion included cultural stumbling blocks: acculturation, prejudice, discrimination, racism, ethnocentrism, cultural blindness, cultural conflict, cultural imposition, stereotyping, in addition to cultural building blocks: cultural sensitivity, knowledge, respect, willingness to modify care, and cultural relativism.

Intercultural Health Care – Spring semester: Discussion, focus sheets, interviews and intercultural service learning experience. This course emphasized the value of human diversity in order to provide safe, high-quality care across the age spectrum. Culture shock and reverse entry are discussed. Students were expected to immerse themselves in a culture other than their own through a faculty lead intercultural experience.

Intercultural Service Learning: (common experiences/activities): Students self-select the location of the immersion intercultural 12-14 day experience. Each student participated in daily reflective journaling, debriefing, practiced nursing within an intercultural site, actively participated in cultural interaction with patients, patient's families, and within the community, and participated in cultural events during the experience. Trip costs vary from $500-$3,000.

Domestic (Arizona, Georgia, Illinois, or Indiana): *n* = 18

International (Belize, India, or Uganda): *n* = 38" (Schmidt, 2016, p. 176–177).

Measurement: 56 senior baccalaureate nursing students completed the TSET and CCCET-SV pretest at the end of their "seminar in nursing" course (Fall semester) and post-test after spring semester course and intercultural SL experience.

Evaluation:

- Statistically significant increases occurred in TSET subscale scores for both groups.
- There were no statistically significant differences in TSE between domestic and international service learning groups.
- When examining changes in TSET subscale scores, the international group experienced statistically significant greater change in Practical Subscale scores.

(*Continued*)

**BOX 3.4**

*Complementing, Connecting, and Scaffolding Courses and Domestic and International Immersion Experiences (Continued)*

- Comparison of CCCET-SV individual item scores (percent and frequency) provided information about provision of cultural-specific care (Subscale 1; 25 items), cultural assessment (Subscale 2; 28 items), and cultural sensitivity (Subscale 3; 30 items) and their changes post-intercultural SL experience.
- Student scores demonstrated a statistically significant increase in CCCET post-test scores for subscale 3 (Cultural Sensitivity). (Subscale 2 and 3 were not appraised).
- When examining *change scores* (CCCET Subscale 3 [Cultural Sensitivity] pretest to posttest), both groups demonstrated statistically significant increases; however statistically significant difference was noted with international groups demonstrating greater change.

(Schmidt, 2012, 2016)

curricula with opportunities for service-learning activities at varying levels of involvement throughout the program. Well-designed service-learning activities serves a twofold purpose of assisting under-served communities while expanding students' cultural competence development through professional and personal interactions in diverse communities.

## Cultural Immersion Abroad

One question frequently posed is whether cultural immersion abroad makes a difference in cultural competence development. "What is optimal?" is yet another frequently asked question. Using a quasi-experimental non-equivalent control group, cross-sectional design, Larsen and Reif (2011, 2016) evaluated the impact of a study abroad experience on baccalaureate students' transcultural competence (Box 3.3). All students completed a community health course; however, study abroad students completed a one-credit cultural preparatory class and their cultural immersion experience. TSE scores increased significantly on all subscales for pretest to post-test for both immersion abroad group and control group; however, the cultural immersion participants had significantly greater positive change scores on each subscale when compared with student non-participants. (Larsen & Reif, 2016). Based on these results, they recommended offering cultural education classes to include immersion experiences for all students and continue measurement and evaluation using the TSET. Results suggest that complementing, connecting, and scaffolding courses have the greatest potential to enhance cultural competence development and produce optimal outcomes.

### Complementing and Scaffolding Courses and Domestic and International Immersion Experiences

Another frequent question is whether TSE changes or confidence development results in behavior change, specifically, cultural competent behaviors and cultural congruent care with diverse communities. Three related questions include: (a) "Is an international experience needed?"; (b) "Does a domestic immersion or domestic service-learning experience change TSE and cultural competence behaviors and attitudes in clinical settings or with patients and communities?"; and 3) What type of cultural learning immersion experience (international or domestic) yields more significant outcomes?"

Schmidt's (2012, 2016) study design combined quantitative descriptive approaches (administration of the TSET and CCCET) and qualitative approaches (reflective journal responses) to evaluate the effectiveness of a domestic and international service learning experience on baccalaureate students' TSE and cultural competence learning. Box 3.4 highlights learning topics, concepts, and activities purposefully interconnected, complementary, and scaffolded between courses in fall and spring semester followed by the domestic or international immersion service-learning experience. Notably, all students demonstrated statistically significant increases in all 3 TSET subscale scores and CCCET-SV Subscale 3 (Cultural Sensitivity) scores. (CCCET subscale 2 and 3 were not appraised for changes but provided information about cultural assessment and provision of cultural-specific care). Reflective journals elaborated on their experience, adding richness to the data and aligned well with the CCC framework (learning in 3 domains and confidence development).

### Cultural Immersion Impact on Post-Graduates' Clinical Practice

Another question often raised is "What is the impact of cultural competence education and TSE development on future cultural competence behaviors and actions with culturally diverse and different clients and communities?" Amerson's series of quantitative and qualitative studies on cultural immersion experiences locally and internationally provided supportive evidence of the CCC theoretical framework, the TSET, and the impact of these experiences on post-graduates' clinical nursing practice (Amerson, 2009, 2010, 2012, 2016; Amerson & Livingston, 2014). TSET data affirmed that all baccalaureate nursing students enrolled within a community health nursing course demonstrated changes (increases) in TSET subscale and total scores regardless of local or international experiences; however due to small sample size in the international group, further analyses could not determine which sections had statistically significant changes.

In a subsequent study and to further evaluate the process of learning cultural competence during international service learning, Amerson & Livingston (2014) utilized reflexive photography, a qualitative research methodology newer to nursing research. Data collected from over 100 photographs and student interviews were analyzed using the NVivo software and according to prescribed rigor of reflexive photography, yielding themes consistent with the CCC model: cognitive, practical, affective, and transcultural self-efficacy. Later, and to further explore how participation in an international service-learning project (Ecuador or Guatemala) during a community health course influenced TSE of 14 baccalaureate nursing students and their subsequent nursing practice, Amerson utilized an explanatory case study approach.

> A constant comparative analysis of telephone interviews generated findings and themes consistent with the CCC model and suggested that: (a) learning occurred in each of the 3 domains (cognitive, practical, and affective) thereby enhancing transcultural self-efficacy; and (b) graduates were able to provide culturally congruent care as a result of their increased TSE. (Amerson, 2012, p. 6)

### Cultural Competence Education, TSE, and Patient Care Outcomes

Although studies linking underlying assumptions of the CCC model with patient care outcomes have been limited, the beginning evidence is supportive and promising. Francisco's study of nurses in an urban, metropolitan hospital serving diverse, at-risk, and under-served communities comparing nurses' TSET scores, Hospital Consumer Assessment of Healthcare Providers and Systems (HCAHPS) survey item scores, and cultural competence educational experiences suggested that there is a relationship between transcultural self-efficacy, cultural competence, formal and informal cultural competence learning experiences of nurses, and patient satisfaction (2013). In addition, higher TSET scores were associated with nurses who had previous education (such as employee education) with opportunities to implement their learning with diverse populations. Higher HCAHPS scores were found on units staffed by nurses with higher TSET scores (Francisco, 2013).

Further studies administering the TSET pre and post cultural competence employee education programs and correlating scores with patient outcome measures such as HCAHPS (specifically the items related to culture) has great potential. Improving patient outcome measures has many long-term implications

**BOX 3.5**

*Cultural Competence Employee Education: Workshop*

Innovation: After conducting a needs assessment, Dolgan (2001) designed, implemented, and evaluated a full-day, seven-hour face-to-face staff development workshop to enhance the cultural competence of obstetrical nurses caring for culturally different and diverse patients and families. Topics and strategies included: a) welcome, workshop overview, and self-assessment; b) icebreakers and self-heritage sharing; c) story-telling; d) debriefing; e) healthcare disparities and demographic changes; f) group activity, multiculturalism; g) diversity quiz; h) case studies; i) cultural similarities and differences; j) strategies for caring for individuals from different cultures; k) admission assessment; l) summary and conclusion. Five case studies (one of dominant U.S. culture; and 4 cultural and/or religious minority cultures prioritized as high needs within the institution) incorporated cultural values and beliefs, ethnomedicine, women's health issues, traditional and folk healing, religion and spirituality.

Measurement: 19 obstetrical nurses employed at an urban hospital in the mid-west United States completed the TSET immediately prior to the start of the workshop and immediately at the end of the workshop.

Evaluation: Analyses using SEST scores generated statistically significant changes from before workshop to after workshop on all three subscales. Additional paired sample *t*-test analyses comparing mean scores for each TSET question demonstrated statistically significant change between pretest and post-test for virtually every item. All items on the Cognitive and Practical subscales changed significantly. As expected, the Affective subscale item relating to self-awareness of one's own cultural heritage and belief systems (item 54) demonstrated no change; and an additional eight of the remaining 29 subscale items yielded no statistically significant changes. SEL calculations (using low, medium, high grouping initial method – See Appendix A, #23) indicated that changes occurred in the expected direction on all subscales (increase).

beyond just individual patients. For example, since HCAHPS scores are currently related to reimbursement in the United States, higher reimbursement will permit increased quality and quantity of continued services, especially for at-risk and under-served communities while generating substantial revenue for healthcare institutions and providers (Jeffreys, 2016a). Several summative evaluation measure examples focused on patient outcomes (access, quality, and cost) following cultural competence employee workshops and incorporating the TSET provide resources for leaders in health care (Jeffreys, 2016c).

Consistent with one of the intended purposes of the TSET, Francisco (2013) proposed that results (such as TSET items least and most confident) can be used to design a cultural competence program for new nurse orientation with the TSET administered pretest and post-test as well as examining patient satisfaction scores for changes. Analyzing TSET and CCCET results to obtain learner baseline information and develop cultural competence education programs based on learner needs and prioritized focus areas or topics, assists in cost-effective, quality programs and outcomes to meet learner, healthcare consumer, and institutional needs.

## Cultural Competence Workshop for Staff Nurses

To enhance the cultural competence of obstetrical nurses caring for culturally different and diverse patients and families, Dolgan (2001) designed, implemented, and evaluated a full-day, seven-hour face-to-face staff development workshop for obstetrical nurses (Box 3.5). Statistically significant TSET subscale mean scores changes from before the workshop to after the workshop occurred on all three subscales. Paired sample *t*-test analyses comparing mean scores for each TSET question demonstrated statistically significant change between pretest and post-test on all 25 Cognitive Subscale items and all 28 Practical Subscale items. As

**BOX 3.6**

*DNP Capstone: Staff Education: Cultural Assessment, Culturally Congruent Care, and Documentation*

Innovation: Four, educational modules delivered in 2, one-hour sessions consisting of lecture, discussion, PowerPoints, simulation, simulation video vignettes (VSim), resources, charts, cultural assessment documentation forms, chart adaptations to facilitate documentation, documentation of culturally influenced interventions.

Measurement: TSET and patient charts pre and post ($n$ = 8) matched. Chart reviews collected over 4 months on 212 medical records at 5 different data points for cultural assessments and culturally influenced interventions.

Evaluation: Statistically significant changes on the TSET Practical and Affective subscales from pretest to post-test with changes on the Cognitive subscale occurring in the expected direction but just missing statistical significance. Statistically significant increases in cultural assessment documentation (from 34% to 66%) and culturally influenced interventions (from 26% to 74%) by nurse practitioners pre and post educational intervention. Statistical significance reached when examining pre-post documentation of cultural assessments and culturally influenced interventions. (Courtney & Wolgamott, 2015, p. 354)

**BOX 3.7**

*Program Evaluation: DNP-FNP Cultural Competence Curricular Enhancements*

Innovation: The innovation consisted of three major initiatives: faculty development, student development, and web-assisted learning environment with cultural competence resources for faculty and students. During the DNP-FNP curriculum development process, expert consultants (transcultural nursing scholar, nurse scientist, and a clinical psychologist) worked individually and as a team with the DNP-FNP project director, DNP-FNP faculty in several initial foundational professional development workshops aimed at weaving cultural competence throughout the curriculum in regard to topics, assignments, resources, content, concept, and strategy mapping aimed at complementary and scaffolded learning congruent with the 3 pillars within the philosophy of the School of Nursing, and outcome measurements. Strong foundational cultural competence was introduced during a formalized orientation program for newly admitted students and included cultural competence content, concepts, and interactive components including self-awareness and reflection. Cultural competence content, concepts, and learner-centered individual and group activities were woven throughout each course, purposely connected to complement and connect courses at the same curricular level and scaffold at higher levels, leading to end-of-program student learning outcomes and end of program outcomes. The web-assisted learning environment was developed in collaboration of the consultants, librarians, web-designers, and faculty with enhancements during the curriculum based on new literature and resources and curricular and student needs.

Measurement: Five post-masters DNP-FNP student cohorts completed the TSET at the orientation prior to any cultural competence educational interventions (pretest), at the end of year 1, end of year 2, and end of year 3 (end of program). Means, standard deviation, and F tests were calculated across each testing time.

Evaluation: "There were significant gains from program start to finish with a scaffolded cultural competence-enhanced curriculum, as demonstrated across all 5 cohorts. Between-group analyses reflected gains for each cohort with a large gain for 3 cohorts: 2, 3, and 5 had 1 *SD* above the mean while cohorts 1 and 4 had an extra-large gain of 2 *SD* above the mean" (Singleton, 2017, p. 520).

expected, the Affective subscale item relating to self-awareness of one's own cultural heritage and belief systems (item 54) demonstrated no change; and an additional eight of the remaining 29 subscale items yielded no statistically significant changes.

Dolgan's recommendations included: (a) implementing and evaluating the cultural competence educational workshop to newly hired maternity unit nurses for the hospital's new maternity center; (b) extending research time frame and track organizational benefits and long-term effects on participants; and (c) building upon proven strategies that conserves resources and produces measurable outcomes. Her expanded innovation, measurement, and evaluation is presented in the next section.

### Cultural Competence Staff Development: Self-Instruction Learning Packet (SILP)

To promote cost-effective, flexible learning opportunities amidst varying work schedules, time constraints, and a busy work environment, Dolgan (2004) developed a Self-Instruction-Learning-Packet (SILP) identical to her seven-hour training class on cultural competence (Box 3.5). Subsequently, Velez (2005, 2016) conducted a longitudinal study to evaluate the effectiveness of the SILP on 20 obstetrical nurses' TSE. SEST scores changed significantly from pretest (pre-SILP) to post-test (completion of SILP) on all 3 subscales and the total TSET. Despite small sample size, and regardless of format (all-day staff education workshop or SILP), statistically significant changes in TSE on all three subscales occurred following a well-structured, literature-based, comprehensive cultural competence educational strategy that combined cognitive, practical, and affective components with specific application case studies for obstetrical nurses working in an urban, midwestern hospital.

### Staff Education to Enhance Cultural Assessment, Culturally Congruent Care, and Documentation: A DNP Capstone

Revisiting the question raised earlier, "What is the impact of cultural competence education and TSE development on future cultural competence behaviors and actions with culturally diverse and different clients and communities?" presents numerous opportunities for simultaneously connecting clinical, research, education, and the workplace (CREW) to make a positive difference in patient care. For their DNP capstone experience, Courtney and Wolgamott (2015) developed, implemented, and evaluated a cultural competence educational program for multidisciplinary healthcare professionals working in a clinic. Specifically aimed to prepare professionals with basic content and skills needed to conduct a cultural assessment, provide cultural-specific and congruent care, and document accordingly, their project also involved the examination of patient chart documentation pre and post educational intervention (Box 3.6).

Despite small sample size, statistically significant changes occurred in TSE Practical and Affective subscales with changes occurring in the expected direction on the Cognitive subscale. Notably, nurse practitioners' behaviors changed with more cultural assessments increasing from 34% to 66% and culturally influenced care from 26% to 74%. Documentation provides a method for communicating to all healthcare team members the culture care decisions and actions based on focused cultural assessment, and documenting effectiveness of culturally influenced care decisions and actions using action modes (nursing skills and nursing process as illustrated in CCC model). The expansion of high quality DNP programs has the potential to make a positive difference in health care, especially targeting underserved populations, and enhancing the quality of care through cultural congruence. Educators have the potential to make a difference in this regard by enhancing cultural competence through existing programs and/or crafting multidimensional strategies throughout new curricula and programs starting with a core foundational framework. For example, Courtney and Wolgamott, were part of Cohort 2 in a grant-funded DNP program with cultural competence enhancements (See next section).

## Train-the-Trainer, Partnerships, Linking CREW

Spear-headed by Dr. Margaret Andrews (2011), the train-the-trainer grant project had several components, including: (a) faculty development, curriculum development, and student development; (b) partnerships with key organizations with similar philosophy and mission commitment to cultural competence; (c) scholarly networks and guest speakers with expertise in culture, cultural theory, psychometrics; (d) Leininger's framework; (e) Jeffreys' CCC framework; (f) train-the-trainer webinars for nurses in clinical practice and nurse educators; (g) online journal; and (h) measurement and evaluation with the TSET (Andrews et al., 2011; Andrews & Collins, 2015; Collins & Andrews, 2016). As mentioned earlier in the chapter, the train-the-trainer format directly reached 3,116 nursing students, nurses, and nurse educators over a 5-year period with cascading effects of the train-the-trainer format. Trained trainers were prepared to be cultural competence advocates, promoters, and resources within their various settings, seeking and creating formal and informal educational opportunities for cultural competence enhancement in self, individuals, and organizations. Statistically significant aggregate changes were noted between TSET pretest and post-test subscale scores. In addition, statistically significant changes occurred on each of the 83 TSET items (Andrews et al, 2011).

Notably, there were many positive outcomes from this grant, however, for the purposes of this chapter discussion thread, the focus is shifted back to the grant's interventions targeting DNP curricular enhancements. Following a faculty development workshop series and meetings with invited transcultural nurse scholar consultants, coordinated curricular enhancements in the DNP curriculum were designed, implemented, measured, and evaluated. Fifty-three post-masters DNP students completed the TSET at program entry prior to cultural competence educational intervention and post-test (after cultural competence enhanced curriculum intervention) and at the end of year one. Statistically significant increases in TSET mean scores occurred on each of the subscales and total TSET score with an overall increase by 27.8% (Creech et al., 2017).

### Program Evaluation: Cultural Competence Enhancements Throughout the Curriculum

In another multiphase, grant-funded study to enhance cultural competence in a DNP program, Singleton (2017) evaluated the enhancement of cultural competence throughout a DNP-Family Nurse Practitioner (FNP) program by tracking 5 student cohorts prior to any cultural competence education (TSET pretest at orientation) and then at the end of each year of the 3-year program (Box 3.7). Conceptualized prior to the DNP-FNP program design phase, the project consisted of three major initiatives: faculty development, student development, and web-assisted learning environment with cultural competence resources for faculty and students. Consistent with other researchers, statistically significant gains on each TSET subscale and total TSET occurred between pretest and post-tests. Further scrutiny of data revealed that

> while the pre-intervention subscale mean scores showed the students to have the most confidence, or self-efficacy, in the affective domain, the postintervention scores showed a balancing of confidence across the 3 domains – affective, cognitive, and practical. This result supports the assumption of the CCC model that TSE is influenced by formalized education and other learning experiences, and that the curriculum offered comprehensive learning that brought the three domains of learning – cognitive, practical, and affective – into closer balance. (Singleton, 2017, p. 520)

Singleton (2017) summarized,

> There were significant gains from program start to finish with a scaffolded cultural competence-enhanced curriculum, as demonstrated across all 5 cohorts. Between-group analyses reflected gains for each cohort with a large gain for 3 cohorts: 2, 3, and 5 had 1 *SD* above the mean while cohorts 1 and 4 had an extra-large gain of 2 *SD* above the mean. The results

> reinforce the importance of looking at the curriculum over several groups to assess the impact on planned learning outcomes before making curricular changes, as cohorts of students may respond differently to the same curriculum. (Singleton, 2017, p. 520)

Similarly, coordinated cultural competence enhancements throughout undergraduate curricula comparing and contrasting several student cohorts (longitudinal and/or cross-sectional samples measurement with TSET) and conducting formative and summative evaluations over time have yielded findings consistent with the CCC model in associate degree programs (Appendix A) and baccalaureate programs (Curtis, Bultas, & Green, 2016; Grund et. al., 2016; Halter et al., 2015). Common enhancement components include steps consistent with *optimal cultural competence* development: self-assessment, active promotion, systematic inquiry, decisive action, innovation, measurement, and evaluation and correspond with resources available (Jeffreys, 2016a, 2016b).

## UTILITY TO NEW AND/OR PRIORITIZED TOPICS, PEDAGOGY, AND TECHNOLOGY

A theory, model, and questionnaire must be durable throughout time and flexible enough to be adaptable to new situations, topics, pedagogy, and technology. Over time (since initial conceptualization and research in 1993), much has changed in the teaching of cultural competence. Changes such as "cultural competence as a human right that is legally and ethically mandated by numerous accrediting agencies," demographic shifts, and rapidly moving populations worldwide has increased the value and need for cultural competence education. New teaching modalities such as standardized patients, simulation, and distance education present new opportunities for comprehensively weaving together cognitive, psychomotor/practical, and affective learning in order to enhance optimal cultural competence development. Cultural competence within the CCC model advocates the diversity of diversity worldview, going beyond what has been traditionally included to include less visible populations such as multiple heritage (multiethnic or mixed race) individuals and families (Jeffreys & Zoucha, 2017a, 2017b, 2017c), LGBTQ individuals and families, religious minorities, new immigrants, and refugees to name a few. The CCC model and its corresponding questionnaires (TSET, CCCET, and CSAT-DD) have been flexible enough to address new and/or less visible topics in society, health care, pedagogy, and technology. Several examples of their utility to new and/or prioritized topics, pedagogy, and technology are visible in the educational innovations listed below:

- Pre/postnatal virtual simulation experience with African American and Amish patients (Weideman et al, 2016)
- Simulation experience with Muslim and Somalian patients/families concerning respiratory failure and systematic infectious process (Norwegian students) (Grossman, Mager, Opheim, & Torbjornsen, 2012).
- Simulation experience with Muslim and Italian Catholic patients/families concerning respiratory failure and systematic infectious process (US students). (Grossman et. al., 2012).
- Standardized patient simulation, Turkish Muslim female immigrant with limited English proficiency in preoperative setting (Ozkara San, 2018)
- Standardized patient simulation, gay couple of mixed backgrounds (ethnicity, race, religion) in an inpatient setting for management of chronic illness (Ozkara San, 2018).

Several main points concerning these innovations will be mentioned. First, innovations were guided by the CCC model, measured TSE pre-intervention and post-intervention, incorporated multidimensional components, and focused on authentic, real-life clinical situations with immediate relevance to learners within a safe, simulated practice environment. Second, the researchers followed recommended standards for the pedagogy and/or technology selected, such as the International Association for Clinical Simulation and Learning (INACSL) Standards of Best Practice: Simulation (INACSL, 2013, 2016), Jeffries Simulation Framework (Jeffries, 2005; 2012; Jeffries, Rodgers, & Adamson, 2015), and Wallace's (2007) best practices in pedagogy using standardized patients. Third, preparatory, prebriefing, and debriefing components incorporated multidimensional components involving cognitive, psychomotor/practical, and affective learning. Fourth, study results demonstrated increases from pretest to post-test on all subscales and total TSET score with the Affective Subscale just missing statistical significance ($p$ = .054) in one study (Ozkara San, 2018), the Practical Subscale missing statistical significance ($p$ < .07) among Norwegian students (Grossman et al., 2012), and all other mean score comparisons demonstrating statistically significant increases. Fifth, researcher recommendations provide advice for educators and researchers interested in designing, adapting, implementing, and evaluating these or similar strategies within a variety of settings.

## CONCLUSION

Nurses and other healthcare professionals are challenged to engage in the ongoing process of cultural competence development of self and others with a desired outcome goal of achieving cultural congruence in clinical, research, education, and workplace (CREW) settings. Understanding the multidimensional process, participating in formalized transcultural education, broadening the view of diversity, engaging in interprofessional and interdisciplinary collaboration locally and worldwide, developing new educational innovations, and disseminating best practices using valid measures and a connecting framework are priorities, challenges, and future directions. The CCC theoretical model, associated questionnaires, innovation spotlight exemplars, and research presented in this chapter are valuable resources to guide new priorities and future directions.

Prepared by the theorist and researcher who is privy to knowledge that may not be accessible to others, this chapter shared insights, evidence-based decision-making, and practical recommendations. A time-sequenced appendix traced the author's initial questions, conceptualization, series of studies, and other scholarly work in theory development and evaluation that lead up to the present and future. A second appendix, based on questions frequently asked or observations noted when conducting and/or reviewing research involving the CCC model and/or the TSET, presents select recommendations from A to Z (Appendix B). They are intended to prompt a starting point for further inquiry, action, and innovation within an evidence-based framework.

Gleaned from 25 years and over 70 studies incorporating the CCC model and/or one of its associated questionnaires (TSET, CCCET, CSAT-DD), innovation spotlight exemplars across various academic levels (ADN through DNP) and clinical staff settings featured course enhancements, curricular enhancements, service-learning, cultural immersion, employee education, workshops, complementing and scaffolding activities, program evaluation, train-the-trainer, partnerships, and utility to new and/or prioritized topics, pedagogy, and technology. Taken all together, these resources provide readers, educators, and researchers with a springboard of evidence-based and theoretically linked teaching-learning strategies to spark new ideas, innovations, and adapt into their clinical, research, education, and/or workplace setting. "Whatever inquiries, actions, and innovations are done (or not done) today will influence the future. Through coordinated group efforts, the goals of culturally congruent health care and multicultural workplace harmony may be achieved" (Jeffreys, 2016a, p. 561).

## REFERENCES

Adams, T. M. (2012). *The evaluation of service-learning as an innovative strategy to enhance BSN students' transcultural self-efficacy*. (Unpublished doctoral dissertation). Alvernia University, Reading, PA.

Adams, T. M., & Nevel, K. (2007). *Appraisal of BSN Students' Transcultural Self-Efficacy using Jeffreys's Transcultural Self-Efficacy Tool*. (Unpublished study).

Adams, T. M., & Nevel, K. M. (2016). TSET Research Exhibit 8.1, Evaluating the effectiveness of a transcultural nursing course on students' transcultural self-efficacy. In M. R. Jeffreys (Ed.), *Teaching cultural competence in nursing and health care: Inquiry, action, and innovation* (3rd ed., pp. 248–252). New York, NY: Springer Publishing.

Amerson, R. (2009). *The influence of international service-learning on cultural competence in baccalaureate nursing graduates and their subsequent nursing practice.* (Unpublished doctoral dissertation). The Graduate School of Clemson University, Clemson, SC. Retrieved from ProQuest. (3389233).

Amerson, R. M. (2010). The impact of service-learning on cultural competence. *Nursing Education Research, 31*(1), 18–22.

Amerson, R. M. (2012). The influence of international service-learning on transcultural self-efficacy in baccalaureate nursing graduates and their subsequent practice. *International Journal of Teaching and Learning in Higher Education, 24*(1), 6–15.

Amerson, R. M. (2016). TSET Research Exhibit 9.2. Evaluating the effectiveness of a community health course and service-learning on students' transcultural self-efficacy. In M. R. Jeffreys (Ed.), *Teaching cultural competence in nursing and health care: Inquiry, action, and innovation* (3rd ed., pp. 302–306). New York, NY: Springer Publishing.

Amerson, R. & Livingston, W. G. (2014). Reflexive photography: An alternative method for documenting the learning process of cultural competence. *Journal of Transcultural Nursing, 25*(2), 202–210.

Andrews, M. M., Cervantez Thompson, T. L., Wehbe-Alamah, H., McFarland, M. R., Hanson, P. A., Hasenau, S. M., et al. (2011). Developing culturally competent work force through collaborative partnerships. *Journal of Transcultural Nursing, 22*(3), 300–306. http://dx.doi.org/10.1177/1043659611404214.

Andrews, M. M., & Collins, J. (2015). Using Culture Care Theory as the organizing framework for a federal project on cultural competence. In M. McFarland & H. Wehbe-Alamah (Eds.), *Leininger's culture care diversity and universality: A worldwide nursing theory* (3rd ed., pp. 537–552). Boston, MA: Jones and Bartlett.

Bandura, A. (1986). *Social foundations of thought and action: A social cognitive theory.* Englewood Cliffs, NJ: Prentice-Hall.

Bandura, A. (1989). Regulation of cognitive processes through perceived self-efficacy. ***Developmental Psychology***, ***25***(5), 729-735.

Browne, M. W., Cudeck, R., Tateneni, K., & Mels G. (2004). CEFA: Comprehensive exploratory factor analysis, version 2.00 [Computer software and manual]. Available: http://quantrm2.psy. ohio-state.edu/browne

Campinha-Bacote, J. (2003). *The process of cultural competence in the delivery of healthcare services: A culturally competent model of care* (4th ed.). Cincinnati, OH: Transcultural C.A.R.E. Associates.

Capell, J., Veenstra, G., & Dean, E. (2007). Cultural competence in healthcare: Critical analysis of the construct, its assessment and implications. *Journal of Theory Construction and Testing, 11*(1), 30–37.

Cervone, D. & Peake, P.K. (1986). Anchoring, efficacy, and action: The influence of judgmental heuristics on self-efficacy judgments and behavior. ***Journal of Personality and Social Psychology***, ***50***, 492-501.

Collins, J. & Andrews, M. M. (2016). TSET Research Exhibit 16.1, Evaluating the impact of a train-the-trainer collaborative project on transcultural self-efficacy perceptions. In M. R. Jeffreys (Ed.), *Teaching cultural competence in nursing and health care: Inquiry, action, and innovation* (3rd ed., pp. 542–544). New York, NY: Springer Publishing.

Courtney, R., & Wolgamott, S. (2015). Using Leininger's theory as the building block for cultural competence and cultural assessment for a collaborative care team in a primary care setting.

In M. McFarland & H. Wehbe-Alamah, (Eds.) *Leininger's culture care diversity and universality: A worldwide nursing theory* (3rd ed., pp. 345–368). Boston, MA: Jones and Bartlett.

Creech, C., Filter, M., Wehbe-Alamah, H., McFarland, M.R., Andrews, M., & Pryor, G. (2017). An intervention to improve cultural competence in graduate nursing education. ***Nursing Education Perspectives***, *38*(6), 333-336.

Curtis, M. P., Bultas, M. W., & Green, L. (2016). Enhancing cultural competency. *Online Journal of Cultural Competence in Nursing and Healthcare, 6*(1), 1–13. http://dx.doi.org/10.9730/ojccnh.org/v6n1a1.

Dolgan, C. M. (2001). *The effects of cultural competency training on nurses' attitudes.* (Unpublished master's thesis). Cleveland State University, Cleveland, OH.

Dolgan, C. M. (2004). *Maternity nursing: Increasing our cultural competence Self-instructional learning packet (SILP).* In J. Velez (2005), *The effects of cultural competency training using self-instruction on obstetrical nurses' awareness, knowledge and attitudes.* (Unpublished master's thesis). Cleveland State University, Cleveland, OH

Douglas, M. K., & Pacquiao, D. (2010). Core curriculum for transcultural nursing and health care. *Journal of Transcultural Nursing, 21*(Supplement 1).

Francisco, S. (2013). The *effects of nurses' cultural competency upon patient satisfaction within BLHC healthcare system.* (Unpublished doctoral dissertation). Argosy University, Chicago, IL.

Gozu, A., Beach, M. C., Price, E. G., Gary, T. L., Robinson, K., Palacio, A., et al. (2007). Self-administered instruments to measure cultural competence of health professionals: A systematic review. *Teaching and Learning in Medicine, 19*(2), 180–190.

Grossman, S., Mager, D., Opheim, H., & Torbjornsen, A. (2012). A bi-national simulation study to improve cultural awareness in nursing students. *Clinical Simulation in Nursing, 8*(8), 341–346.

Grund, F., Halter, M. M., Fridline, M., See, S., Young, L., & Reece, C. (2016). TSET Research Exhibit 4.4, Evaluating the effectiveness of cultural educational offerings on students' transcultural self-efficacy. In M. R. Jeffreys (Ed.), *Teaching cultural competence in nursing and health care: Inquiry, action, and innovation* (3rd ed., pp. 120–123). New York, NY: Springer Publishing.

Halter, M., Grund, F., Fridline, M., See, S., Young, L., & Reece, C. (2015). Transcultural self-efficacy perceptions of baccalaureate nursing students. *Journal of Transcultural Nursing, 26*(3), 327-335.

Harper, M. G. (2008). *Evaluation of the antecedents of cultural competence.* Unpublished doctoral dissertation, University of Central Florida, Orlando, FL.

Hoyer, G. (2016). TSET Research Exhibit 7.1, Exploring transcultural self-efficacy perceptions of nursing education administrators and faculty related to lesbian, gay, bisexual, transgender (LGBT) issues. In M. R. Jeffreys (Ed.), *Teaching cultural competence in nursing and health care: Inquiry, action, and innovation* (3rd ed., pp. 222–223). New York, NY: Springer Publishing.

International Nursing Association for Clinical Simulation and Learning (INACSL). (2013). Standards of best practice: Simulation. *Clinical Simulation in Nursing, 9*(6), ii–iii. http://dx.doi.org/10.1016/j.ecns.2013.05.008

International Nursing Association for Clinical Simulation and Learning (INACSL). (2016). Standards of best practice: Simulation[SM]. *Clinical Simulation in Nursing, 12* (Supplement), s48–s50. http://dx.doi.org/10.1016/j.ecns.2016.10.001

Jeffreys, M.R. (1993). The relationship of self-efficacy and select academic and environmental variables on academic achievement and retention. Unpublished doctoral dissertation, New York: Teachers College, Columbia University.

Jeffreys, M. R. (1994). *Transcultural self-efficacy tool (TSET).* Unpublished manuscript.

Jeffreys, M. R. (2000). Development and psychometric evaluation of the Transcultural Self-Efficacy Tool: A synthesis of findings. *Journal of Transcultural Nursing, 11*(2), 127–136.

Jeffreys, M. R. (2002). A transcultural core course in the clinical nurse specialist curriculum. ***Clinical Nurse Specialist: The Journal for Advanced Nursing Practice***, *16*(4), 195-202.

Jeffreys, M. R. (2006). *Teaching cultural competence in nursing and healthcare*. New York, NY: Springer Publishing.

Jeffreys, M. R. (2010). *Teaching cultural competence in nursing and health care: Inquiry, action, and innovation* (2nd ed.). New York, NY: Springer Publishing.

Jeffreys, M. R. (2011). *Graduate student data – MS program results: Transcultural Self-Efficacy Tool (TSET)*. Unpublished report.

Jeffreys, M. R. (2016a). *Teaching cultural competence in nursing and health care: Inquiry, action, and innovation* (3rd ed.). New York, NY: Springer Publishing.

Jeffreys, M. R. (2016b). *The Cultural Competence Education Resource Toolkit* (3rd ed.). New York, NY: Springer Publishing.

Jeffreys, M. R. (2016c). Exhibit 13.3. Innovations in cultural competence education: Summative evaluation – Sample for measuring changes in patient outcomes (access, quality, and cost). In M. R. Jeffreys (Ed.), *Teaching cultural competence in nursing and health care: Inquiry, action, and innovation* (3rd ed., pp. 443–450). New York, NY: Springer Publishing.

Jeffreys, M. R. (2017). FITNESS for culturally congruent care. *Journal of Transcultural Nursing, 28*(5), 523.

Jeffreys, M. R., & Dogan, E. (2010). Factor analysis of the Transcultural Self- Efficacy Tool (TSET). *Journal of Nursing Measurement, 18*(2), 120–139.

Jeffreys, M. R., & Dogan, E. (2012). Evaluating the influence of cultural competence education on students' transcultural self-efficacy perceptions, *Journal of Transcultural Nursing, 23*(2), 188–197.

Jeffreys, M. R., & Dogan, E. (2013). Evaluating cultural competence in the clinical practicum, *Nursing Education Perspectives, 34*(2), 88–94.

Jeffreys, M. R., & Smodlaka, I. (1996). Steps of the instrument design: An illustrative approach for nurse educators. *Nurse Educator, 21*(6), 47–52.

Jeffreys, M. R., & Smodlaka, I. (1998). Exploring the factorial composition of the Transcultural Self-Efficacy Tool. *International Journal of Nursing Studies, 35*, 217–225.

Jeffreys, M. R., & Smodlaka, I. (1999a). Construct validation of the Transcultural Self-Efficacy Tool. *Journal of Nursing Education, 38*, 222–227.

Jeffreys, M. R., & Smodlaka, I. (1999b). Changes in students' transcultural self-efficacy perceptions following an integrated approach to culture care. *Journal of Multicultural Nursing and Health, 5*(2), 6–12. [Erratum, 2000, *6*(1) 20].

Jeffreys, M. R., & Zoucha, R. (2017a). Revisiting "The Invisible Culture of the Multiracial, Multicultural Individual: A Transcultural Imperative". *Journal of Cultural Diversity*, *24*(1), 3–5.

Jeffreys, M. R., & Zoucha, R. (2017b). The Invisible Culture of the Multiracial, Multicultural Individual: A Transcultural Imperative: A Reprint from 2001. *Journal of Cultural Diversity*, *24*(1), 6–10.

Jeffreys, M. R., & Zoucha, R. (2017c). Book Review: Mixed-race Youth and Schooling: The Fifth Minority. *Journal of Cultural Diversity*, *24*(1), 11–12.

Jeffries, P. R. (2005). A framework for designing, implementing, and evaluating simulations used as teaching strategies in nursing. *Nursing Education Perspectives, 26*(2), 96–103.

Jeffries, P. R. (2012). *Simulation in nursing education: From conceptualization to evaluation* (2nd ed.). New York, NY: National League for Nursing.

Jeffries, P. (2015). *The NLN Jeffries Simulation Theory.* Washington, DC: National League for Nursing.

Jeffries, P. R., Rodgers B., & Adamson, K. (2015). NLN Jeffries Simulation Theory: Brief narrative description. *Nursing Education Perspectives, 36*(5), 292–293.

Krentzman, A. R., & Townsend, A. L. (2008). Review of multidisciplinary measures of cultural competence for use in social work education. *Journal of Social Work Education, 44*(2), 1–25.

Larsen, R., & Reif, L. (2011). Effectiveness of cultural immersion and culture classes for enhancing nursing students' transcultural self-efficacy. *Journal of Nursing Education, 50*(6), 350–354.

Larsen, R., & Reif, L. (2016). TSET Research Exhibit 9.1. Evaluating the effectiveness of an immersion experience on cultural competence. In M. R. Jeffreys (Ed.), *Teaching cultural competence in nursing and health care: Inquiry, action, and innovation* (3rd ed., pp. 299–301). New York, NY: Springer Publishing.

Leininger, M. (1991). *Culture care diversity and universality: A theory of nursing*. New York, NY: National League for Nursing.

Leininger, M. M. (2002). Part I. The theory of culture care and the ethnonursing research method. In M. M. Leininger & M. R. McFarland (Eds.), *Transcultural nursing: Concepts, theories, research, and practice* (3rd ed., pp. 71–98). New York, NY: McGraw-Hill.

Leininger, M., & McFarland, M. R. (2006). *Culture care diversity and universality: A worldwide nursing theory* (2nd ed.). Sudbury, MA: Jones and Bartlett Publishers.

Lin, C. J., Lee, C. K., & Huang, M. C. (2017). Cultural competence of healthcare providers: A systematic review of assessment instruments. *Journal of Nursing Research, 25*(3), 174–186.

Loftin, C., Hartin, V., Branson, M., & Reyes, H. (2013). Measures of cultural competence in nurses: An integrative review. *The Scientific World Journal, 2013*, 1–10. http://dx.doi.org/10.1155/2013/289101

Marion, L., Douglas, M., Lavin, M. A., Barr, N., Gazaway, S., Thomas, E., et al. (2016). Implementing the new ANA Standard 8: Culturally congruent practice. *Online Journal of Issues in Nursing*, 22(1). http://dx.doi.org/10.3912/OJIN,Vol22No01PPT20.

McFarland, M. R. & Wehbe-Alamah, H. B. (2015). *Leininger's culture care diversity and universality: A worldwide nursing theory*. Sudbury, MA: Jones & Bartlett.

McFarland, M.; & Wehbe-Alamah, H. (2018). *Leininger's Transcultural Nursing: Concepts, theories, research, and practice* (4th ed.). New York: McGraw-Hill.

Ozkara San, E. (2018). *Effect of the diverse standardized patient simulation (DSPS) cultural competence education strategy on nursing students' transcultural self-efficacy perceptions*. (Unpublished doctoral dissertation). The City University of New York Graduate College, New York, NY.

Purnell, L. D. (2013). *Transcultural health care: A culturally competent approach* (4th ed.). Philadelphia, PA: FA Davis.

Rogers-Walker, M. (2014). *Examining the relationship between participation in service-learning and the levels of transcultural self-efficacy reported by associate of science in nursing students*. Unpublished doctoral dissertation, Capella University.

Rogers-Walker, M. (2016). TSET Research Exhibit 9.3. *Examining the relationship between participation in service-learning and the levels of transcultural self-efficacy reported by associate of science in nursing students*. In M. R. Jeffreys (Ed.), *Teaching cultural competence in nursing and health care: Inquiry, action, and innovation* (3rd ed., pp. 307–310). New York, NY: Springer Publishing.

Sagar, P. L. (2014). *Transcultural Nursing Education Strategies*. New York, NY: Springer Publishing.

Schmidt, L. (2012). *An evaluation of the impact of an intercultural service learning experience on the development of transcultural self-efficacy of nursing students* (Doctoral dissertation). Indianapolis, IN: Indiana University.

Schmidt, L. (2016). Exhibit 6.3. *Evaluating the effectiveness of a domestic and internationals service-learning experience on cultural competence as measured by the Transcultural Self-Efficacy Tool (TSET) and Cultural Competence Clinical Evaluation Tool (CCCET)*. In M. R. Jeffreys (Ed.), *Teaching cultural competence in nursing and health care: Inquiry, action, and innovation* (3rd ed., pp. 174–180). New York, NY: Springer Publishing.

Shen, Z. (2015). Cultural competence models and cultural competence assessment instruments in nursing: A literature review. ***Journal of Transcultural Nursing***, 26(3), 308-321

Singleton, J. K. (2017). An enhanced cultural competence curriculum and changes in transcultural self-efficacy in Doctor of Nursing Practice students. *Journal of Transcultural Nursing, 28*(5), 516–522.

Sudman, S. & Bradburn, N. M. (1982). *Asking questions: A practical guide to questionnaire design.* San Franscisco, CA: Jossey-Bass.

Velez, J. (2005). *The effects of cultural competency training using self-instruction on obstetrical nurses' awareness, knowledge and attitudes.* (Unpublished master's thesis). Cleveland State University, Cleveland, OH.

Velez, J. (2016). TSET Research Exhibit 13.1, Evaluating the effects of cultural competency training using self-instruction learning packets. In M. R. Jeffreys (Ed.), *Teaching cultural competence in nursing and health care: Inquiry, action, and innovation* (3rd ed., pp. 452–454). New York, NY: Springer Publishing.

Wallace, P. (2007). *Coaching standardized patients: For use in the assessment of clinical competence.* New York, NY: Springer Publishing Company.

Weideman, Y. L., Young, L., Lockhart, J. S., Grund, F. J., Fridline, M. M., & Panas, M. (2016). A virtual community: Building capacity through collaboration. *Journal of Professional Nursing, 32*(5S), S48–S53.

## APPENDIX A
## Jeffreys' Cultural Competence and Confidence (CCC) Theory and Research Timeline

**Precursor – Dissertation Study Results – (1993)** [1]

Results of a dissertation study indicated nursing students were least confident (efficacious) about skills related to communication and cultural topics (Jeffreys, 1993).

**Questions Raised** [2]

1. Why were students least confident about items related to cultural issues?
2. How would students have responded to items that further delineated the various dimensions of culture?
3. If students are less confident about general communication skills, (and cultural issues) how will cultural assessments be performed (or will they be performed)?
4. What teaching interventions are needed to prepare culturally diverse students to provide culturally competent care to many different diverse patients and groups?

**Initial Idea** [3]

Develop a composite of students' needs, values, attitudes, and skills related to transcultural nursing care and assess changes following education interventions.

**Preliminary Literature Review** [4]

Conceptual and empirical literature (books, articles, conference proceedings, and ERIC documents) in the areas of:

1. Transcultural nursing
2. Cultural issues in nursing care
3. Self-efficacy theory, research, and measurement (as used in psychology, education, and nursing)
4. Instrumentation

**Synthesis Appraisal and Decision** [5]

1. Conceptual and empirical interdisciplinary literature indicated that self-efficacy is an influencing factor in learning and performance of domain-specific tasks or skills.
2. Self-efficacy measures must be tailored to the domain or situation being explored (Bandura, 1986).
3. No self-efficacy tool had been designed specifically for multicultural undergraduate nursing students who must learn to provide culturally competent care for diverse patients representing many different cultural groups.

**Decision**: Develop a reliable and valid instrument to meet specific current and future purposes.

**Initial Purpose and Objectives** 6

***Initial Purpose***: to measure and evaluate students' self-efficacy perceptions (confidence) for performing general transcultural nursing skills among diverse (and culturally different) client populations.

***Objectives:***

1. Develop a composite of learner needs, values, attitudes, and skills.
2. Assess teaching intervention effectiveness.
3. Identify nursing skills perceived as more difficult or stressful by learners (least confident).
4. Identify differences between learner groups.
5. Identify changes in self-efficacy perceptions over time.

**Grant Proposal – (1993)** 7

***Design and Evaluation of the Transcultural Self-Efficacy Tool (TSET)***

**Exploration of Conceptual and Practical Support, Resources, and Feasibility – (1994)** 8

1. Dr. Madeleine Leininger (phone meeting)
2. Psychometric expert/statistician (in-person and phone meetings, e-mail)
3. Chairperson and institutional grants office (in-person and phone meetings, e-mail)

**Literature Review – Focus on Tool Development, TSET Purpose and Objectives** 9

Conceptual and empirical literature (books, articles, conference proceedings, and ERIC documents) in the areas of:

1. Transcultural nursing
2. Cultural issues in nursing care
3. Self-efficacy theory, research, and measurement (as used in psychology, education, and nursing)
4. Instrumentation

**Synthesis Appraisal and Decision – General Content Areas and Subscales** 10

1. Transcultural nursing and cultural competence development is multidimensional, involving cognitive, psychomotor, and affective learning. ***Decision***: *Taxonomy of Educational Objectives* (Cognitive, Psychomotor, and Affective) would be used as a guide for categorizing items into one of the 3 domains.
2. Self-efficacy theory emphasizes that there may be distinct dimensions within a specific domain, necessitating separate subscales to measure each dimension. (Bandura, 1989). ***Decision***: Categorize items into 3 separate subscales consistent with 3 learning domains.

Additional literature-supported considerations and decisions:

1. Beginning learners have limited knowledge about transcultural nursing skills.
   ***Decision***: Knowledge level on the taxonomy was targeted. Subscale would be named ***Cognitive Subscale*** and ask respondents to rate how knowledgeable they felt about the ways in which cultural factors may influence nursing care among clients of different cultural backgrounds.
2. Provision of cultural congruent care begins with cultural assessment (a psychomotor or practical skill of communication/interview) (Leininger, 1991).
   ***Decision***: Subscale would be named ***Practical Subscale*** and ask respondents to rate their level of confidence about interviewing clients of different cultural backgrounds to learn about their cultural values and beliefs.
3. Affective learning is considered the most important in developing professional values and attitudes, is the least and most difficult to measure, and often takes longest to change.
   ***Decision***: The ***Affective Subscale*** would utilize a multilevel approach incorporating professional values, transcultural nursing literature, and the taxonomy. To best accomplish this, an Affective Subscale blueprint would be carefully designed to address values, attitudes, and beliefs concerning cultural awareness, acceptance, appreciation, recognition, and advocacy in an ascending order (least to most difficult) as suggested by the taxonomy and consistent with Bandura's theoretical framework.
4. ***Subscale sequence***: Instrumentation guidelines supported putting least threatening items first and most threatening last to prevent anchoring bias (Sudman & Bradburn, 1982). It was assumed that students would be least threatened by questions concerning their knowledge, more threatened by questions about applying that knowledge, and most threatened by questions arousing affect.
   ***Decision***: Present Cognitive Subscale first and Affective Subscale last.

**Synthesis Appraisal and Decision – Item Development, Directions, Length** 11

Based on consensus in the educational instrumentation literature and with specific considerations for self-efficacy tools the following preliminary decisions were proposed:

1. ***General item content:*** Specific to cultural care issues or transcultural nursing ***and*** appropriate for entry-level nursing students.
2. ***Individual item content:*** a) address only 1 issue; b) clear and succinct; ***and*** c) avoid redundancy between items.
3. ***Item structure:*** Close-ended and positively phrased (Consistent with self-efficacy tools).
4. ***Item sequence***: Cluster items sequentially as they occur (e.g., pregnancy, birth) or least stressful to more stressful or complex.
5. ***Directions to emphasize individual efficacy appraisal***: a) personalized items and directions using second pronoun; and b) highlighting/bolding and underlining important words.

6. ***Length***: approximately 20 to 30 items on each subscale to capture the targeted domain/dimension and instrument purpose and objectives with the least number of unique items while avoiding redundancy ***and*** to permit psychometric testing for reliability and validity as well as subscale scoring (e.g., mean) for further statistical analyses (such as pretest and post-test).

Synthesis Appraisal and Decision – **Scaling and Scoring** 12

***Rating scale***: Bandura advocates 10-point rating scale for self-efficacy tools with anchors at each end yet some other researchers developed shorter self-efficacy scales and/or with Likert-type rating.

***Decision***: Design two forms of the TSET for pilot-testing: one with 10-point scale with 2 anchors (not at all confident to totally confident) and one with 6-point Likert-type scale (1 = not at all confident; 2 = uncertain; 3 = a little confident; 4 = somewhat confident; 5 = almost certain; and 6 = totally confident).

***Scoring***: Bandura and other self-efficacy researchers advocated/utilized scoring measures that included self-efficacy strength (SEST) and frequently included self-efficacy level (SEL) specific to each dimension of self-efficacy within the task domain. SEST was calculated by item means within a subscale. SEL pertained to % of items at minimum confidence level (usually at or above 20% on a 100% confidence) and placed respondents in low, medium, or high SEL groupings.

***Decision***: SEST scores would be calculated by adding item ratings within a subscale and dividing by number of items, resulting in subscale mean or subscale SEST score. SEL scores would be calculated next in the following manner: Low (students who selected a 1 or 2 response on 80% or more of the subscale; High (students who selected a 9 or 10 response on 80% or more of the subscale items; and Medium (students who selected responses ranging from 3 to 8 on 80% of the subscale items or who did not fall into low or high group).

**Blueprint and TSET Draft** 13

1. Common themes and topics concerning transcultural nursing and culture were listed.
2. Individual items were developed for each theme and topic.
3. Each item was categorized within appropriate category/subscale: Cognitive, Practical, or Affective.
4. Each item was appraised for content, structure, clarity, brevity, and other considerations as per the proposed item development plan.
5. Items were revised accordingly.
6. Cognitive Subscale items were sequenced conceptually and/or sequentially (e.g., pregnancy, birth)
7. Practical Subscale items first included items related to general communication (language preference, level of comprehension, etc.) with more complex and sensitive interview topics later (discrimination and bias, etc.)
8. Affective Subscale items were presented in an ascending order of complexity or stressfulness (least to most) as per the item development blueprint plan.

**Content Expert Review** [14]

1. 6 doctoral prepared experts certified in transcultural nursing.
2. Written information identified instrument purpose, objectives, and brief background for reviewers.
3. Experts rated the content appropriateness of proposed 93 items to transcultural nursing.
4. Rating scale ranged from 0 (not appropriate) to 4 (most appropriate).
5. Qualitative comments were invited about any aspect of the questionnaire.

**Psychometric Expert Review** [15]

1. Doctoral prepared psychologist with expertise in educational measurement and diverse students.
2. Same written information shared with content expert reviewers identified instrument purpose, objectives, and brief background overview for psychometric expert.
3. Expert reviewed directions, sentences, items, format, words for any potential ambiguity or issue that would potentially interfere with type of responses desired, intended statistical analyses, or validity.
4. Expert was queried about controversial issue of measurement scales (10-point, 6-point, other).
5. Feasibility of data processing, data management, and timeline were collaboratively explored.

**Synthesis Appraisal and Decision – Revised Draft – (1994)** [16]

***Content validity experts***

1. Pre-established criteria for revisions (based on majority of experts) were to: a) exclude items rated as 0 or 1; b) revise items rated as 2; and c) include items rated as 3 or 4.
2. 13 of 93 items were deleted (5 Cognitive, 6 Practical, and 2 Affective).
3. One Affective Subscale item was expanded into 4 distinct items as per experts' comments and suggestions
4. One Practical Subscale item was revised to be more specific.
5. Affirmed exclusive categorization within designated subscale (items fit exclusively with one subscale as presented)
6. Instrument directions were revised for clarity based on experts' recommendations

***Psychometric expert***

1. Affirmed proposed revisions based on content validity experts' ratings and qualitative comments.
2. Affirmed proposed revisions congruent with feasibility of responses, data processing, management, and analyses.
3. Affirmed researcher's proposed plan to pilot 10-point and 6-point rating scale.
4. Discussed issues concerning questionnaire length and subscale sequencing and possible influence on reliability and validity.

***Decision***: Revised draft would contain 3 subscales presented in the following sequence Cognitive (25 items), Practical (28 items) and Affective (30 items) however two different response scales would be piloted. To examine effect of instrument length, 2 student groups would complete the entire 83-item TSET (one with 10-point scale, one with 6-point scale), 6 groups would complete only one of the TSET subscales (half completing 10-point scale and half completing 6-point scale). Conduct study to pilot 2 forms of the TSET and determine preliminary reliability and validity estimates.

**Study 1 – Pretest – (Fall 1994)** 17

294 associate degree students enrolled in a clinical nursing course in a college within an urban public university system

***Results***:

1. Cronbach $\alpha$ for internal consistency was .97 and .98 (total 83-item TSET) with subscale range .90 to .98.
2. Split-half reliability ranged .76 to .93 (total 83-item TSET and subscales).
3. Test-retest (2 weeks between administration) ranged .63 to .84 ($p < .001$).
4. 6-point rating scale responses demonstrated less disparity than 10-point scale.
5. Mean ratings for 3 subscales were more alike on 6-point scale than on 10-point scale.
6. Mean ratings were lowest on first subscale (Cognitive) and highest on third subscale (Affective).

**Synthesis Appraisal and Decision** 18

1. ***TSET Response Option Scale:*** Item response distribution and subscale means were more disparate on 10-point scale, suggesting that 10-point scale could detect more subtle differences. A 10-point scale was also advocated by Bandura (1986). A future purpose of the TSET would be to detect differences between groups and changes following educational interventions.
   ***Decision***: 10-point scale is more valid and reliable and should be used in TSET with anchors labeled from 1 (not confident) to 10 (totally confident) as piloted.
2. ***TSET Length:*** Coefficient $\alpha$ was similarly high whether students completed 3 subscales (83 items) or just one subscale. Bandura advocated separate subscales for different dimensions of self-efficacy. Self-efficacy is situation-specific and multidimensional, necessitating separate subscales for different dimensions. Transcultural scholars agree that cultural competence and cultural congruent care is multidimensional, involving knowledge, skills, and affective components. Similarly, educational experts advocate integration of cognitive, psychomotor, and affective components to deepen learning.
   ***Decision***: TSET shall contain all 83-items as categorized within one of three designated subscales to tap into 3 domains of learning and TSE dimensions.

3. ***TSET Subscale Sequence***: "Although it was originally hypothesized that students would be most confident about their attitudes (Affective Subscale) and least confident about their knowledge (Cognitive Subscale), it was uncertain whether the anchoring effect had influenced these results. The anchoring effect refers to the phenomenon that initial self-evaluation responses will significantly influence later self-evaluations, resulting in artificially high or low scores and decreasing validity (Cervone & Peake, 1986)" (Jeffreys, 2000, p. 130).
   ***Decision***: Conduct a second pretest with the Affective Subscale presented first, and Cognitive Subscale presented last using 10-point or 6-point scale for additional comparison.

**Study 1 – Second Pretest – (Spring 1995)** 19

74 associate degree students enrolled in a clinical nursing course within an urban public university system college.

***Results***:

1. Cronbach $\alpha$ for internal consistency was .97 (total 83-item TSET) with subscale range .91 to .98.
2. 6-point rating scale responses had less disparity than 10-point scale.
3. Mean ratings for 3 subscales were more alike on 6-point scale than on 10-point scale.
4. Mean ratings were lowest on the Cognitive Subscale and highest on the Affective Subscale.
5. Means were higher overall and skewed toward the upper range in comparison with first pretest.

**Synthesis Appraisal and Decision** 20

Although subscale sequencing was reversed from first pretest study sequence, mean ratings continued to be lowest on the Cognitive Subscale and highest on the Affective Subscale yet means were skewed overall to the upper range of possible scores, limiting ability to detect subtle changes in future uses with pretest and post-test studies. This finding suggests that an anchoring effect may have occurred when the Affective Subscale was presented first.

***Decision***: Empirical results of second pretest support presentation of Cognitive Subscale first and Affective Subscale last.

**Final TSET Version Confirmed – (1995)** 21

As initially proposed and presented in 1994 (post-content validity expert review) and based on empirical results of first and second pretest analyses, final TSET format would contain: a) 83 items; b) 3 subscales presented in the following sequence: Cognitive, Practical, Affective; and c) 10-point rating scale with anchors labeled 1 (not confident) to 10 (totally confident).

(See Jeffreys & Smodlaka, 1996 for more details).

**Study 2 – Construct Validity: Factor Analysis** 22

1,260 culturally diverse undergraduate nursing students enrolled in one of 2 traditional baccalaureate clinical courses or 5 associate degree clinical courses within a Northeastern US public university system.

***Results***:

1. Cronbach $\alpha$ for internal consistency was .98 (total 83-item TSET) with subscale range .96 (Cognitive and Affective) and .97 (Practical).
2. Mean ratings were lowest on the Cognitive Subscale and highest on the Affective Subscale.
3. Interitem correlation matrix indicated that all items correlated between .30 and .70.
4. Intercorrelations between subscale means ranged from .53 (Cognitive and Affective) to .62 (Cognitive and Practical) and .68 (Practical and Affective) with $p < .001$.
5. Principal Component Analysis (PCA) with varimax rotation and pre-established criteria of: a) factor loading of .50 or higher; b) eigenvalues greater than 1.00; c) contain at least 3 items whose difference in loading on any other factors would be more than .30 yielded 9 factors:
   - Recognition
   - Kinship and social factors
   - Professional nursing care
   - Cultural background and identity
   - Life-cycle transitional phenomena
   - Awareness of cultural gap
   - Communication
   - Self-awareness
   - Appreciation
6. 70 items loaded exclusively on one of the 9 factors, accounting for 62% of the variance.
7. Cronbach $\alpha$ for the 9 factors ranged from .87 to .95.
8. Items clustering together made sense conceptually and was consistent with the underlying framework.
9. Notably, all items within a factor came from a single subscale of the TSET.

(See Jeffreys, 2000, 2016a; Jeffreys & Smodlaka, 1998 for more details).

**Synthesis Appraisal and Decision** 23

Findings suggest that the TSET:

1. Demonstrates internal consistency
2. Assesses the multidimensional nature of TSE
3. Taps the three dimensions of learning (cognitive, practical, and affective) as evidenced by high internal consistency of factors and items loading exclusively on one factor and one subscale only

4. Learning in the cognitive, practical, and affective dimensions are paradoxically distinct but interrelated
5. Factors (item clusters) are congruent with the underlying conceptual framework and associated literature (transcultural nursing, self-efficacy, education, and psychometrics)
6. Contains 83 unique items within the content domain (previously affirmed by content validity experts and further substantiated by interitem correlation matrix results between .30 and .70).

***Decision***: Expand TSET psychometric studies to explore ability to detect differences between groups and changes within groups following educational interventions. Because the self-efficacy literature and Bandura's seminal work reported self-efficacy strength (SEST) scores and self-efficacy level (SEL) scores to capture different aspects of self-efficacy, both scores would be calculated for each subscale. SEST referred to the subscale mean whereas in Bandura's seminal work, SEL referred to number of items perceived with more than 20% confidence and would be coded in the following manner: Low (students who selected a 1 or 2 response on 80% or more of the subscale; High (students who selected a 9 or 10 response on 80% or more of the subscale items; and Medium (students who selected responses ranging from 3 to 8 on 80% of the subscale items or who did not fall into low or high group).
(See Jeffreys & Smodlaka, 1998 for more details).

**Study 3 – Construct Validity: Predictive Validity, Contrasted Group, Cross-Sectional** 24

566 culturally diverse nursing students enrolled in a first semester or last semester clinical nursing course within 5 associate degree programs within a Northeastern US public university system.

***Results***:

1. Cronbach $\alpha$ for internal consistency was .98 (total 83-item TSET) with subscale range .95 to .97.
2. On all items, student selected responses ranging from 1 (not confident) to 10 (totally confident).
3. For both novice and advanced students, mean ratings (self-efficacy strength [SEST] scores were lowest on the Cognitive Subscale and highest on the Affective Subscale.
4. SEST mean scores were lower for novice (first semester) students than for advanced (last semester) students on all subscales.
5. *t*-test analyses with subscale SEST scores indicated statistically significant differences between novice and advanced students on the Cognitive and Practical subscales ($p < .05$); Affective subscale differences just missed statistical significance ($p < .06$).
6. Using the predetermined SEL coding for low (respondents selecting a 1 or 2 response on 80% or more of subscale items), the greatest percentage of low SEL occurred on the Cognitive Subscale (29%) followed by the Practical Subscale (23%) and the Affective Subscale (22%).

7. Using the predetermined SEL coding for high (respondents selecting a 9 or 10 response on 80% or more of subscale items), the greatest percentage of high SEL occurred on the Affective Subscale (39%) followed by the Practical Subscale (22%) and the Cognitive Subscale (19%).
8. The majority of students fell into the Medium SEL category for the Practical Subscale (54%) and Cognitive Subscale (51%) while on the Affective Subscale the percentage of medium SEL scores equaled that of high SEL (39%).
9. Chi-square analyses indicated that low, medium, and high SEL groups were influenced significantly by semester (first or fourth/last) on all subscales.
10. Using multiple regression with SEST scores as the dependent variable, age, gender, ethnicity, language, and income were not statistically significant predictors on any of the subscales. For the Practical and Affective Subscales, semester (first/novice versus fourth/last) was the only statistically significant predictor while previous healthcare experience was the statistically significant contributor in predicting Cognitive SEST scores.

(See Jeffreys, 2000, 2016a; Jeffreys & Smodlaka, 1999a for more details).

**Study 4 – Construct Validity: Predictive Validity, Contrasted Group, Longitudinal** 25

51 associate degree nursing students in a college within an urban public university system who completed the TSET pretest at the beginning of their first semester clinical nursing course and post-test during their last clinical course in fourth semester.

***Results***:

1. Cronbach $\alpha$ for internal consistency was .97 and .98 (total 83-item TSET) with subscale range .92 to .97.
2. On all items, student selected responses ranging from 1 (not confident) to 10 (totally confident).
3. During both semesters, mean ratings (self-efficacy strength [SEST] scores were lowest on the Cognitive Subscale and highest on the Affective Subscale.
4. SEST mean scores were lower in the first semester than in the fourth semester on all subscales.
5. *t*-test analyses with subscale SEST scores indicated statistically significant differences between first and fourth semester on all subscales ($p < .001$).
6. Using the predetermined SEL coding for low (respondents selecting a 1 or 2 response on 80% or more of subscale items), the greatest percentage of pretest low SEL occurred on the Cognitive Subscale (41%) followed by the Practical Subscale (33%) and the Affective Subscale (16%). On post-test, the greatest percentage of low SEL occurred on the Practical and Affective subscale (6%; $n = 3$) followed by the Cognitive (4%; $n = 2$).

7. Using the predetermined SEL coding for high (respondents selecting a 9 or 10 response on 80% or more of subscale items), the greatest percentage of pretest high SEL occurred on the Practical and Affective Subscale (16%) followed by the Cognitive Subscale (2%; $n = 1$). On post-test, the greatest percentage of high SEL occurred on the Affective subscale (43%) followed by the Practical (35%) and Cognitive (28%).
8. The majority of students fell into the Medium SEL category during both pretest and post-test on all subscales with the percentage of medium scores increasing on the Cognitive (57% to 69%) and Practical (51% to 59%); however, decreased on the Affective (69% to 51%) due to greater percentage in Affective high SEL group.
9. In the majority of cases, students' SEL scores increased (in cases of pretest low or medium scorers); or remained the same (cases of pretest medium or high scorers). (Please note that remaining in the same SEL score category does not mean that students' SEST scores or item responses did not change; this level of detail was not examined).
10. No decrease in pretest medium scorers occurred on any of the subscales; however, one pretest high scorer (Affective Subscale) decreased SEL score to a medium level and on the Practical Subscale, one high scorer dropped to the low group and three high scorers decreased to a medium level.
11. *t*-test analyses yielded statistically significant SEL score differences between the first semester and fourth semester on all subscales.

(See Jeffreys 2000, 2016a; Jeffreys & Smodlaka, 1999b for more details).

**Disseminate Synthesized Findings, Theoretical Framework, and Recommendations – 2000** 26

In addition to summarizing processes of TSET design and evaluation, Jeffreys, 2000 article was the first published article to: present thirteen underlying assumptions of TSE*, proposed future research and educational applications, and included a concluding note to educators and researchers interested in requesting a copy of the TSET. *14th assumption added in 2005 (See 29 and 30)

(See Jeffreys, 2000 for more details).

**Disseminate Utility of Theory for Graduate Education and Practice Settings** 27

Jeffreys, M. R. (2002). A transcultural core course in the clinical nurse specialist curriculum. *Clinical Nurse Specialist: The Journal for Advanced Nursing Practice. 16*(4), 195–202.

Jeffreys, M. R. (2005). Clinical nurse specialists as cultural brokers, change agents, and partners in meeting the needs of culturally diverse populations. *Journal of Multicultural Nursing and Health, 11*(2), 41–48.

**Expanded Utility by Other Educators and Researchers** 28

1. Ongoing questions, requests, and correspondence from educators and researchers around the world and in various health disciplines, and within different settings revealed a critical gap in educational resources specifically focused on the teaching-learning process of cultural competence.
2. Increasing requests for the TSET, such as review, administration in a study, translations.
3. Researchers completing studies using the TSET, reporting findings consistent with CCC framework.
4. Several TSET researchers using SEL score calculations found few in low group using the 20% minimum SEL scoring method. The 20% benchmark was initially selected based on Bandura's work with phobics and academically low-achieving children who usually did not meet these benchmarks prior to therapeutic intervention.

***Decision***: Fill the gap in evidence-based educational resources specifically focused on the teaching-learning process of cultural competence by writing a book. Included would be a visual diagram of the theoretical framework and a chapter detailing its components, psychometric history of TSET development and evaluation, research updates, and innovative teaching-learning strategies for academia, healthcare institutions, and professional associations. To address the SEL scoring issue, conduct a new literature search and consult with an educational measurement expert.

Cultural Competence and Confidence Model – **Visual Diagram and TSE Pathway – (2005)** 29

1. The CCC model's visual diagram succinctly illustrates major components of the learning process, providing a visual (big picture/panoramic) framework and cognitive map for understanding the multidimensional process of cultural competence development.
2. A close-up view of TSE, cultural competence, and culturally congruent care is depicted through the TSE Pathway, thereby tracing the proposed influences of TSE on a learner's actions, performance, and persistence for learning tasks associated with cultural competence development and culturally congruent care.
3. Taken together, the panoramic view and the close-up view of the TSE Pathway encourages viewers to seriously contemplate all components by condensing and expanding upon each area, within the context of the connection between all its parts. (This is consistent with a holistic view).

**Book 1 - *Teaching Cultural Competence in Nursing and Health Care: Inquiry, Action, and Innovation* - (2006) – AJN Book of Year Award** 30

Book's major highlights for advancing theory, innovation, measurement, and evaluation (TIME):

1. First comprehensive published discussion about CCC framework, visual model, and TSE Pathway.
2. Definition of cultural competence formally added as #1 model assumption, making 14 assumptions in total.
3. TSET background and updates incorporating findings from other researchers in academia and health care.
4. Guide to study design, data interpretation, and avoiding pitfalls. Recommended that SEST scores always be calculated for each subscale and that SEL scores, if used, are an additional, supplementary approach for analyzing data. After literature review and statistical consultation, several different grouping methods were proposed such as involving percentages or standard deviations to compute low, middle, and high groups
5. A wide selection of educational activities, including vignettes and case examples, adaptable for diverse learners in academia, healthcare institutions, and professional associations.
6. Tables, assessment tools, and diagrams to assist educators and researchers.

**Expanded Utility by Other Educators and Researchers** 31

1. Increase in correspondence from educators and researchers around the world and in various health disciplines revealing that there is a growing demand for more educational resources for cultural competence.
2. User-friendly evidence-based strategies for making a difference are sparse.
3. Increasing requests for the TSET, such as review, administration in a study, translations.
4. Researchers completing studies using the TSET, reporting findings consistent with CCC framework.
5. Consultation and workshop requests generate more interest in model, TSET, and utility in clinical practice.
6. No tool available to measure cultural competence behaviors in clinical settings.

***Decision***: Expand studies and seek grant-funding.

**Series of Expanded Studies – Literature Review, Grant Proposals, Instrumentation: TSET, CCCET, CSAT-DD – (2006-2010)** 32

***Purposes:***

1. TSET (See # 33-38)
2. CCCET (See # 39-43)
3. CSAT-DD (See # 39-43)
4. CCC Model – expansion and further validation (See #45 and #47)

**Study 5 – Construct Validity: Factor Analysis** 33

272 culturally diverse undergraduate nursing students enrolled in an associate degree clinical course at an urban college within a Northeastern US public university system.

***Results***:

1. Cronbach $\alpha$ for internal consistency was .99 (total 83-item TSET) with subscale range .97 (Cognitive and Practical) and .98 (Affective).
2. Mean ratings were lowest on the Cognitive Subscale and highest on the Affective Subscale.
3. Interitem correlation matrix indicated that all items correlated between .30 and .70.
4. Common Exploratory Factor Analysis (CEFA) using the Comprehensive Exploratory Factor Analysis software developed by Brown, Cudek, Tateneni, and Mels (2004) and following a series of steps detailed in Jeffreys and Dogan (2010) yielded 4 factors:
   - Knowledge and Understanding
   - Interview
   - Awareness, Acceptance, and Appreciation
   - Recognition
5. 69 items loaded exclusively on one of the 4 factors.
6. Cronbach $\alpha$ for the 9 factors ranged from .94 to .98.
7. Items clustering together made sense conceptually and was consistent with the underlying framework.
8. All items within a factor came from a single subscale of the TSET.
9. Notably, Factor 1 incorporated all 25 items on the Cognitive Subscale.

(See Jeffreys & Dogan, 2010 for more details).

**Study 6 – Construct Validity: Predictive Validity, Contrasted Group, Cross-Sectional** 34

147 culturally diverse nursing students enrolled in a first semester or last semester clinical nursing course at an urban college within a Northeastern US public university system.

***Results***:

1. Cronbach $\alpha$ for internal consistency was .97 (total 83-item TSET) with subscale range .97 to .98.
2. Statistically significant intercorrelations between all subscale combinations was consistent with Bandura's expectations that a) self-efficacy tools should have different subscales to measure confidence for different dimensions within a content domain and b) that subscales should be distinct yet moderately intercorrelated.
3. For both novice and advanced students, mean ratings (self-efficacy strength [SEST] scores were lowest on the Cognitive Subscale and highest on the Affective Subscale.

4. SEST mean scores were lower for novice (first semester) students than for advanced (last semester) students on all subscales.
5. *t*-test analyses with subscale SEST scores indicated statistically significant differences between novice and advanced students on the Cognitive subscale ($p < .05$); Practical and Affective subscale differences changed in the expected direction (increased) but was not statistically significant.
6. Using ANOVA with SEST scores as the dependent variable, gender, race/ethnicity, ability to speak another language besides English fluently, and birth in the United States were not statistically significant predictors on any of the subscales. Overall, ANOVA supported that the strongest significant predictor for subscale scores was semester (first vs. fourth) rather than demographic variables. Previous healthcare experience was also statistically significant for Cognitive and Affective subscales. On the Practical Subscale, English as primary language was the single significant demographic predictor.

(See Jeffreys & Dogan, 2012 for more details).

**Study 7 – Construct Validity: Predictive Validity, Contrasted Group, Longitudinal**

35

36 associate degree nursing students in a college within an urban public university system who completed the TSET pretest at the beginning of their first semester clinical nursing course and post-test during their last clinical course in fourth semester.

***Results***:

1. Cronbach $\alpha$ for internal consistency was .97 and .98 (total 83-item TSET) with subscale range .97 to .98.
2. Intercorrelations among pretest, post-test, and change in SEST scores by subscales yielded statistically significant intercorrelations between all combinations.
3. During both semesters, mean ratings (self-efficacy strength [SEST] scores were lowest on the Cognitive Subscale and highest on the Affective Subscale.
4. SEST mean scores were lower in the first semester than in the fourth semester on all subscales.
5. *t*-test analyses with subscale SEST scores indicated statistically significant differences between first and fourth semester on all subscales ($p < .05$).
6. Using ANOVA with SEST scores as the dependent variable, gender, race/ethnicity, English as primary language, ability to speak another language besides English fluently, and birth in the United States and previous healthcare experience were not statistically significant predictors on any of the subscales. The only statistically significant predictor was semester (first vs. fourth) rather than demographic variables, implying that cultural competence educational interventions throughout the curriculum influenced TSE perceptions. (See Jeffreys & Dogan, 2012 for more details).

**Study 8 – Construct Validity: Predictive Validity, Transcultural Course, Longitudinal** 36

9 graduate nursing students in a college within an urban public university system who completed the TSET pretest at the beginning of their 15-week required core transcultural nursing course and post-test at the end of the semester.

***Results***:

1. Cronbach $\alpha$ for internal consistency was .98 and .99 (total 83-item TSET) with subscale range .91 to .99.
2. On both pretest and post-test, mean ratings (self-efficacy strength [SEST] scores were lowest on the Cognitive Subscale and highest on the Affective Subscale.
3. SEST mean scores increased from pretest to post-test on all subscales.
4. *t*-test analyses with subscale SEST scores indicated statistically significant differences between pretest and post-test on the Practical Subscale ($p < .05$).

(Jeffreys, 2011; See Jeffreys, 2002 for course overview).

**Study 9 – Construct Validity: Predictive Validity, Graduate Clinical Course, Longitudinal** 37

14 graduate nursing students in a college within an urban public university system who completed the TSET pretest at the beginning of their 15-week required clinical practicum course (CNS-adult health) and post-test at the end of the semester.

***Results***:

1. Cronbach $\alpha$ for internal consistency was .99 and .96 (total 83-item TSET) with subscale range .94 to .99.
2. On both pretest and post-test, mean ratings (self-efficacy strength [SEST] scores were lowest on the Cognitive Subscale and highest on the Affective Subscale.
3. SEST mean scores increased from pretest to post-test on all subscales.
4. *t*-test analyses with subscale SEST scores indicated statistically significant differences between pretest and post-test on the Cognitive Subscale and Practical Subscale ($p < .05$).

(Jeffreys, 2011).

**Synthesis Appraisal and Decision** 38

1. Conceptual and empirical interdisciplinary literature indicated that self-efficacy is an influencing factor in learning and performance of domain-specific tasks or skills.
2. The TSET and its 83-items had been validated via content validity experts and numerous studies by author and other researchers.
3. Evidence-based research models and educational practices that promote transcultural nursing require valid research methods for evaluating cultural competence performance in clinical settings.

4. Legal, ethical, and accreditation mandates demand theoretically based, valid, comprehensive tools to assess aspects of culturally specific care within the clinical practicum or workplace; yet no relevant ones existed.

**Decision**: Develop a reliable and valid instrument adapted from the TSET for evaluating the extent of culturally specific care provided for a diverse clientele, the frequency of cultural assessments, and the development of culturally sensitive and professionally appropriate attitudes, values, and beliefs. Develop a user-friendly tool to collect data about the clinical practicum/agency site, specifically focusing on descriptions of diverse client populations and clinical problems.

**Cultural Competence Clinical Evaluation Tool (CCCET) Initial Purpose and Objectives**

39

***Initial Purpose***: Develop a reliable and valid instrument adapted from the TSET to meet specific current and future objectives in clinical practicum courses and clinical workplace settings.

***Objectives:***

1. Develop a composite of learner needs, values, attitudes, skills, and behaviors.
2. Identify types of cultural-specific care provided more frequently.
3. Identify types of cultural-specific provided less frequently.
4. Identify cultural assessments performed more frequently.
5. Identify cultural assessments performed less frequently.
6. Identify differences within groups.
7. Identify differences between groups.
8. Identify at-risk individuals.
9. Compare similarities and difference between student or employee and teacher/preceptor or agency evaluator ratings.
10. Evaluate effectiveness of specific teaching interventions.
11. Assess changes in cultural competent behaviors, cultural specific care provision, assessment, skills, and attitudes over time.

**Clinical Setting Assessment Tool – Diversity and Disparity: Initial Purpose and Objectives**

***Initial Purpose***: Develop a survey tool to collect data about the clinical practicum/agency site, specifically focusing on descriptions of diverse client populations and clinical problems.

***Objectives:***

1. Describe demographic characteristics of client population within clinical practicum/agency site.
2. Describe type of clinical focus areas or problems within clinical practicum/agency site.
3. Evaluate amount and type of expose of student/learner/nurse to culturally diverse clients and targeted clinical focus areas.

**Exploration of Conceptual and Practical Support, Resources, and Feasibility – (2006)** 40

1. Transcultural nursing scholars/previous content validity experts (e-mail, phone, in-person discussion)
2. Psychometric expert/statistician (phone meetings, e-mail)
3. Chairperson and institutional grants office (in-person and phone meetings, e-mail)

**CCCET and CSAT-DD Draft, Psychometric Expert Review, and Content Validity** 41

*CCCET:*

1. Adapted from the psychometrically valid TSET.
2. All 83 items remained the same, sequenced, organized, and presented as in TSET.
3. Consistent with TSET, uses a 10-point rating scale.
4. Three subscales measuring different dimensions of clinical cultural competence behaviors:
   - Subscale 1 (Provision of Cultural-Specific Care), 25 items
   - Subscale 2 (Cultural Assessment), 28 items
   - Subscale 3 (Cultural Sensitivity), 30 items
5. Directions modified slightly to correspond with subscales and purpose.
6. 10-point rating ranging from 1 to 10 per each item as follows:
   - Subscale 1 – extent of culturally specific care provision from 1 (not at all) to 10 (totally)
   - Subscale 2 – frequency of cultural assessment from "never" (1) to "always" (10)
   - Subscale 3 – developed or further developed from "not at all (1) to "to a great extent" (10)
7. Additional response option of selecting "A" (clinical area not available) or "B" (diverse clients not available)
8. Review by psychometric expert/statistician affirmed final format and plan for data analyses.
9. Review by three transcultural nursing experts yielded a Content Validity Index (CVI) of 0.91.

*CSAT-DD*

1. Cover page gathers information about the type of agency (e.g., private, public) and whether the instructor/preceptor/agency evaluator completed a college level course and/or continuing education (CE) units in transcultural nursing or cultural competence in health care.
2. Part I (15 items) gathers information about the demographic make-up of the client population (age, ethnicity, languages spoken, religion, etc.) as well as identifying the most prevalent characteristics represented.
3. Part II (28 items) asks respondents to identify the five most frequent clinical focus areas evident in the clinical setting. (28 items corresponded with 28 focus areas of Healthy People 2010).
4. Review by psychometric expert/statistician affirmed final format and plan for descriptive data analyses.

(See Jeffreys, 2016a; b for more details)

**Study 10 – CCCET and CSAT-DD Undergraduate Students** 42

161 culturally diverse undergraduate nursing students enrolled in one of 18 second-semester 15-week, 9-credit medical-surgical associate degree clinical course sections at an urban college within a Northeastern US public university system who completed the CCCET-Student Version (CCCET-SV) at the end of the semester and whose clinical instructors independently completed a CCCET-Teacher Version (CCCET-TV) for each student at the end of the semester. (student and instructor did not see each other's ratings)

***Results***:

1. Cronbach $\alpha$ for internal consistency was .99 (total 83-item CCCET-SV) with subscale range .97 to .98.
2. Cronbach $\alpha$ for internal consistency was .95 (total 83-item CCCET-TV) with subscale range .85 to .98.
3. Although $\alpha$ coefficients were excellent, small sample size (due to A and B responses warranted exclusion from the overall coefficient analyses) was an unavoidable limitation.
4. Teacher ratings were predominantly higher than student ratings on Subscale 1 and predominantly lower on Subscales 2 and 3.
5. Subscale 1 differences between student and teacher item mean ratings, ranged from -1.39 to 0.12.
6. Subscale 2 differences between student and teacher item mean ratings ranged from -.05 to 1.35.
7. Subscale 3 differences between student and teacher item mean ratings ranged from 0.16 to 2.17.
8. On Subscale 3, the greatest change occurred on the two items dealing with advocacy.
9. For the most part, the rank ordered results were consistent with the course objectives and emphasis, curriculum, the underlying assumptions of the CCC model, and related literature.
10. Conceptual fit of findings provided beginning evidence for validity.

***CSAT-DD***

1. 42% of clinical instructors had completed a college level course in transcultural nursing or cultural competence in health care.
2. 63% of clinical instructors had completed CE units related to transcultural nursing or cultural competence and health care.
3. Part I aggregated data substantiated that diversity across all expected categories for each of the fifteen client characteristics was evident.
4. The clinical settings provided exposure to demographically diverse clients, although the predominant reported characteristics represented the predominant groups in the nearby communities and the predominant type of agencies.

5. Part II aggregated responses confirmed that all 28 clinical focus areas were represented in the clinical area.
6. The most common areas included chronic kidney disease, diabetes, heart disease and stroke, cancer, respiratory diseases, and disability and secondary conditions
7. The predominant focus areas corresponded to the medical-surgical clinical topics.

(See Jeffreys, 2016a; Jeffreys & Dogan, 2013 for more details)

**Study 11 – CCCET and CSAT-DD Graduate Students** 43

Twenty-four students independently completed the CCCET at the end of their graduate level (MS) clinical practicum during the three targeted semesters. To allow matching of CCCET-Teacher Version (TV) and CCCET-Student Version (SV), preceptors completed the CCCET-TV for each student at the end of the clinical practicum, placing the completed CCCET-TV in an envelope, sealing, and then giving to the student for return to the course coordinator. The student's CCCET-SV was placed in an envelope prior to sealing and returning to the researcher.

***Results***:

1. Cronbach $\alpha$ for internal consistency ranged from .97 to .99 on CCCET-SV subscales.
2. Cronbach $\alpha$ for internal consistency was .96 and .97 on CCCET-TV Subscales 1 and 2; too few cases were available to calculate CCCET-TV Subscale 1.
3. Although $\alpha$ coefficients were excellent, small sample size (due to A and B responses warranted exclusion from the overall coefficient analyses) was an unavoidable limitation.
4. Subscale 1 average differences between student and preceptor item mean ratings equaled -1.75.
5. Subscale 2 average differences between student and preceptor item mean ratings equaled -1.04.
6. Subscale 3 average differences between student and preceptor item mean ratings equaled -09.
7. The most frequent provision of cultural specific care areas corresponded with areas emphasized greatly within the didactic and clinical course and within advanced practice nursing role development.
8. The most changed attitudes, values, and beliefs corresponded with issues related to health disparities and healthcare disparities (access, quality, and cost) such as inadequacies in the nation's healthcare system, socioeconomic factors, discomforts entering a culturally different world, and advocacy.

***CSAT-DD***

1. 67% of the preceptors had completed courses or CE units related to cultural competence and health care.
2. Part I aggregated data substantiated that diversity across all expected categories for each of the fifteen client characteristics was evident.

3. The clinical settings provided exposure to demographically diverse clients, although the predominant reported characteristics represented the predominant groups in the nearby communities and the predominant type of agencies.
4. Part II aggregated responses confirmed that all 28 clinical focus areas were represented in the clinical area.
5. The predominant focus areas corresponded to the clinical areas of expertise appropriate for an adult health or geriatric CNS (heart disease and stroke, diabetes, respiratory diseases, disability and secondary conditions, and health communication).

(See Jeffreys & Dogan, Exhibit 6.2 in Jeffreys, 2016a).

**Synthesis Appraisal and Decision**

44

***Summary of findings from TSET, CCCET, CSAT-DD***

1. Repeated psychometric testing of the TSET continues to demonstrate consistently high reliability and validity consistent with the underlying conceptual framework of the Cultural Competence and Confidence (CCC) model.
2. Research findings consistently support that the TSET detected differences in TSE perceptions within and between groups, such as pre and post educational intervention.
3. The strong psychometric properties (validity and reliability) and comprehensiveness of the TSET (content validation) provided a strong conceptual and psychometric framework for the CCCET.
4. Findings demonstrated that the CCCET-SV and CCCET-TV were psychometrically valid and reliable.
5. High Cronbach $\alpha$ coefficients on both versions (total instruments and subscales) provided beginning evidence for internal consistency.
6. The high congruency between student and teacher/preceptor ratings obtained in two separate studies of undergraduate and graduate students provide beginning evidence that the CCCET can be an effective, comprehensive, and systematic means for assessing learning and performance of behaviors, skills, and values deemed necessary for cultural competence.
7. The CCCET can be used for multiple formative and summative evaluation purposes to guide individual, course, curricular, or employee education program innovations and teaching-learning strategies.
8. The CSAT-DD collected data about the clinical practicum/agency site, specifically focusing on descriptions of diverse client populations (Part I) and clinical problems (Part II), confirming that clinical placement sites met course and program objectives.

***Decision***: Disseminate updated research about TSET and new tools (CCCET and CSAT-DD), updates about CCC model, and create a toolkit to assist other researchers and educators interested in designing, implementing, and evaluating teaching-learning innovations for cultural competence development in a variety of settings. Provide a forum to showcase other researchers applying CCC model and/or associated instruments and provide ideas for educational strategies that work or don't work. Prepare book and toolkit proposal.

**Book 2 – *Teaching Cultural Competence in Nursing and Health Care: Inquiry, Action, and Innovation*** (2010) (2nd edition) and ***Cultural Competence Education Resource Toolkit*** 45

Book's major highlights for advancing theory, innovation, measurement, and evaluation (TIME):

1. *Optimal cultural competence* (OCC) introduced as a new challenge to reach beyond competence (a minimum expectation) toward the potential for "more," consistent with lifelong learning and cultural competence development as ongoing.
2. Introduced the 7 (nonlinear) steps essential for OCC: self-assessment; active promotion; systematic inquiry; decisive action; innovation; measurement; and evaluation.
3. Theoretical assumptions empirically supported and those under study identified.
4. Digital *Cultural Competence Education Resource Toolkit* introduced, with 21 distinct resources (evaluation and assessment tools, questionnaires, and activities) for incorporating the 7 essential steps of OCC.
5. Transcultural Self-Efficacy Tool – Multidisciplinary Healthcare Provider (TSET-MHP) version introduced with word "nurse" and "nursing" changed to fit with multidisciplinary healthcare personnel.
6. New questionnaires, CCCET and CSAT-DD described and available for review in toolkit with CCCET versions for students, teachers, preceptors, employees, and agency evaluators.
7. TSET updates incorporating findings from other researchers in academia and health care supplemented with abstracts and exhibits detailing educational innovation, measurement, and evaluation.
8. Chapters detailing employee orientation, staff education, continuing education with contributing authors.
9. Chapters detailing multidimensional strategies for undergraduates and graduates with contributing authors.
10. Recommended that SEST scores always be calculated for each subscale and that SEL scores, if used, are an additional, supplementary approach for analyzing data, noting that standard setting research, using very large samples, will provide empirical evidence for grouping approach selected. In lieu of a very large sample, low-medium-high groupings can be implemented, and data appraised with limitations acknowledged.

**Expanded Utility by Other Educators and Researchers** 46

1. Increase in correspondence from educators and researchers around the world and in various health disciplines revealing that there continues to be a demand for more educational resources for cultural competence education using an interactive, user-friendly approach.
2. Increasing requests for TSET, such as review, administration in a study, translations.
3. More researchers completing studies using the TSET, reporting findings consistent with CCC framework.
4. Consultation and workshop requests generate more interest in model, TSET, CCCET, CSAT-DD and utility in clinical practice.

***Decision***: Disseminate updated research about TSET and new tools (CCCET and CSAT-DD), updates about CCC model, and update. Provide a forum to showcase other researchers applying CCC model and/or associated instruments and provide ideas for educational strategies that work or don't work. Expand book to include contributions from international researchers, TCN scholars, and educators. Prepare book and toolkit proposal.

**Book 3– *Teaching Cultural Competence in Nursing and Health Care: Inquiry, Action, and Innovation*** (2016) and ***Cultural Competence Education Resource Toolkit*** (3rd edition).

47

Book's major highlights for advancing theory, innovation, measurement, and evaluation (TIME):

1. *Optimal cultural competence* (OCC) formally introduced to the theory and added to the core, with 7 (nonlinear) steps essential for OCC: self-assessment; active promotion; systematic inquiry; decisive action; innovation; measurement; and evaluation.
2. CCC model's visual diagram revised to illustrate OCC's placement at the center core of the model
3. Visual diagram added to show ongoing movement between 7 steps essential for OCC.
4. Contributions from other researchers incorporating model and/or TSET and/or CCCET
5. New features added for enhanced user-friendly utility in a variety of settings. Features include snapshot scenarios and vignettes in conversational tone to demonstrate theory and questionnaires in action.

**Expanding Understanding of Theory and Utility through Creative Performance – (2016)**

48

As one of 4 Transcultural Nursing Society (TCNS) scholar panelists at 2016 International TCNS Conference, Cincinnati, Ohio, author enacted a 12-minute creative performance (story-telling, acting, props, costumes) to act out components of CCC model, tell the story of its beginnings, tie in to present day, and stimulate audience interest in future innovative applications.

**Synthesized Appraisal and Updates – (2018)**

49

***Evidence-based Updates and Universal Utility of Jeffreys' Cultural Competence and Confidence (CCC) Framework for Nursing Education (and Beyond) through TIME***

Process of preparing manuscript for *Annual Review of Nursing Research* (ARNR) involved review of over 70 studies and numerous documents providing educators and researchers with an ensemble of resources.

**To be written .........**

50

Innovation and collaboration invited......

## APPENDIX B

## Jeffreys' Cultural Competence and Competence (CCC) Theoretical Framework and Transcultural Self-Efficacy Tool (TSET): Select Recommendations for Educators and Researchers A to Z

The A–Z list of select recommendations was compiled to assist educators and researchers who wish to:

- Contemplate cultural competence education research possibilities
- Avoid research design and data interpretation pitfalls
- Apply the CCC model as a theoretical framework
- Contribute to the growing psychometric history of the TSET
- Adapt educational innovation spotlights and exemplars
- Expand the repertoire of evidence-based innovations for academic and workplace settings
- Embark on new directions for cultural education topics, pedagogy, and technology
- Explore CCC theory, innovation, measurement, and evaluation (TIME)

The recommendations are based on questions frequently asked or observations noted when conducting and/or reviewing research involving the CCC model and/or the TSET. They are intended to prompt a starting point for further inquiry, action, and innovation within an evidence-based framework. While some recommendations are generally applicable to many types of studies, some recommendations are specific to the CCC model and TSET. Both general and specific issues warrant consideration.

- ***Acknowledge authors and other names appropriately***
  Misspellings of author, model, or questionnaires complicate literature searches and lead to missed and/or inaccurate information. Similarly, incorrect reference citations miss contributions of others.
- ***Appraise all TSET subscales always***
  TSE is multidimensional, and cultural competence is multidimensional involving cognitive, practical, and affective components. Administering 1 or 2 subscales misses the holistic perspective.
- ***Ask the right questions***
  Asking "what are the changes in TSE" acknowledges that increases, decreases, or no changes could occur. For example, within self-efficacy framework, overly confident (supremely efficacious) individuals are at-risk for poor outcomes. Supremely efficacious (overly confident individuals) view tasks as unimportant, see no need to prepare, and may not see a need to perform the task, therefore cultural assessments and cultural congruent

care may never be rendered, jeopardizing patient outcomes or causing multicultural workplace conflict. In this example, following a cultural competence learning event, lowering of TSE perceptions to more realistic and resilient is desirable. Individuals with resilient TSE view obstacles as challenges, actively seek out additional resources, and expend extra energy aimed at cultural congruence and optimal cultural competence in all settings.

- ***Begin at the beginning with baseline data***
  To determine effectiveness of something or change in something, pretest is needed to establish baseline.
- ***Contemplate the CCC model comprehensively***
  Superficial, swift perusal of the CCC model will miss many of the key components intricately woven and interconnected from its origins in nursing, transcultural nursing, education, and psychology (self-efficacy). This will be counterproductive to creating a strong foundation for a study or educational innovation. The model's visual diagram and its accompanying TSE pathway illustration are resources to assist in remembering and understanding key components of the theory.
- ***Complement, connect, and scaffold courses, course components, and curricula***
  Disconnected learning activities do not add depth or breadth.
- ***Determine demographic data collection and purpose***
  Demographic data will help determine whether the actual sample is truly representative of the targeted sample, can be used to compare and contrast TSE perceptions between samples and strategies, permitting the expansion of scientific knowledge, to examine within-group differences based on demographic factors, and to help substantiate the underlying assumptions and directional conceptual relationships proposed in the CCC model and TSE Pathway. "Significant differences in TSE perceptions based on demographic variables can be desirable if differences are consistent with the underlying theoretical framework. For example, the CCC model purports that novice learners will have lower self-efficacy perceptions than advanced learners. Demographic data distinguishing between novices and advanced learners must therefore be collected and analyzed. In contrast, lack of statistically significant differences in TSE perceptions based on such variables as race, ethnicity, language, religion, or socioeconomic status supports the underlying theoretical assumption that all learners (despite race, ethnicity, etc.) benefit from transcultural nursing educational experiences" (Jeffreys, 2016a, p.150).

- ***Employ evidence-based best practices***
  Evidence-based best practices concerning cultural competence education, clinical topic, population, education, self-efficacy, pedagogy, and technology should guide decision-making in innovation and research.
- ***Formulate feasible innovation and research plans***
  Ideas that aren't feasible won't get done. Searching the literature for creative ways to enhance feasibility, such as grant funding or partnerships can transform the impossible into the possible.
- ***Get generationally and geographically diverse groups***
  Generalizability can be expanded by comparing results and CCC model assumptions within and between similar and different groups.
- ***Highlight key points – don't hide key points***
  Succinct synthesis points provide quick access to key points that can be missed in lengthy narratives.
- ***Initiate IRB approval prior to initiating educational innovation and research.***
  "Because IRB approval must be obtained before a study is initiated and because every educational intervention has the potential to make a difference (positive or negative) in the process of cultural competence development, nurse educators must seriously consider the benefits and take the extra step in obtaining IRB approval. Educators must also be aware that guidelines concerning outcomes assessment, IRB approval processes and procedures, educator roles and responsibilities, mandated certifications to conduct human subject research, and organizational leadership may change; therefore, seeking out updated information ahead of planned research is advantageous" (Jeffreys, 2016a, p. 151).
- ***Join others in joint collaborative partnerships***
  Shared expertise and resources can generate new ideas, innovations, and jumpstart positive change.
- ***Keep to the data; Know difference between statistical and practical significance***
  Don't make gigantic leaps in data interpretation. Recognizing that statistically insignificant results can have practical significance and recognizing that statistically significant results do not always yield meaningful findings or practical significance are equally important. Know rationale for data analyses selected.
- ***Limit limitations, learn from the literature***
  Avoid mistakes and limitations that are acknowledged in the literature. Don't repeat other's mistakes and limitations if avoidable. Acknowledging anticipated unavoidable limitations with rationale for why advantages outweigh disadvantages strengthens a study.

- ***Make multidimensional teaching-learning strategies***
  Cultural competence is an ongoing, multidimensional learning process that integrates transcultural skills in all three dimensions (cognitive, practical, and affective), involves TSE (confidence) as a major influencing factor, and aims to achieve culturally congruent care. The most comprehensive learning involves the integration of cognitive, practical, and affective dimensions." (Assumptions 1 and 7) (Jeffreys, 2016a, pp. 75–76).
- ***Name names and titles consistently and list numbers neatly in narrative, tables, and figures***
  Tables with columns neatly aligned, consistency in decimal places, presenting numbers in sequence that makes sense and follows publication guidelines enhances readability, comparison, and utility of findings.
- ***Operationalize variables consistent with model***
  A unique feature of the CCC model includes clearly defined conceptual definitions for variables and concepts within the theory. The corresponding questionnaire (TSET, TSET-MHP, or CCCET) provide direct, valid, psychometrically tested quantitative measures to operationalize variables.
- ***Organize study around CCC framework at the onset***
  Comprehensive understanding of the CCC framework can assist with organizing study components at the onset, during implementation of the study, and to aid in data analysis and interpretation. Observing assumptions and conceptual fit of data contributes to ongoing validation of assumptions and model.
- ***Prioritize purposes of research or innovation***
  Too many purposes or variables can be overwhelming. Narrowing purpose(s) and planning sequenced projects to develop an evidence-based repertoire of educational innovations has much potential.
- ***Question quality of innovation and research***
  Every innovation and research study benefits from a critical appraisal using pre-established guidelines for research rigor generally and within the targeted, specific area studied, methodology, and so on. Quality improvements and advancement of nursing theory and research cannot occur without quality analysis.
- ***Quote assumptions exactly and query paraphrased statements for accurate meaning***
  The CCC model presents 14 assumptions. Quoting exactly (and providing a citation) assures that alternate statements do not change the intended meaning. Sometimes, even changing one word or a punctuation mark can change a meaning entirely or even slightly.

- ***Repeat reliability measures***
  Reliability should be assessed each time an instrument is administered. To determine internal consistency, Cronbach $\alpha$ has been most frequently evaluated and ongoing measures will contribute to the psychometric history of the TSET and CCCET.
- ***Score the TSET by calculating subscale means (Self-Efficacy Strength [SEST] scores)***
  Subscale means (SEST) scores is the primary scoring method. Add subscale item responses and divide by number of items. This permits easy comparison within and between subscales and within and between studies.
- ***Select Self-Efficacy Level (SEL) scoring for subscales and total TSET as supplementary***
  SEL scoring, or grouping SEST scores into low, medium, and high groups is supplementary and can add richness to data interpretation. Design and study purpose may determine appropriateness of additional selection. Several recent studies have selected the quartile method for grouping: 25% in low, 50% in medium, 25% in high. (Grund et al., 2016; Halter et al., 2015; Ozkara San, 2018).
- ***Select SEST total TSET (mean) score as a supplementary scoring option***
  Add all 83 item responses and divide by 83 for the mean score. This should be used as supplementary to SEST subscale score analyses and not as a substitute.
- ***Test theoretical tenets (assumptions)***
  Many of the testable assumptions of the CCC model have been validated. Expanding studies to include new topics, pedagogies, and technologies for clinical, academic, and workplace settings will provide opportunities to validate the theory more broadly.
- ***Use intellectual property with permission***
  Follow copyright rules and ethical principles consistent with professional codes of ethics. Check with author or copyright holder concerning procedure(s) for reprinting, adapting, translating, copying, administering, or other forms of "using" published and unpublished intellectual materials such as illustrations, models, graphs, questionnaires, handouts, electronic slides, videos, and so on.
- ***Validate innovations with experts***
  Review by content experts, such as those with clinical, transcultural, pedagogical, technological, and statistical expertise will enhance the educational innovation and study design and enhance the confidence by which outcomes are interpreted.

- ***Widen worldview to make invisible populations visible***
  Expand innovations and research to meet the healthcare needs of marginalized and invisible populations, such as multiple heritage (multiethnic and mixed race) individuals and families, LGBT individuals and families, religious minorities, new immigrants, refugees, and so on, with new pedagogy and technology such as simulation, distance education, and standardized patients.
- ***Expect and explicate ethical practices in all parts of the research process***
  The protection of human subjects and strategies to assure ethical practices in all parts of the research process should always be required and acknowledged in published or presented work.
- ***Yearn to continue program of research and teaching scholarship***
  Innovation creativity is enhanced through intrinsic motivation for topic of interest. Desire and motivation to engage in the ongoing process of developing optimal cultural competence in self and in others is easily recognizable, even in written work, that can inspire others. Genuine passion can inspire others.
- ***Zip together all components***
  All health professionals need to actively engage in the ongoing, multidimensional process of developing optimal cultural competence in self and others. Understanding the multidimensional process, participating in formalized transcultural education, broadening the view of diversity, engaging in interprofessional and interdisciplinary collaboration locally and worldwide, and disseminating best practices using valid measures and a connecting framework are priorities, challenges, and future directions. The CCC theoretical model, associated questionnaires, educational innovations, and research are valuable resources to guide new priorities and future directions. "Whatever inquiries, actions, and innovations are done (or not done) today will influence the future. Through coordinated group efforts, the goals of culturally congruent health care and multicultural workplace harmony may be achieved" (Jeffreys, 2016a, p. 561).

# APPENDIX C
## Studies Involving Jeffreys' Cultural Competence and Confidence (CCC) Theoretical Framework and/or the Transcultural Self-Efficacy Tool (TSET)

Studies are grouped according to primary purpose(s) of study in the following categories:

- Educational Intervention – Academic
- Educational Intervention – Staff
- Course Evaluation
- Program Evaluation
- Instrumentation
- Perceptions (TSE)
- Relationship (of TSE to other variables)

**Educational Intervention – Academic**


Adams, T. M. (2012). *The evaluation of service-learning as an innovative strategy to enhance BSN students' transcultural self-efficacy*. (Unpublished doctoral dissertation). Alvernia University, Reading, PA.

Amerson, R. M., (2012). The influence of international service-learning on transcultural self-efficacy in baccalaureate nursing graduates and their subsequent practice. *International Journal of Teaching and Learning in Higher Education, 24* (1), 6-15.

Amerson, R. & Livingston, W. G. (2014). Reflexive photography: An alternative method for documenting the learning process of cultural competence. *Journal of Transcultural Nursing*, 25 (2), 202-210.

Andrews, M. M. et al., (2011). Developing a culturally competent workforce through collaborative partnerships. *Journal of Transcultural Nursing, 22* (3), 300-306.

Andrews, M. M., & Collins, J. (2015). Using Culture Care Theory as the organizing framework for a federal project on cultural competence. In M. McFarland & H. Wehbe-Alamah, (Eds.) *Leininger's culture care diversity and universality: A worldwide nursing theory* (3rd Edition, p. 537-552). Boston, MA: Jones and Bartlett.

Collins, J. & Andrews, M. M. (2016). TSET Research Exhibit 16.1, Evaluating the impact of a train-the-trainer collaborative project on transcultural self-efficacy perceptions. In M. R. Jeffreys (Ed.), *Teaching cultural competence in nursing and health care: Inquiry, action, and innovation* (3rd ed., pp. 542-544). New York: Springer Publishing.

Creech, C., Filter, M., Wehbe-Alamah, H., McFarland, M.R., Andrews, M., & Pryor, G. (2017). An intervention to improve cultural competence in graduate nursing education, *Nursing Education Perspectives, 38*(6), 333-336.

Czanderna, H. K. (2013). A *Qualitative Study on the Impact of a Short-Term Global Healthcare Immersion Experience in Bachelor of Science Nursing Students*. (Doctoral dissertation). The University of Kansas, Lawrence, KS. Retrieved from ProQuest Dissertations and Thesis. (Accession Order No. UMI 3587761)

Grossman, S., Mager, D., Opheim, H., & Torbjornsen, A. (2012). A bi-national simulation study to improve cultural awareness in nursing students. *Clinical Simulation in Nursing, 8* (8), 341-346.

Grund, F., Halter, M. M., Fridline, M., See, S., Young, L., & Reece, C. (2016). TSET Research Exhibit 4.4, Evaluating the effectiveness of cultural educational offerings on students' transcultural self-efficacy. In M. R. Jeffreys (Ed.), *Teaching cultural competence in nursing and health care: Inquiry, action, and innovation* (3rd ed., pp. 120-123). New York: Springer.

Halter, M., Grund, F., Fridline, M., See, S., Young, L., & Reece, C. (2015). Transcultural self-efficacy perceptions of baccalaureate nursing students. *Journal of Transcultural Nursing, 26*(3), 327-335.

Larsen, R., & Reif, L. (2011). Effectiveness of cultural immersion and culture classes for enhancing nursing students' transcultural self-efficacy. *Journal of Nursing Education, 50* (6), 350-354.

Larsen, R., & Reif, L. (2016). TSET Research Exhibit 9.1. Evaluating the effectiveness of an immersion experience on cultural competence. In M. R. Jeffreys (Ed.), *Teaching cultural competence in nursing and health care: Inquiry, action, and innovation* (3rd ed., pp. 299–301). New York: Springer Publishing.

Matejka, M., & Gulbransen, K. A. (2008). *The impact of a cultural immersion experience with low technology on nursing students' transcultural self-efficacy.* Paper presented at Sigma Theta Tau International Nursing Research Congress in Singapore, July 9, 2008.

Matejka, M. & Gilbransen, K. (2010). *The impact of a cultural immersion experience on students' development of cultural competence* (Poster Presentation). Transcultural Nursing Society International Conference (2010), Atlanta, GA & Red Deer College Nursing Research Conference (2011), Red Deer, Canada.

Meedzan, N.L. (2012). *The impact of a cultural immersion teaching experience on transcultural self-efficacy in baccalaureate nursing students.* (Oral presentation). Transcultural Nursing Society's 38th Annual Conference, October 17-20, 2012, Orlando, Florida.

Ochs, J. H. (2017). *Evaluating an innovative pedagogy for teaching transcultural nursing in an online format.* (Poster). Virginia Henderson Global Nursing e-Repository. Item http://hdl.handle.net/10755/603770.

Ozkara San, E. (2018). *Effect of the diverse standardized patient simulation (DSPS) cultural competence education strategy on nursing students' transcultural self-efficacy perceptions.* (Unpublished doctoral dissertation). The City University of New York Graduate College, New York, NY.

Polchert, M. J. (2014). Cultural competence and confidence in nursing students: A triangulated approach to evaluate domains of learning. (Oral presentation), April 4, 2014, Sigma Theta Tau International, Nursing Education Research Conference, Virginia Henderson Global Nursing e-Repository. Item http://hdl.handle.net/10755/316830.

Schmidt, L. (2012). *An evaluation of the impact of an intercultural service learning experience on the development of transcultural self-efficacy of nursing students* (Doctoral dissertation). Indianapolis, IN: Indiana University.

Schmidt, L. (2016). Exhibit 6.3. *Evaluating the effectiveness of a domestic and internationals service-learning experience on cultural competence as measured by the Transcultural Self-Efficacy Tool (TSET) and Cultural Competence Clinical Evaluation Tool (CCCET).* In M. R. Jeffreys (Ed.), *Teaching cultural competence in nursing and health care: Inquiry, action, and innovation* (3rd ed., pp. 174-180). New York: Springer Publishing.

Weideman, Y.L., Young, L., Lockhart, J. S., Grund, F.J., Fridline, M. M. & Panas, M. (2016). A virtual community: Building capacity through collaboration. *Journal of Professional Nursing, 32*(5S), S48-S53.

**Educational Intervention – Staff**

Andrews, M. M. et al., (2011). Developing a culturally competent workforce through collaborative partnerships. *Journal of Transcultural Nursing, 22* (3), 300-306.

Andrews, M. M., & Collins, J. (2015). Using Culture Care Theory as the organizing framework for a federal project on cultural competence. In M. McFarland & H. Wehbe-Alamah, (Eds.) *Leininger's culture care diversity and universality: A worldwide nursing theory* (3rd Edition, p. 537-552). Boston, MA: Jones and Bartlett.

Bloch, C. (2012). *Cultural competency intervention program for healthcare workers.* (Doctoral dissertation). Azusa Pacific University, Azusa, CA. Retrieved from ProQuest Dissertations and Thesis. (Accession Order No. UMI 3548294).

Bloch, C. (2016). TSET Research Exhibit 13.2, Evaluating the effectiveness of a cultural competency intervention program for health care workers. In M. R. Jeffreys (Ed.), *Teaching cultural competence in nursing and health care: Inquiry, action, and innovation* (3rd ed., pp. 454-455). New York: Springer.

Collins, J. & Andrews, M. M. (2016). TSET Research Exhibit 16.1, Evaluating the impact of a train-the-trainer collaborative project on transcultural self-efficacy perceptions. In M. R. Jeffreys (Ed.), *Teaching cultural competence in nursing and health care: Inquiry, action, and innovation* (3rd ed., pp. 542-544). New York: Springer Publishing.

Courtney, R., & Wolgamott, S. (2015). Using Leininger's theory as the building block for cultural competence and cultural assessment for a collaborative care team in a primary care setting. In M. McFarland & H. Wehbe-Alamah, (Eds.) *Leininger's culture care diversity and universality: A worldwide nursing theory* (3rd Edition, p. 345-368). Boston, MA: Jones and Bartlett.

Dolgan, C.M. (2001). *The effects of cultural competency training on nurses' attitudes.* (Unpublished master's thesis). Cleveland State University, Cleveland, OH.

Platter, B. (2005, October). *Clinical nurse cultural competency pre and post transcultural nursing education.* (Paper presentation), Transcultural Nursing Society Conference, New York, NY.

Velez, J. (2005). *The effects of cultural competency training using self-instruction on obstetrical nurses' awareness, knowledge and attitudes.* (Unpublished master's thesis). Cleveland State University, Cleveland, OH.

Velez, J. (2016). TSET Research Exhibit 13.1, Evaluating the effects of cultural competency training using self-instruction learning packets. In M. R. Jeffreys (Ed.), *Teaching cultural competence in nursing and health care: Inquiry, action, and innovation* (3rd ed., pp. 452-454). New York: Springer.

**Course Evaluation**

Adams, T. M., & Nevel K. (2007). *Appraisal of BSN Students' Transcultural Self-Efficacy using Jeffreys's Transcultural Self-Efficacy Tool.* (Unpublished study).

Adams, T. M., & Nevel, K. M. (2016). TSET Research Exhibit 8.1, Evaluating the effectiveness of a transcultural nursing course on students' transcultural self-efficacy. In M. R. Jeffreys (Ed.), *Teaching cultural competence in nursing and health care: Inquiry, action, and innovation* (3rd ed., pp. 248-252). New York: Springer.

Amerson, R. (2009). *The influence of international service-learning on cultural competence in baccalaureate nursing graduates and their subsequent nursing practice.* (Unpublished doctoral dissertation). The Graduate School of Clemson University, Clemson, SC. Retrieved from ProQuest. (3389233).

Amerson, R. M. (2010). The impact of service-learning on cultural competence. *Nursing Education Research, 31* (1), 18-22.

Amerson, R. M. (2016). TSET Research Exhibit 9.2. Evaluating the effectiveness of a community health course and service-learning on students' transcultural self-efficacy. In M. R. Jeffreys (Ed.), *Teaching cultural competence in nursing and health care: Inquiry, action, and innovation* (3rd ed., pp. 302–306). New York: Springer Publishing.

Durant, M. A. (2017). *The impact of innovative transcultural activities on undergraduate-level healthcare science students' perceived self-efficacy and cultural competence.* (Unpublished doctoral capstone project). American Sentinel University, Aurora, CO.

Jeffreys, M. R. (2011). *Graduate student data – MS program results: Transcultural Self-Efficacy Tool (TSET).* Unpublished report.

Nicely, S. & Stricklin, S. M. (2017). Enhancing cultural competence: The impact of a short-term study-away experience on regional campus students. *Journal of Nursing and Health Care, 3*(1), 1-5.

Rogers-Walker, M. (2014). *Examining the relationship between participation in service-learning and the levels of transcultural self-efficacy reported by associate of science in nursing students.* Unpublished doctoral dissertation, Capella University.

Rogers-Walker, M. (2016). TSET Research Exhibit 9.3. *Examining the relationship between participation in service-learning and the levels of transcultural self-efficacy reported by associate of science in nursing students.* In M. R. Jeffreys (Ed.), *Teaching cultural competence in nursing and health care: Inquiry, action, and innovation* (3rd ed., pp. 307–310). New York: Springer Publishing.

**Program Evaluation**

Allen, J., Brown, L., Duff, C., Nesbitt, P., & Hepner, A. (2013). Development and evaluation of a teaching and learning approach in cross-cultural care and antidiscrimination in university nursing students. *Nurse Education Today, 33*, 1592-1598.

Burrell, P. (2010). *Perceived cultural competency of nursing students.* (Unpublished study).

Burrell, P. (2016). TSET Research Exhibit 7.3, Evaluating the effectiveness of cultural competence threads throughout a baccalaureate curriculum. In M. R. Jeffreys (Ed.), *Teaching cultural competence in nursing and health care: Inquiry, action, and innovation* (3rd ed., pp. 228-230). New York: Springer.

Creech, C., Filter, M., Wehbe-Alamah, H., McFarland, M.R., Andrews, M., & Pryor, G. (2017). An intervention to improve cultural competence in graduate nursing education, *Nursing Education Perspectives, 38*(6), 333-336.

Curtis, M. P., Bultas, M. W., & Green, L. (2016). Enhancing cultural competency. *Online Journal of Cultural Competence in Nursing and Healthcare, 6*(1), 1-13. doi:10.9730/ojccnh.org/v6n1a1.

Ferguson, P. (2007). *Transcultural self-efficacy in graduating nursing students.* (Doctoral dissertation). Illinois State University. IL. Retrieved from ProQuest Dissertations and Thesis. (Accession Order No. UMI 3280900).

Jeffreys M. R., Dogan E. (2012). Evaluating the influence of cultural competence education on students' transcultural self-efficacy perceptions. *Journal of Transcultural Nursing, 23* (2) 188–197.

Mesler, D. M. (2014). A comparative study of cultural competence curricula in baccalaureate nursing programs. *Nurse Educator, 39* (4), 193-198.

Rudnick, L. E. (2004). *Nursing students' perceived self-efficacy to provide culturally competent nursing care: An educational outcomes assessment study.* (Doctoral dissertation). Wilmington College, NJ. Retrieved from ProQuest Dissertations and Thesis. (Accession Order No. UMI 3156560).

Shattel, M. M., Nemitz, E. A., Crosson, N., Zackeru, A. R., Starr, S., Hu, J., & Gonzales, C. (2013). Culturally competent practice in a pre-licensure baccalaureate nursing program in the United States: A mixed-methods study. *Nursing Education Perspectives, 34* (6), 383-389.

Singleton, J.K., & Slyer, J. T. (2016). TSET Research Exhibit 7.2, Evaluating the enhancement of cultural competence throughout a Doctor of Nursing Practice (DNP) program. In M. R. Jeffreys (Ed.), *Teaching cultural competence in nursing and health care: Inquiry, action, and innovation* (3rd ed., pp. 224-227). New York: Springer.

Singleton, J. K. (2017). An enhanced cultural competence curriculum and changes in transcultural self-efficacy in Doctor of Nursing Practice students. *Journal of Transcultural Nursing, 28*(5), 516-522.

Stegman, B. C. (2013). *Cultural competence integration in the nursing curriculum.* Dissertations. 274. http://irl.umsl.edu/dissertation/274.

**Perceptions (TSE)**

Blackstock, S. (2003). *An examination of senior nursing students' perceptions of culturally competent nursing practices and their self-efficacy in delivering quality healthcare to culturally diverse patients.* (Doctoral dissertation). The University of North Carolina, Greensboro, NC. Available from ProQuest Dissertations and Theses database. (UMI No.3093858).

Forgacs, E. (2001). The transcultural nursing self-efficacy perceptions of graduating nursing students. (Unpublished master's thesis). Regis College, Weston, MA.

Hoyer, G. (2013). *Transcultural self-efficacy of nursing education leaders and faculty related to non-binary sexual identities.* (Doctoral dissertation). Eastern Michigan University, Ypsilanti, MI. Available from ProQuest Dissertations and Theses database. (UMI No.3619027).

Hoyer, G. (2016). TSET Research Exhibit 7.1, Exploring transcultural self-efficacy perceptions of nursing education administrators and faculty related to lesbian, gay, bisexual, transgender (LGBT) issues. In M. R. Jeffreys (Ed.), *Teaching cultural competence in nursing and health care: Inquiry, action, and innovation* (3rd ed., pp. 222-223). New York: Springer.

Hyun, D. J. J. (2012). *Development and evaluation of a teaching and learning approach in cross-cultural care and antidiscrimination in university nursing students.* (Unpublished doctoral dissertation). St. Paul University, Manila, Philippines.

Kim, S-H. (2013). Transcultural self-efficacy and educational needs for cultural competence in nursing of Korean nurses. *Journal of Korean Academy of Nursing, 43* (1), 102-113.

Li, J., He, Z., Luo, Y., & Zhang, R. (2016). Perceived transcultural self-efficacy of nurses in general hospitals in Guangzhou, China. *Nursing Research, 65*(5), 371-379.

Lim, J., Downie, J., & Nathan, P. (2004). Nursing students' self-efficacy in providing transcultural care. *Nurse Education Today, 24*, 428-434.

MacQuarrie, D. (2004). *Assessment of student nurses' transcultural self-efficacy perceptions when caring for culturally diverse clients.* (Unpublished master's thesis). McMaster University, Hamilton, ON.

Malliarou, M., Oikonomou, A., Nika, S., & Sarafis, P. (2017). Greek military nurses readiness to provide transcultural care to immigrants. *British Journal of Medicine and Medical Research, 19*(6), 1-11.

Mayfield, C. L. (2014). *Transcultural self-efficacy perceptions of associate degree nursing students at a greater Minnesota college setting.* (Unpublished master thesis). Minnesota State University, Moorhead, MN.

Olaivar, O. K. (2014). *Transcultural self-efficacy perceptions of nurse practitioners in Fresno, California.* (Unpublished master's thesis). California State University, Fresno, CA. Available from ProQuest Dissertations and Theses database. (UMI No. 1553972).

Sarafis, P. A., & Malliarou, M. (2013). Cultural self-efficacy of baccalaureate nursing students in a Greek University. *Iranian Journal of Nursing and Midwifery Research, 18* (6), 446-450.

Sarafis, P. A., & Malliarou, M. (2016). TSET Research Exhibit 4.2, Evaluating the transcultural self-efficacy perceptions of baccalaureate students in Greece. In M. R. Jeffreys (Ed.), *Teaching cultural competence in nursing and health care: Inquiry, action, and innovation* (3rd ed., pp. 107-110). New York: Springer Publishing.

**Relationship** (of TSE to other variables)

Farber, J. (2015). *The Relationship between Cultural Experiences and Perceived Transcultural Self-Efficacy of Nurse Faculty*. (Unpublished doctoral dissertation), Widener University, Chester, PA.

Francisco, S. (2013). The *effects of nurses' cultural competency upon patient satisfaction within BLHC healthcare system.* (Unpublished doctoral dissertation). Argosy University, Chicago, IL.

Fridline, M. (2016). TSET Research Exhibit 4.5, Using CART analysis to examine the relationship of demographic variables to transcultural self-efficacy perceptions of baccalaureate nursing students. In M. R. Jeffreys (Ed.), *Teaching cultural competence in nursing and health care: Inquiry, action, and innovation* (3rd ed., pp. 124-127). New York: Springer.

Kontzamanis, E. (2013). *An investigation of the relationship between nursing faculty attitudes toward culturally diverse patients and transcultural self-efficacy*. (Unpublished doctoral dissertation). The City University of New York (CUNY) Graduate College, NY, NY. Available from ProQuest Dissertations and Theses database. (UMI No. 3561605).

Lee, K.E. & Kim, N. S. (2017). Factors affecting transcultural self-efficacy among nursing students. *Journal of Health Informatics and Statistics, 42*(1), 1-9.

Nokes, K. M., & Gilmartin, M. J. (2015). Are personality characteristics of Clinical Nurse Leader graduate nursing students related to culturally competent nursing care? *Journal of Nursing Education and Practice, 5*(5), DOI: 10.5430/jnep.v5n5p1. http://dx.doi.org/10.5430.jnep.v5n5p1.

Schroeder, P. A. (2012). *The influence of cultural immersion on transcultural self-efficacy for nursing students at private faith-based baccalaureate nursing programs.* (Doctoral dissertation). The University of South Dakota, Vermillion SD. Retrieved from ProQuest Dissertations and Thesis. (Accession Order No. UMI 3524460).

Toney, D. A. (2004). *Exploring the relationship between levels of cultural competence and the perceived level of quality care among registered nurses caring for culturally diverse patients.* (Doctoral dissertation). Capella University, Minneapolis, MN. Available from ProQuest Dissertations and Theses database. (UMI No. 3132753).

**Instrumentation**

Bayik, A., Basalan Iz, F., (2007). *The reliability and validity of transcultural self- efficacy tool in Turkish community*. (Unpublished study). Ege University School of Nursing, Izmir/Turkey.

Bayik, Temel, A., & Basalan, Iz, F. (2016). TSET Research Exhibit 4.1. The Reliability and Validity of the Transcultural Self-Efficacy Tool–Turkish (TSET–Turkish). In M. R. Jeffreys (Ed.), *Teaching cultural competence in nursing and health care: Inquiry, action, and innovation* (3rd ed., pp. 104–107). New York: Springer Publishing.

Chen, J. (2014). *Development and Validation of Chinese Version of Transcultural Self-Efficacy Tool.* (Unpublished doctoral dissertation). Tongji University, Shanghai, China.

Chen, J. (2016). TSET Research Exhibit 4.3, Exploring the validity of the Transcultural Self-Efficacy Tool (TSET)-Chinese with staff nurses in China. In M. R. Jeffreys (Ed.), *Teaching cultural competence in nursing and health care: Inquiry, action, and innovation* (3rd ed., pp. 110-112). New York: Springer Publishing.

Jeffreys, M. R., & Dogan, E. (2010). Factor analysis of the Transcultural Self- Efficacy Tool (TSET). *Journal of Nursing Measurement, 18* (2), 120-139.

Jeffreys, M. R. & Dogan, E. (2013). Evaluating cultural competence in the clinical practicum, *Nursing Education Perspectives, 34*(2), 88-94.

Jeffreys, M. R. & Dogan, E. (2016a). Exhibit 6.1, Disseminating findings via a professional conference: Sample conference abstract. In M. R. Jeffreys (Ed.), *Teaching cultural competence in nursing and health care: Inquiry, action, and innovation* (3rd ed., pp. 168-169). New York: Springer.

Jeffreys, M. R. & Dogan, E. (2016b). Exhibit 6.2, Evaluating cultural competence in the clinical practicum: Graduate nursing education. In M. R. Jeffreys (Ed.), *Teaching cultural competence in nursing and health care: Inquiry, action, and innovation* (3rd ed., pp. 170-173). New York: Springer.

Jeffreys, M. R. & Dogan, E. (2016c). Exhibit 6.4, Evaluating cultural and clinical diversity and disparity in the clinical setting. In M. R. Jeffreys (Ed.), *Teaching cultural competence in nursing and health care: Inquiry, action, and innovation* (3rd ed., pp. 184-185). New York: Springer.

Jeffreys, M. R., & Smodlaka, I. (1996). Steps of the instrument design: An illustrative approach for nurse educators. *Nurse Educator, 21*(6), 47-52.

Jeffreys, M. R., & Smodlaka, I. (1998). Exploring the factorial composition of the Transcultural Self-Efficacy Tool. *International Journal of Nursing Studies, 35*, 217-225.

Jeffreys, M. R., & Smodlaka, I. (1999a). Changes in students' transcultural self-efficacy perceptions following an integrated approach to culture care. *Journal of Multicultural Nursing and Health,* 5(2), 6-12.

Jeffreys, M. R., & Smodlaka, I. (1999b). Construct validation of the Transcultural Self-Efficacy Tool. *Journal of Nursing Education, 38*(5), 222-227.

Sarafis, P. A., *Igoumenidis* M., Tzavara, C., & Malliarou, M. (2014). Reliability and validity of the transcultural self-efficacy tool questionnaire (Greek version). *Journal of Nursing Measurement,* 22(2), E41-E51.

CHAPTER 4

# The Hispanic/Latino Immigrant Cancer Survivor Experience in the United States

## *A Scoping Review*

Joan Such Lockhart, Melinda G. Oberleitner, and David A. Nolfi

**ABSTRACT**

Cancer is the leading cause of death among U.S.-born Hispanic/Latinos. Issues confronting these cancer survivors and their families are complex and include physical, psychological, social, spiritual, and financial concerns from the time of diagnosis throughout the remainder of the survivor's life. However, cancer survivors who are also immigrants living in the United States often face additional challenges being a cancer survivor related to cultural beliefs, language, access to care, and socioeconomic status. Therefore, this chapter describes the results of a scoping review of research published over the past decade and focused on cancer survivors who are adult immigrants of Hispanic/Latino ethnicity living in the United States. This method provided a rigorous and transparent method for mapping published research retrieved through three major databases and for identifying existing gaps. Of the 951 references that were initially identified, 18 studies from 2008 to 2017 met the inclusion criteria. Four major themes were identified through thematic analysis: (1) survival patterns ($n$ = 2); (2) barriers ($n$ = 5); (3) decision-making ($n$ = 2); and (4) quality of life (QOL; $n$ = 9). Results


http://dx.doi.org/10.1891/0739-6686.37.119

offer evidence to guide informed, patient-centered care and culturally appropriate interventions tailored to the needs of Hispanic/Latino immigrants. Finally, findings can be used by nurses to guide future oncology research about this vulnerable and underserved population of cancer survivors.

## INTRODUCTION

Cancer is the second leading cause of death in the United States. Due to rapid advancements in the understanding of cancer biology, early detection and diagnostic capabilities, and availability of more individualized treatment options, the death rate from cancer has declined from a high of 215.1 per 100,000 population in 1991 to 158.6 in 2015, a drop of over 26%, or more than 2.3 million fewer deaths from cancer (Siegel, Miller, & Jemal, 2018). Concomitant with the decline in death rates from cancer, the number of cancer survivors is increasing exponentially. As of January 1, 2016, more than 15.5 million Americans with a history of cancer, almost 5% of the population, were alive (American Cancer Society [ACS], 2018). Due to continued advances in the discovery of precision treatment options and integration of sophisticated supportive care during the acute treatment phase and beyond, the number of cancer survivors is expected to grow to 20.3 million by 2026 and to 26.1 million by 2040 in the United States alone (Bluethmann, Mariotto, & Rowland, 2016).

The National Coalition for Cancer Survivorship, the National Cancer Institute's (NCI) Office of Cancer Survivorship, and others adopted the definition of cancer survivorship in the mid-1990s as the period from the time of diagnosis through the rest of the cancer survivor's life. Issues confronting cancer survivors and their families are complex and include physical, psychological, social, spiritual, and financial concerns from the time of diagnosis throughout the remainder of the survivor's life (Hewitt, Greenfield, & Stovall, 2005). In an effort to bring attention to the myriad needs of cancer survivors and support a goal of developing a comprehensive public health effort to address cancer survivorship, a National Plan for Cancer Survivorship: Advancing Public Health Strategies was developed through a partnership between the Centers for Disease Control and the Lance Armstrong Foundation (2004). Among the specific objectives of the National Action Plan are to "establish a solid base of applied research and scientific knowledge on the ongoing physical, psychological, social, spiritual, and economic issues facing cancer survivors" and to "ensure all cancer survivors have adequate access to high-quality treatment and post-treatment follow-up services" (ES-2).

Cancer incidence and outcomes from cancer vary significantly among racial and ethnic groups. Racial and ethnic groups that are more likely than the general population to have higher incidence and mortality rates from cancer include African Americans/Blacks, Asian Americans, Hispanic/Latinos, American Indians, Alaska Natives, and underserved Whites (Kennedy, Kidd, McDonald, & Biddle, 2015; Pinheiro, Callahan, Jin, & Morris, 2016; Singh & Hiatt, 2006). Among members of immigrant groups, foreign-born immigrants in the United States are, in general, diagnosed with cancer less frequently than U.S.-born members of the same ethnic group due, in part, to lifestyle factors such as lower smoking and obesity rates among foreign-born immigrants (Kennedy et al, 2015; Pinheiro et al., 2016; Singh & Hiatt, 2006). However, research on another group of immigrants, undocumented or unauthorized immigrants, reveals findings of concern as undocumented immigrants have worse clinical outcomes than that of the general population (Castro-Echeverry et al., 2013). As of 2015, the Pew Research Center estimated there were 11 million unauthorized immigrants living in the United States; the majority of undocumented immigrants are Hispanic/Latinos (Krogstad, Passel, & Cohn, 2018). As a group, undocumented immigrants are less likely to have access to consistent primary and preventive care services, are less likely to be insured, and are more likely to visit urgent care centers and emergency departments for their healthcare needs (Bustamante et al., 2010). These barriers to routine care with consistent providers who are able to monitor patients for issues associated with acute or chronic conditions result in poorer health outcomes, especially as related to cancer. For example, undocumented immigrants are more likely to be diagnosed with cancer in advanced stages, which negatively impacts survival outcomes (Castro-Echeverry et al., 2013).

Ethnic minorities, a term often applied to population groups of color, are predicted to be the majority in the United States by 2050 (U.S. Census Bureau, 2005). Members of ethnic minority and medically underserved population groups are affected disproportionately by cancer (Institute of Medicine, 1999). Due to expected growth in populations in ethnic minority communities and also as a result of aging, by the year 2030, projections are there will be as much as a 99% increase in cancer among minorities compared to a projected increased cancer incidence of 31% among Whites (Smith, Smith, Hurria, Hortobagyi, & Buchholz, 2009). Barriers, including lack of health insurance (Grant et al., 2015) and other obstacles, lead to disparities in cancer prevention, early detection, and optimal treatment, especially for members of ethnic minority groups. For example, according to the ACS (2018), Hispanics and Blacks continue to be the most likely groups to be uninsured at 16% and 11%, respectively, compared to 6% of the non-Hispanic White (NHW) population. Members of ethnic minorities, including immigrants, are significantly more likely to be diagnosed with cancer when the cancer is in a more advanced stage, making the cancer more difficult and more expensive to treat, resulting in less successful outcomes (ACS, 2018).

Hispanics/Latinos represent the largest and fastest growing racial/ethnic minority group in the United States, comprising about 17% of the country's population in 2014. Estimates are that the Hispanic/Latino population in the United States will double by 2050 (Colby & Ortman, 2014). The term "Hispanic" refers to individuals of Mexican, Cuban, Puerto Rican, South or Central American, Dominican, or other Spanish descent; the majority of Hispanics in the United States are of Mexican origin (64%; U.S. Census Bureau, 2014). Federal government standards mandate race and ethnicity to be separate concepts; therefore, persons identifying with Hispanic origin may be of any race and may have various combinations of racial ancestry.

Cancer is the leading cause of death among U.S. Hispanic/Latinos (ACS, 2015). Cancer rates in Hispanic/Latinos vary by country of origin and by subpopulations, and variations in cancer risk have been validated between Hispanics and NHW (Siegel et al., 2015). Hispanics are especially vulnerable to disparities in care compared to other racial and ethnic groups. Hispanics are less likely to have health insurance and are more likely to be affected by poverty and lower levels of education, which may impact access to health care and information about health. In addition, there is high prevalence of strong risk factors associated with the development of cancer, such as obesity, among Hispanics (National Center for Health Statistics, 2015). It has also been recognized that there is significant diversity within Hispanic populations in terms of degree of acculturation and nativity status, which may mask important differences in cancer incidence and mortality in subethnic groups (Siegel et al., 2015).

When compared to other racial/ethnic groups, which share comparable socioeconomic characteristics, Hispanics/Latino immigrants tend to exhibit overall better cancer-related health indicators in some studies. The term "Hispanic paradox" refers to this phenomenon. The Hispanic paradox may be a result of cultural and lifestyle factors common to Latino immigrants who are living in Hispanic enclaves in which foreign-born immigrants retain lifestyle practices favored in their countries of origin such as healthier eating and sexual/reproductive behaviors, support of extended family, and a distinct genetic heritage. It is speculated that health advantages of foreign-born Hispanic immigrants erode over time in subsequent generations for those who are born and live in the United States, as members of successive generations become more acculturated or assimilated into a less healthy "Western" or "Americanized" lifestyle (ACS, 2015; Stern et al., 2016).

The concept of culture and its relationship or influence on cancer remains poorly defined, and cultural beliefs may also serve as barriers to some groups accessing effective health care (Kagawa-Singer, Dadia, Yu, & Surbone, 2010). Results of emerging research on culture and cancer reveal the important impact of cultural influences on patients' and communities' perceptions of their risk for cancer, trust in health professionals and institutions which provide cancer screening, detection, diagnosis and treatment, and cultural factors which may impact individuals' adherence to recommended treatments for cancer (Kagawa-Singer et al., 2010).

Important research priorities identified in a 2008 survey of oncology nurses included symptom management and the potential uses of technology to improve management of disease and treatment-related symptoms. However, when compared to rankings from the 2008 survey of oncology nurses on research priorities, results of a 2013 survey indicated that focus areas on minority and underserved populations moved up in the rankings in terms of research importance. Specifically, screening research in minorities and screening and early detection in underserved or underinsured populations were among the top five positions in the priority rankings: survivorship issues overall were represented in eight of the top 20 ranked research priorities (LoBiondo-Wood et al., 2014).

### Purpose and Research Questions

This chapter describes the results of a scoping review of the literature focused on research conducted over the past decade on cancer survivors who are adult immigrants of Hispanic/Latino ethnicity and who reside in the United States. Specific research questions included:

1. From a research perspective, what is known about Hispanic/Latino immigrants in the United States who are cancer survivors?
2. How can this information be used to provide informed, patient-centered care and evidence-based interventions which are tailored to the needs of Hispanic/Latino immigrants living in the United States who have been diagnosed with cancer?

## METHODS

The scoping study methodology by Arksey and O'Malley (2005) was used to conduct a review of the literature about Hispanic immigrant cancer survivors and summarize their findings. This framework outlines five stages of the review process: (1) identify a research question; (2) identify relevant studies; (3) select studies; (4) chart data from selected studies, and (5) collate, summarize, and report findings (Arksey & O'Malley, 2005). An advantage of using this methodology is that it allows a comprehensive and transparent review of the literature in a relatively short period compared to a systematic review.

The authors searched the CINAHL, PubMed, and Scopus databases using combinations and variations of keywords and subject headings for concepts such as cancer survivors, immigrants, and emigrants (although Scopus does not have its own subject headings, it includes searchable subject headings borrowed from other databases). The author (D.A.N.) who was an experienced health science librarian with expert searching techniques guided the database search. When possible, explode functions were used for subject headings (to find narrower headings) and truncation for keyword terms (to find variant word endings). Table 4.1 includes lists of terms used for each database, and readers may contact the corresponding author to obtain full search strategies. The searches were run in January 2018, and the authors limited the results to English-language articles published between 2008 through 2017. Additionally, the CINAHL and Scopus searches were limited to exclude articles indexed to Medline, which is a subset of PubMed.

Recognizing the diversity of terminology used to describe Hispanic/Latino populations and the ambiguous usage of certain terms (e.g., Latin American includes Spanish, French, and Portuguese speakers), the authors decided to use Hispanic/Latino population as an inclusion criterion instead of a search term. Similarly, because test searches showed that many database records failed to describe geographic settings clearly, the authors decided to use "United States" as an inclusion criterion instead of a search term. The authors used reference software to record search results, store studies, and locate full text. The authors also used a web-based project management system to coordinate all phases of the project.

### Inclusion/Exclusion Criteria

Study selection was based on the following inclusion criteria: cancer survivors (all types and stages), adult (18 years and older), any gender, immigrant/

**TABLE 4.1**
*Search Terms*

| Keywords | Subject Headings |
|---|---|
| Aliens | Cancer patients |
| Asylum seekers | Cancer survivors |
| Cancer diagnosis | Emigrants and immigrants |
| Cancer patient | Emigration and immigration |
| Cancer | Immigrants |
| Emigrants | Neoplasm staging |
| Immigrants | Neoplasms |
| Refugees | Refugees |
| Survival | Survivors |
| Survivors | Survivorship |

foreign born, Hispanic/Latino ethnicity ("Cuban, Mexican, Puerto Rican, South or Central American, or other Spanish culture or origin regardless of race"; U.S. Census Bureau, 2018), and living in the United States. Because the authors found many examples of studies that included several populations, one final consideration was that a majority of the study samples contained within each study (more than 50%) must meet the inclusion criteria of adult Hispanic/Latino cancer survivor. Exclusion criteria were studies about children, U.S. born, families of cancer survivors, and healthcare professionals. The authors also excluded studies when they could not determine the immigrant status of the sample populations.

Figure 4.1 shows each stage of the study selection process following the Preferred Reporting Items for Systematic Reviews and Meta-Analyses guidelines (Moher, Liberati, Tetzlaff, & Altman, 2009). Two of the authors who were

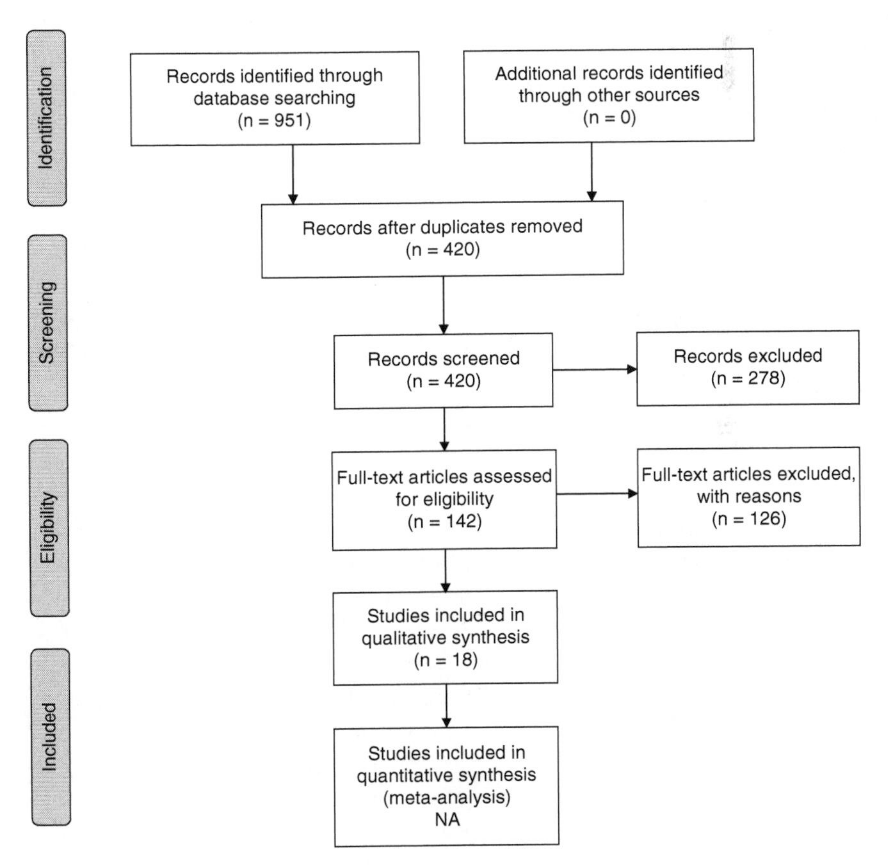


**FIGURE 4.1** Preferred Reporting Items for Systematic Reviews and Meta-Analyses flow diagram.

experienced oncology nurse researchers (J.S.L. and M.G.O.) followed a logical study selection process: (1) independently reviewing the titles and/or abstracts of each study retrieved through the database searches, using the inclusion criteria, and examining the full text to clarify questions; (2) comparing their selected studies with each other and discussing any differences (using full text) until 100% consensus was reached. This process resulted in a final sample of 18 studies that met the inclusion criteria.

Next, the researchers read the full text version of the sample studies, extracted key data from each study, and organized them using a table (chart) format with the following headings: (1) author(s) and publication date; (2) study purpose; (3) study design; (4) sample and setting; (5) data collection; and (6) study findings and recommendations. Attention was paid to retrieving descriptors about the sample population such as demographics, birth country, number of years living in the United States, and cancer type. Table 4.2 illustrates the charting of sample study data according to author/year, study design and purpose, study population and setting, methods, and findings. Extracted data were analyzed using descriptive statistics and/or thematic analysis across the 18 sample studies.

## FINDINGS

### Demographic Description of Sample Studies

Findings for this scoping review begin with a summary of descriptive data extracted from the sample studies and organized by categories such as publication date, study design, sample characteristics, and data collection methods. This section is followed by a thematic analysis conducted across all included studies.

The final 18 sample studies were conducted in the United States and published from 2008 to 2017, with most studies ($n$ = 5) published in 2013. The publication dates were fairly evenly distributed across the decade with no studies published in 2010 or 2012. The sample studies were published in 12 different journal titles; more than one study was included in three of the journals: *Journal of Cancer Education* ($n$ = 4); *Journal of Psychosocial Oncology* ($n$ = 3); and *Supportive Cancer Care* ($n$ = 2). Only one study reflected authors who were affiliated with schools of nursing (Campesino et al., 2009) and published in a journal dedicated to nursing, *Advances in Nursing Science*.

While both qualitative ($n$ = 7) and quantitative designs ($n$ = 11) were reported in these studies, nearly two-thirds (61.1%) of the studies relied on quantitative methods. Qualitative designs were simply described as being exploratory in nature; two studies mentioned using a grounded theory approach during analysis. Most quantitative designs were nonexperimental ($n$ = 9) and included

**TABLE 4.2**

*Charting of Sample Studies (N = 18)*

| Author(s), Year | Study Design and Purpose | Study Population and Setting | Methods | Findings |
|---|---|---|---|---|
| Buki et al. (2008) | Qualitative:<br>Examine experiences of immigrant breast cancer survivors along survivorship continuum, from diagnosis to long-term survivorship | 18 immigrant Latina breast cancer survivors<br>Ages 35–67 years ($M$ = 51.22)<br>Lived in the United States average 19.18 years | Separate focus groups with women in the acute, re-entry, and long-term survivorship stages<br>Grounded theory analysis | Treatments tailored for each survivorship stage more likely to be effective than generic interventions; distinct cultural experiences identified |
| Campesino, Ruiz, Glover, and Koithan, (2009) | Qualitative:<br>Identify consequences of recent immigration legislation enacted in Arizona in terms of barriers created to accessing cancer treatment and follow-up care; seek in-depth understanding of cancer care experiences in illegal Latina immigrants with breast cancer | 10 Mexican immigrant cancer survivors; migrated to the United States within past 7–15 years<br>Ages 36–64 years ($M$ = 48, $SD$ = 4.8)<br>Nine residing illegally in the United States; one legal resident<br>Due to illegal status, most ineligible for state-sponsored health insurance; paying out of pocket for cancer care treatments; over 60% reported yearly household income of $20,000 or less | Semi-structured interviews to explore distress related to economic perceptions/ experiences in cancer care delivery; framed stories as counter-narratives | Majority described significant psychological distress related to economic situation; experienced interruption or cessation of cancer care due to inability to pay; added to their burdens of living with cancer; healthcare professionals need to employ targeted interventions for cancer patients experiencing financial burdens. |

(Continued)

**TABLE 4.2**
*Charting of Sample Studies (N = 18) (Continued)*

| Author(s), Year | Study Design and Purpose | Study Population and Setting | Methods | Findings |
|---|---|---|---|---|
| Carrion, Nedjat-Haiem, Martinez-Tyson, and Castaneds (2013) | Qualitative: exploratory<br>Identify factors facilitating completion of advanced care planning (ACP) and decision-making patterns | Three groups of 15 Latinas with cancer in central Florida; 15 in each group of Columbian, Puerto-Rican, and Mexican; Years in the United States by group range: 1 to over 31 years | Purposive in-depth, open-ended, semi-structured interview using grounded theory approach and thematic analysis conducted in Spanish | Knowledge gap existed regarding ACP among women in the study. Differences between the three groups a result of migration/immigration history, income, education, English language proficiency, and other factors. Differences contribute to their readiness, receptiveness, and willingness to engage in ACP. |
| Carrion Nedjat-Haiem, and Martinez-Tyson (2013) | Qualitative: exploratory<br>Explore beliefs and treatment decisions of foreign-born Latino men diagnosed with cancer | 15 Latino men diagnosed with cancer within the past 5 years in central Florida<br>Nine men with prostate cancer<br>Two men with brain cancer<br>Two men with colorectal cancer<br>Two men with lung cancer<br>Years in the United States range: 1 to 31+ years | In-depth, semi-structured interviews and thematic analysis; interviews conducted in Spanish | Treatment decisions based on the men's fear of dying; Latino men's preferences related to communication about diagnostic information warrant additional research themes: cancer diagnosis synonymous with death; diagnostic-related communication; reliance on physicians for treatment decisions; limited information and informal advanced care planning; support received and role changes. |

| | | | | |
|---|---|---|---|---|
| Carrion, Nedjat-Haiem, Macip-Billbe, and Black (2017) | Qualitative: exploratory<br>Perceptions of coping to understand the meaning of the experience with the cancer within the participant's social and cultural contexts | 60 immigrant and migrant Latino men and women diagnosed with cancer within past 5 years; recruited from community-based organizations, clinics, and churches<br>Median age: 55 years<br>80% of women diagnosed with breast cancer; 94% of men had prostate cancer<br>Years in the United States: range 1 to over 31 years | 60- to 90-minute semi-structured interviews asking open-questions pertaining to coping. | Emerging themes associated with the development of coping strategies included positive reframing, family support, religion and spirituality, and support from healthcare providers. When medical and helping professionals provided tangible support, participants engaged in meaning-based coping. Provides insight into existing coping strategies utilized by Latinos. |
| Changrani et al. (2008) | Quantitative: (RCT)<br>Examines viability of Online Cancer Support Groups (OSGs) for Hispanic immigrants with breast cancer and effectiveness of OSGs. | 68 Spanish-dominant speaking women with breast cancer (experimental group [EG] *n* = 48; usual care group [CG] *n* = 20)<br>Women from 12 Latin American Countries<br>Age: EG mean 46.2 years<br>CG mean 50.8 years<br>Years in the United States:<br>EG mean 14 years<br>CG mean 24.2 years | RCT<br>Groups facilitated by trained bilingual facilitators<br>Four scales used to study the effectiveness of psychosocial interventions targeting breast cancer patients: depression, personal growth, QOL, and pain | OSGs are acceptable to and feasible for immigrant minorities, including those with limited English proficiency; no significant change in outcomes pre–post but trends noted |

(*Continued*)

**TABLE 4.2**
*Charting of Sample Studies (N = 18) (Continued)*

| Author(s), Year | Study Design and Purpose | Study Population and Setting | Methods | Findings |
|---|---|---|---|---|
| Costas and Gany (2013) | Quantitative<br>Describe the depressive symptoms in a sample of African Caribbean and Latino cancer patients; examine differences in specific symptoms between the two groups | 44 immigrant Afro-Caribbean and 145 Latino underserved cancer patients recruited from five New York City hospitals | Nested cohort<br>Retrospective<br>Latino and Afro-Caribbean<br>Depressive symptoms measured to screen and obtain severity score | Similar levels of positive screen for depression among cancer patients; more Latinos reported depressed mood, more intense depression/anxiety and being diagnosed with depression. |
| Costas-Muniz et al. (2013) | Quantitative: correlation<br>Examine rate of awareness cancer stage and desire for cancer treatment information and determine demographic and medical correlates of lack of cancer knowledge | 271 underserved Latino cancer patients recruited from four cancer clinics in New York City<br>Mean age = 55 years<br>Years in the United States: range <5 to 20 years | Cross-sectional needs assessment in preferred language | Being an immigrant with limited English proficiency and monolingual in Spanish were predictors for stage unawareness and less desire/need for cancer information; 65% had no stage knowledge; 15% wanted information. |

| | | | | |
|---|---|---|---|---|
| Costas-Muniz et al. (2015) | Quantitative: correlation<br>Examine association between somatic and nonsomatic depressive symptoms, QOL, and self-reported adherence to cancer-related medical appointments and treatments, delays, and interruptions among a cohort of underserved, immigrant minority cancer patients. | 622 diverse immigrant adult cancer patients undergoing outpatient treatment at 10 hospital-based cancer clinics in New York City<br>Mean age = 55.5 years<br>53.5% Latinos; breast cancer (42%) | Survey:<br>Sociodemographic, health-related questions assessing missed appointments and delays/or interruptions, and QOL and depression scales | Positive depression screen, poor physical and emotional well-being significant predictors of missed appointments and delays and/or interruptions of treatment. |
| D'Orazio, Meyerowitz, Stone, Felix, and Muderspach (2011) | Quantitative<br>Describe and identify cancer-related, contextual, and dispositional variables that predict depression, affect, and QOL | 54 women recruited from the Los Angeles County/University of Southern California Gynecological Clinic; cervical cancer survivors<br>Lived in the United States: 5–38 years<br>Mean = 16.9 years<br>Age: 30–75 years (Mean = 50.48) | Data from medical chart; measurement of level of acculturation, depression, affect, QOL, coping, social support strategies, social support. | Patients experiencing high levels of depression, negative affect, and low levels of positive affect; most common type of life stress reported: immigration-related stress; reported adequate amounts of social support. |

(*Continued*)

**TABLE 4.2**
*Charting of Sample Studies (N = 18) (Continued)*

| Author(s), Year | Study Design and Purpose | Study Population and Setting | Methods | Findings |
|---|---|---|---|---|
| Galvan, Buki, and Garces (2009) | Qualitative<br>Explore QOL issues in Latina breast cancer survivors focus on social support experiences | 22 immigrant Latina women with breast cancer at various stages<br>Mean age = 51 years | Demographic and interview guide<br>Focus groups; individual interviews<br>Emotional, informational, instrumental support needs assessed. | Provided five recommendations to improve QOL in this medically underserved population<br>Types of support important by stage of diagnosis<br>Participants who perceived they received social support reported less psychological distress and better adjustment to diagnosis of breast cancer than those who did not perceive social support |
| Gany et al. (2011) | Quantitative<br>Impact of a multi-lingual, multi-disciplinary team targeting social and economic determinants of cancer treatment adherence among at-risk Hispanic immigrants. | 328 Hispanic patients recruited at 10 hospital-based clinics in New York<br>37% of sample resided in mainland United States for 10 years or less<br>90 males/238 females | Trained bilingual facilitators assessed needs via intake needs assessment survey in the patient's preferred language.<br>Nested cohort | Most commonly identified needs: financial support, food support, and transportation assistance<br>Patients characterized as "high need" were significantly younger and were likely to be more recent immigrants; high-need patients were more likely to have immigrated from Mexico. |

| | | | | |
|---|---|---|---|---|
| Gany et al. (2013) | Quantitative<br>Explore patient knowledge of cancer diagnosis among underserved immigrant/migrant minorities. | 434 immigrant/migrant female/male cancer patients recruited in a hospital-based cancer clinic in New York City<br>58% from Puerto Rico<br>68% female<br>68% ages 50–69 years<br>61% lived in the United States 15 years or fewer | Retrospective chart review for diagnosis; demographic and self-reported diagnosis and treatment information | Most (87%) preferred to speak a language other than English in the healthcare setting. 16% had incorrect knowledge of cancer Multivariate analysis indicated that both preference for non-English language and a "below the belt cancer"(bladder, colorectal, penile, gynecological, prostate, and testicular cancer) diagnosis predictive of incorrect knowledge of cancer diagnosis. |
| Gomez, Guendelman, Harley, and Gomez (2015) | Quantitative<br>Examination of stage of diagnosis and survival after cervical cancer and associations with Hispanic nativity to explore whether the socioeconomic status (SES) of the neighborhood and residence in a Hispanic enclave modify the association of nativity with stage and survival | 9,219 patient records of Hispanic women aged 21 years and older from the California Cancer Registry between 1994 and 2009<br>68.7% foreign-born | Retrospective analysis of cancer registry | 75% of immigrant cases lived in low SES, high enclave neighborhoods. Women at highest risk for diagnosis with advanced stage cervical cancer were foreign-born living in low SES–low enclave neighborhoods followed by women in low SES–high enclave neighborhoods; ethnic enclaves may offer protective effects by buffering against acculturation.<br>More foreign-born women diagnosed at an older age and lived in lower SES–high enclave neighborhoods; more U.S.-born women died from cervical cancer but proportions of overall deaths were comparable. |

(Continued)

**TABLE 4.2**

*Charting of Sample Studies (N = 18) (Continued)*

| Author(s), Year | Study Design and Purpose | Study Population and Setting | Methods | Findings |
|---|---|---|---|---|
| Gonzales Hurtado-de-Mendoza, Santoyo-Olsson, and Napoles (2016) | Quantitative<br>Assess the relationship among Latina immigrants with breast cancer and test whether two culturally relevant coping strategies (fatalism or acceptance) mediate this relationship. | 150 Spanish-speaking Latina immigrants within 1 year of breast cancer diagnosis<br>67% Mexican<br>Mean age = 50.1 years<br>Most women had low education and acculturation levels.<br>Most diagnosed with invasive breast cancer with all having undergone surgery. | Randomized control trial<br>Surveys measured emotional support, fatalism, acceptance, and emotional well-being and QOL<br>Assessed in person at baseline and via telephone at 6 months | Emotional support may increase well-being among Spanish-speaking Latina cancer survivors by reducing cancer fatalism.<br>Emotional support was negatively associated with fatalism and positively associated with acceptance. |
| Lopez-Class et al. (2011) | Qualitative<br>Examine cultural, social, and healthcare system factors that impact QOL and experiences of Latina immigrant breast cancer survivors | 28 Latina breast cancer survivors from the Latin American Cancer Research Coalition<br>Largely monolingual in Spanish<br>Most (68%) lived in the United States 10 or more years<br>All diagnosed and treated in the United States | Interviews conducted in Spanish followed by select focus groups with guide to expand upon themes.<br>Thematic content analysis | Latina breast cancer survivors adhere to certain cultural values and face unique issues as immigrants, potentially influencing overall QOL and doctor–patient communication.<br>Survivorship experiences appear to be shaped by cultural beliefs and experiences as immigrants. |

| | | | | |
|---|---|---|---|---|
| Moreno et al. (2016) | Quantitative<br>Examine association of dispositional expressivity (i.e., the propensity to experience and express emotions strongly) with cancer-specific coping through avoidance and emotional approach to predict intrusive thoughts and depressive symptoms in Latinas with breast cancer. | 95 recently diagnosed Latina breast cancer patients receiving treatment at a large safety net hospital associated with UCLA Medical Center<br>93% immigrants<br>75% reported income of $20,000 or less annually<br>88% spoke primarily Spanish<br>59% did not graduate from high school<br>Mean age = 52 years<br>Mean years since immigration = 24.13 years | Standardized assessments via telephone interview at two time intervals: within 18 months of diagnosis and 3 months later<br>Assessed dispositional expressivity, coping, intrusive thoughts, depressive symptoms, demographic and cancer-related variables.<br>Path Model Analysis | More recent immigration associated with greater dispositional expressivity, which was associated with coping with the cancer experience using both greater avoidance and emotional approach strategies.<br>Findings suggest Latina breast cancer patients who have a propensity to experience and express emotions strongly may be initially overwhelmed by their cancer-related emotions and consequently turn to avoidance oriented behaviors. |
| Schupp, Press, and Gomez (2014) | Quantitative<br>Evaluation of the impact of nativity and neighborhood-level Hispanic enclave on prostate cancer survival in Hispanics | 35,427 Hispanic men diagnosed with invasive prostate cancer; records from the California Cancer Registry from 1995 through 2008<br>Foreign-born 56% | Retrospective data analysis<br>Block group-level neighborhood measures derived from U.S. Census data. | Hispanic immigrants living in ethnic enclaves had significantly higher survival rates after diagnosis with prostate cancer than U.S.-born Hispanics even though immigrants often have lower SES.<br>For men living in low ethnic enclave areas, survival was comparable between U.S.-born and foreign-born Hispanics.<br>Findings suggest, among Hispanic men, prostate cancer survival varies by nativity and acculturation-related factors. |

*Note*. *M* = mean; QOL = quality of life; *SD* = standard deviation; RCT = randomized controlled trial.

correlational ($n$ = 2), path model analysis ($n$ = 1), and retrospective analyses ($n$ = 6); two studies tested interventions; and two studies were reports derived from larger studies (Campesino et al., 2009; Moreno et al., 2016).

Sample sizes varied widely between the qualitative and quantitative studies and within each design category. For example, studies that were qualitative in nature reported sample sizes (based on our inclusion criteria) ranging from 10 to 60 participants. Quantitative studies had sample sizes ranging from 54 to 35,427 subjects; studies that used retrospective analysis methods reported the higher sample sizes. Both male and female cancer survivors were included as study participants; almost two-thirds of the studies ($n$ = 11, 61.1%) focused solely on women and two studies focused on men. Five additional studies included both genders in their samples. All study participants were adults who were at least 18 years of age or older; most studies reported age distributions that extended past 80 years of age. A few studies reported ages as "means" that ranged from 46.2 to 55 years of age or reported ages as "medians" of 51 to 55 years. While some studies reported participants' ages based on their age at cancer diagnosis, other studies listed their age at the time of study data collection.

Study settings were often located within major cities across the United States and within states where large numbers of foreign-born Hispanic/Latino immigrants migrated such as New York City, Central Florida, Texas, California, and Arizona. Some settings established health care initiatives dedicated to meeting the cancer care needs of underserved populations living in a region and who had socioeconomic issues; their patients also included Hispanic/Latino immigrants.

Various types of cancer were reported in the sample studies, with breast ($n$ = 15) and prostate ($n$ = 6) cancers being the most frequently represented cancer diagnoses among study participants. Of the 15 studies that included women with a breast cancer diagnosis, over half of them ($n$ = 8, 53.3%) focused solely on breast cancer; conversely, prostate cancer was the single diagnosis studied in one-third (33.3%) of the six studies that mentioned prostate cancer. Other types of cancers reported in sample studies included gastrointestinal/stomach ($n$ = 5), lung ($n$ = 4), gynecological ($n$ = 3), cervical ($n$ = 3), colorectal ($n$ = 2), ovarian ($n$ = 2), blood/leukemia ($n$ = 2), head and neck/throat ($n$ = 2), brain ($n$ = 2), skin ($n$ = 2), lymphoma ($n$ = 1), and thyroid ($n$ = 1). Two studies included "other" as a cancer diagnosis category without further description.

All study participants were cancer survivors (based on our inclusion criteria definition presented earlier).They had been diagnosed prior to participating in their respective studies and represented survivors whose cancer was at various stages (or no stage noted). Participants also reported either awaiting treatment or having undergone surgical and/or medical (radiation, chemotherapy, immunotherapy, etc.) treatments for their cancer prior to the study.

All (or more than 50% of sample participants) included in the 18 sample studies were foreign-born immigrants from the Hispanic/Latino culture, either self-identified or identified through national birth records. Study immigrants had lived in the United States anywhere from 1 year to over 43 years at the time of data collection. While many studies did not specifically address the immigrant status of their participants, one study (Campesino et al., 2009) specifically focused on their sample of "undocumented" (illegal) immigrants with one legal immigrant as an exception

The reported birth countries/countries of origin for participants varied, with Mexico (North America) being the most frequent country represented in 12 studies (66.7%). Studies generally described Hispanic/Latino participants as being from geographic regions such as Mexico, Central America, South America, and/or the Spanish Caribbean. Specific birth countries that were identified by geographic region and/or country included in the sample studies were Central America (El Salvador, $n$ = 3; Guatemala, $n$ = 2; Honduras, $n$ = 1; Panama, $n$ = 1); South America (Columbia, $n$ = 6; Venezuela, $n$ = 3; Peru, $n$ = 2; Chile, $n$ = 2; Bolivia, $n$ = 2; Ecuador, $n$ = 2; Paraguay, $n$ = 1; Argentina, $n$ = 1); and the Spanish Caribbean (Puerto Rico, $n$ = 6; Cuba, $n$ = 3; Dominican Republic, $n$ = 5).

Data collection methods varied by study design. For example, all the qualitative studies utilized interviews, focus groups, or a combination of both interviews and focus groups; most data were collected face to face, while two studies used the telephone. Interviews were commonly conducted in the language preferred by participants, which was in almost all cases, Spanish. Spanish researchers were often used to collect data and to back-translate interviews and other data for analysis. Conversely, studies that used quantitative designs relied on surveys and/or standardized tools that had also been translated into Spanish. Five studies retrieved their data from existing databases and/or medical records.

## Thematic Analysis

Four primary themes were identified through thematic analysis of the charted study elements: (1) survival patterns; (2) barriers; (3) decision-making; and (4) QOL. Various subthemes were also included within these themes and are illustrated in Table 4.3 with their respective citations.

### Theme 1: Survival Patterns

*Nativity and Neighborhood Enclave*

As stated earlier, the Hispanic paradox or the "healthy immigrant effect" postulates that foreign-born Hispanic immigrants, especially those living in ethnic enclaves, have a greater survival advantage when compared to U.S.-born immigrants because of their healthier lifestyles as well as strong family and community/

**TABLE 4.3**
*Thematic Analysis from Sample Studies (N = 18)*

| Theme | Subthemes | Study References |
|---|---|---|
| Survival patterns (*n* = 2) | Nativity and neighborhood enclave | Gomez et al. (2015)<br>Schupp et al. (2014) |
| Barriers (*n* = 5) | Immigration legislation | Campesino et al. (2009) |
| | Survivor stage and cultural beliefs | Buki et al. (2008) |
| | Lack of knowledge | Gany et al. (2013)<br>Costas-Muniz et al. (2013) |
| | Treatment adherence | Gany et al. (2011) |
| Decision-making (*n* = 2) | Treatment decisions | Carrion, Nedjat-Haiem, and Martinez-Tyson (2013) |
| | Advanced care planning | Carrion, Nedjat-Haiem, Martinez-Tyson, and Castaneda (2013) |
| Quality of life[a] (*n* = 9) | Quality of life (overall) | Lopez-Class et al. (2011)<br>Costas-Muniz et al. (2015)<br>D'Orazio et al. (2011) |
| | Depression | Costas and Gany (2013) |
| | Coping | Carrion et al. (2017)<br>Moreno et al. (2016)<br>Changrani et al. (2008)<br>Gonzales et al. (2016) |

[a]Studies grouped in the quality of life (QOL) theme were assigned by their primary variable. Many of the studies encompassed more than one QOL variable.

neighborhood support for healthy behaviors. However, some researchers have been concerned this survival advantage is due to underreporting of cancer deaths in immigrants, as some may choose to return to family and healthcare providers in their native countries once diagnosed with a life-threatening disease such as cancer. The terms "salmon bias" and "reverse migration bias" refer to this phenomenon (Turra & Elo, 2008).

The impact of nativity and neighborhood characteristics on cancer outcomes such as incidence and survival in Hispanic/Latinos has been increasingly examined in recent years. For example, cervical cancer incidence rates among Hispanic/Latino women are higher than women in several other ethnic groups; however, studies show considerably lower mortality rates from cervical cancer for foreign-born Hispanic/Latino women overall. Reasons for an immigrant survival advantage in women diagnosed with cervical cancer are not fully understood;

however, understanding how individual- and neighborhood/community-related determinants impact survival after a diagnosis of cervical cancer is crucial to identifying and targeting interventions to improve health outcomes (Gomez et al., 2015).

Gomez et al. (2015) examined stage at diagnosis and survival after diagnosis of Hispanic/Latino women (foreign-born [$n$ = 6,334] and U.S.-born [$n$ = 2,885], diagnosed with cervical cancer and examined the impact of nativity and residence in a Hispanic enclave on clinical outcomes. Foreign-born women diagnosed with cervical cancer were more likely to be diagnosed at an older age and to live in a low-socioeconomic (SES), high-enclave neighborhood; however, once adjusted for age at diagnosis, marital status, and neighborhood SES, age was the major contributor to the differences between foreign-born and U.S.-born women. Longitudinal studies are needed to further refine contributors, individual- or community-related, to late-stage diagnosis of cervical cancer in Hispanic immigrants.

In the Gomez et al.'s (2015) study, when examining survival outcomes related to cervical cancer, once individual factors such as stage at diagnosis were statistically controlled, foreign-born women had a survival advantage over U.S.-born Hispanic women. The researchers also noted the association of nativity and neighborhood SES on survival varied by Hispanic enclave. Survival benefits were noted among foreign-born women, while those women, foreign-born or U.S.-born, who lived in low-SES neighborhoods had lower survival rates. The researchers also examined whether loss to follow-up or the "salmon bias" or "reverse migration bias" was a possible factor in the higher survival rates among foreign-born immigrants. In this study, the "salmon bias" effect was unlikely to explain the survival benefit of foreign-born women (Gomez et al., 2015).

The Hispanic paradox continues to be used as a hypothesis to explain patterns of health outcomes in Hispanics which are comparable to or better than other ethnic groups, especially among foreign-born Hispanic immigrants, despite the lower overall SES of Hispanics, in general. Survival of Hispanic males when diagnosed with prostate cancer is another apparent example of the Hispanic paradox. Prostate cancer is the most commonly diagnosed cancer among Hispanic males (ACS, 2015). When compared to the outcomes of NHW males, Hispanic males are more likely to be diagnosed with prostate cancers, which are in more advanced stages at the time of diagnosis, have higher prostate-specific antigen levels, and higher tumor grade yet, in some studies, Hispanic males have lower death rates from prostate cancer (Hoffmann et al., 2001; Hsu, Mas, Miller, & Nkhoma, 2007; Latini et al., 2006). Deaths from prostate cancer in NHW males and in U.S.-born Hispanics exceed death rates from prostate cancer in foreign-born Hispanics (Du et al., 2006; Esbach, Stimpson, Kuo,

& Gooewin, 2007; Singh & Siahpush, 2001; White, Coker, Du, Eggleston, & Williams, 2011).

Schupp et al. (2014) investigated prostate cancer survival outcomes among Hispanics by nativity (U.S.-born and foreign-born) and ethnic enclave in California. Foreign-born men comprised 56% of the sample, were more likely to be slightly older at time of diagnosis and to be diagnosed at a more advanced stage and grade. Foreign-born Hispanic men were more likely to live in high-ethnic enclave neighborhoods and less likely to live in neighborhoods with higher SES. In terms of survival outcomes, overall, foreign-born Hispanic men living in high-ethnic enclave neighborhoods had better prostate cancer survival outcomes than U.S.-born Hispanics. However, prostate cancer survival for foreign-born men living in low-ethnic enclave areas was comparable to outcomes for U.S.-born Hispanics. It remains unclear why Hispanics living in the United States, despite living in poorer SES conditions overall, experience better health outcomes in some areas, such as prostate cancer survival in foreign-born immigrants, when compared to NHWs. As in the cervical cancer study described above, the researchers in the prostate cancer study were able to statistically disprove the "salmon bias" or "reverse migration bias" effect in this sample. Additional studies are warranted to examine the protective factors associated with living in ethnic enclaves to inform interventions to improve outcomes for cancer survivors (Schupp et al., 2014).

### Theme 2: Barriers

As previously mentioned, immigrants often encounter barriers related to health care, especially when faced with a cancer diagnosis. Five sample studies in this scoping review addressed various barriers encountered by Hispanic/Latino immigrants as cancer survivors related to immigration legislation (Campesino et al., 2009), survivor stage and cultural beliefs (Buki et al., 2008), lack of knowledge (Costas-Muniz et al., 2013; Gany et al., 2013), and treatment adherence (Gany et al., 2011). These latter three studies were authored by similar researchers and were conducted in New York City through Memorial Sloan-Kettering's Cancer Center's Cancer Portal Project (CPP). The CPP is comprised of 10 hospital-based clinics that provide cancer care for many immigrants with a focus on socioeconomic and psychosocial support services. Each of these studies will be discussed in more detail in the following section.

#### *Immigrant Legislation*

Campesino et al. (2009) explored the impact of state-wide immigration legislation that had been implemented in Arizona on undocumented immigrant breast cancer survivors ($N$ = 10) from Mexico, specifically, their ability to access their cancer treatments and follow-up care. This study was part of a larger mixed methods study (sequential, triangulated, and qualitative design) that focused on racial and ethnic discrimination in cancer care. The women's cancer care experiences were captured through their personal stories or testimonials (counter-narratives), a method used in critical race theory (Delgado & Stefancic, 2001). Interviews were conducted in Spanish by a Mexican American researcher; interviews were translated into English for analysis using open coding.

All 10 participants were born in Mexico, spoke only Spanish; all but one participant had been living in the United States illegally for 7–15 years (Campesino et al., 2009). Their ages ranged from 36 to 64 years with a mean age of 48 years. The women had been diagnosed with breast cancer (all stages) within 4 years prior to data collection and had undergone surgical treatment and/or chemotherapy or radiation. Findings revealed that almost all the women (75%) reported having substantial psychological distress due to the financial impact that the legislation had on their access to healthcare services. In fact, the cancer care that they had been receiving either stopped or was interrupted due to their economic challenges. The legislation added an additional burden upon these breast cancer survivors who were already experiencing challenges being undocumented immigrants who lacked health insurance. The authors urge healthcare professionals to use targeted interventions for medically underserved cancer survivors such as the study participants who experienced financial burdens. They emphasize the need for nurses to assume a leadership role in shaping healthcare policies for immigrant cancer survivors.

*Survivor Stage and Cultural Beliefs*

Cultural beliefs influenced the experiences of diverse Latina immigrant breast cancer survivors ($N$ = 18) who shared their personal accounts at three stages during their survivorship, beginning with an acute stage (diagnosis and treatment during Year 1), to a recovery stage (Years 1–3), and then a long-term survivorship stage (4 years postdiagnosis; Buki et al., 2008). Most of these women originated from Central America ($n$ = 8) with others representing South America ($n$ = 5), Mexico ($n$ = 3), and the Dominican Republic ($n$ = 1). On average, they had lived in the United States for about 20 years (mean = 19.18) and ranged in age from 35 to 67 years (mean = 51.22 years). Using focus groups, the researchers captured the women's experiences based on their respective stages in the survivorship continuum. Data analysis revealed five themes that varied in prominence and based on their stage: (1) perceptions of psychological well-being; (2) impact of diagnosis on well-being; (3) impact of treatment on well-being; (4) need for social support; and (5) development of new attitudes (Buki et al., 2008, pp. 165–166). While the immigrants' accounts of their cancer experiences were similar to other U.S.-born cancer survivors, it was evident that their experience illustrated unique challenges influenced by their Latina cultural beliefs. For many of these women, a cancer diagnosis meant death. The authors recommended the use of interventions tailored to the needs of these Latina immigrant breast cancer survivors and also to their respective survivorship stages.

*Lack of Knowledge*

In a retrospective analysis of patients' electronic medical records, Gany et al., (2013) investigated the self-reported knowledge levels of immigrant cancer survivors ($N = 434$) regarding their cancer diagnoses. Most of these newly diagnosed survivors (4 months prior to data collection) were females (68%), age 50–69 years, and preferred using a non-English language (87%) with professionals in the healthcare settings. Latinos from Puerto Rico comprised over half of the study sample (58%) with 61% of the total sample residing in the United States for 15 years or fewer. While breast cancer was the most frequently reported diagnosis (29%), other cancers included cervical, colorectal, lung, and others. Results revealed that 16% of the immigrants had incorrect knowledge about their cancer diagnosis. Most importantly, immigrants' preferences for using a non-English language and being diagnosed with a cancer located "below the belt" (i.e., bladder, colorectal, gynecological, penile, prostate, and testicular) predicted their having incorrect knowledge about their cancer diagnosis. The authors emphasized how language can pose a barrier for immigrant cancer survivors' treatment and health education.

Language was also viewed as a barrier for immigrant cancer survivors ($N = 271$) in a correlation study conducted by Costas-Muniz et al. (2013) who examined the demographic and medical correlates of immigrants' cancer stage knowledge and their desire for more information. The Latina participants were females with a mean age of 55 years and diagnosed with breast, gynecologic, and gastrointestinal cancers. Most of the women had lived in the United States for 6–20 years and were born in the Dominican Republic (35.1%), Puerto Rico (24.4%), Ecuador (10.1%), and Mexico (9.8%). Data were obtained from the women's clinic-based needs assessment surveys. Results indicated that most of the women (65%) had no knowledge of their cancer stage and over one-third of the women (38%) were not aware of their cancer's metastatic status. In addition, only a few of the immigrants (15%) wanted more information about their cancer and/or cancer treatment. In fact, being an immigrant whose language was limited to Spanish only predicted their lack of knowledge and desire for information. Similar to the prior study by Gany et al. (2013), Costas-Muniz et al. (2013) emphasize how language poses a barrier for Latina immigrant cancer survivors, especially related to their cancer care and decision-making.

*Treatment Adherence*

Social and economic determinants of cancer treatment adherence was the focus of a nested cohort investigation by Gany et al. (2011) that involved Hispanic male and female immigrants (*N* = 328) diagnosed with various cancer types with the majority being breast cancer (*n* = 114); the other types of cancers were gastrointestinal, gynecological, head and neck, lung, prostate, leukemia, and lymphoma. Most immigrants were born in the Dominican Republic (*n* = 90), Puerto Rico (*n* = 72), and Mexico (*n* = 62), while many others (*n* = 104) hailed from 12 other Central and South American countries; 37% of all study participants reported having lived in the United States for a decade or less. Participants' diverse ages ranged from 18 to over 80 years, with most (*n* = 157) in the 50–69 age group. Most participants were women (*n* = 238). Study data were obtained from patients' intake needs assessment surveys facilitated by bilingual clinic staff. Results indicated that Hispanic cancer survivors who had more recently immigrated to the United States and who were considerably younger were considered as "high-need" patients. Needs that were commonly expressed by the immigrants included help with basic support such as their transportation, food, and finances.

**Theme 3: Decision-Making**

Two qualitative studies explored the effect of culture on health and/or treatment-related decision making in immigrant Hispanic/Latino male and female cancer survivors (Carrion, Nedjat-Haiem, Martinez-Tyson, 2013; Carrion, Nedjat-Haiem, Martinez-Tyson, & Castaneda, 2013). Both studies were published in 2013 and authored by common researchers. Study participants were recruited from various community-based settings such as clinics, churches, cultural centers, and support groups in Central Florida.

*Treatment Decisions*

Carrion, Nedjat-Haiem, and Martinez-Tyson (2013) explored cultural factors that influenced the treatment decisions of 15 Latino immigrant men who were born in Mexico (*n* = 2), South America (Columbia [*n* = 9]; Venezuela [*n* = 2]), and Cuba (*n* = 2), diagnosed with various types of cancer (prostate, *n* = 9; brain, *n* = 2; lung, *n* = 2; 31–71 years of age [median 55.4 years]), and had been living in the United States from 1 to over 31 years (median 27 years). Data were collected using audiotaped face-to-face semi-structured interviews conducted in Spanish and translated into English; a random sample of six interviews was back-translated into Spanish to ensure accuracy of translation. Data were analyzed using thematic analysis with deductive and inductive codes and constant comparison techniques.

The study findings revealed five major themes: (1) suddenness of the diagnosis and fear of dying; (2) diagnosis-related communication; (3) reliance on physicians for treatment decisions; (4) limited information and informal advanced care planning (ACP); and (5) support received and role changes (Carrion, Nedjat-Haiem, & Martinez-Tyson, 2013, pp.731–734). Receiving an unexpected cancer diagnosis was perceived by the men as a "shock" and immediately led them to believe that they would die from the disease. This reaction was especially true when they were symptom-free. Their emotional reactions were often coupled with concerns about the financial effect that their cancer diagnosis would have on their families and the possible pain and suffering they might experience if/when they eventually succumbed from cancer.

The men expressed mixed reactions to the direct approach that their physicians used when they told them about their cancer diagnosis (Carrion, Nedjat-Haiem, & Martinez-Tyson, 2013). While some men valued their doctors' forthright communication styles, others perceived it as impersonal and disconnected. Some men found it challenging to make treatment decisions during this emotional experience and with the information that was available to them at that time. While the men depended on the expertise of their physicians for advising them about treatment options for their cancer, they wished they had more time to discuss this topic with others before they committed to a treatment. The men had different views regarding their need for completing ACP. While some men felt that it was too early for them to pursue this topic, others either completed a living will and designated a health surrogate ($n = 2$) or were, at least, considering it. Conversations shared by the men reflected their willingness to talk about their health-related needs with their physicians and the willingness of their physicians to discuss options congruent with their culture. The men talked about the support that they received from their family and friends after being diagnosed with cancer and how this support made them feel optimistic in light of their challenges. Finally, some participants were concerned about the various role changes that resulted from their diagnosis and treatment, especially related being cared for by others and not being the financial provider for the family.

Although the participants' cancer stages were not reported, the authors noted the influence of the Latino culture on the men's treatment decision-making: reliance on health provider decisions (physicians) despite having limited information, the importance of family, and the value of sustaining their gender roles during illness (Carrion, Nedjat-Haiem, & Martinez-Tyson, 2013). The men's limited understanding about cancer and the health care system did not reflect their having been in the United States for nearly two decades ($n = 9$). The authors recommend that healthcare professionals who care for immigrant Latino men explore their communication choices before discussing a diagnosis.

*Advance Care Planning*

The second study about decision-making explored aspects that assisted 45 immigrant Latina women complete ACP (i.e., living will, healthcare surrogate, enduring power of attorney) and explored their decision-making patterns (Carrion, Nedjat-Haiem, Martinez-Tyson, & Castaneda, 2013). The women were born in Mexico ($n$ = 15), Columbia ($n$ = 15), and Puerto Rico ($n$ = 15), had been living in the United States for 1 to over 31 years (median), and had been diagnosed with various types of cancers (breast, $n$ = 231; skin, $n$ = 13; ovarian, $n$ = 31; other, $n$ = 25) within 5 years of data collection. Breast cancer was the most frequently cited cancer diagnosis across all three Latina subgroups.

The findings revealed four themes: (1) lack of knowledge of ACP; (2) a shared ACP decision approach; (3) lack of information and informal ACP; and (4) decision-making, a key concern (Carrion, Nedjat-Haiem, Martinez-Tyson, & Castaneda, 2013, pp. 1235–1237). While a little more than half of the women ($n$ = 23) reported that they had heard of ACP and understood its meaning, many of them ($n$ = 13) were unable to correctly explain ACP, especially its association with insurance and finances. Women who seemed to understand the term (ACP) felt that they were not ready to complete it. Nine women who completed some portion of ACP did this in advance and chose to share this decision with others, such as their physicians, spouses or family members. About half of the participants ($n$ = 23) claimed that they received no information about ACP from their healthcare professionals, while others said that they understood the uncertainty of their cancer diagnosis but had discussed their preferences in the event of their death with their families. The women felt it was important to make ACP decisions, especially for their families.

The authors noted that, in general, Latina cancer survivors in their study lacked knowledge about ACP and preferred making ACP decisions with their families (Carrion, Nedjat-Haiem, Martinez-Tyson, & Castaneda, 2013). Differences were noted between their knowledge of ACP and their actually completing ACP. The reading level and language of the ACP documents were not appropriate for many immigrants. The authors recommended that healthcare professionals become trained in communicating about ACP with culturally diverse patients and utilize culturally appropriate ACP documents. Future research is needed to explore ACP decision-making among Latinos with cancer and to develop evidence-based interventions that promote ACP communication in this population.

**Theme 4: QOL**

QOL was the focus in half ($n$ = 9) of the 18 sample studies involving Hispanic/Latino immigrant cancer survivors. Over two-thirds (66.7%) of these studies measured QOL as a general concept (Costas-Muniz et al., 2015; D'Orazio et al.,

2011; Galvan et al., 2009; Gonzales et al., 2016; Lopez-Class et al., 2011), but QOL comprised the main variable in only one study (Lopez-Class et al., 2011).

Most of these studies examined variables that were concepts related to the psychosocial well-being dimension of QOL such as coping (Carrion et al., 2017; Changrani et al., 2008; D'Orazio et al., 2011; Gonzales et al., 2016; Moreno et al., 2016) and depression (Changrani et al., 2008; Costas & Gany, 2013; Costas-Muniz et al., 2015; D'Orazio et al., 2011; Moreno et al., 2016).

Two studies addressed the social well-being component of QOL, specifically social support (D'Orazio et al., 2011; Galvan et al., 2009). While most studies addressed multiple QOL concepts, others focused on just one QOL element such as coping ($n$ = 5) or depression ($n$ = 5). Only two of the sample studies (Changrani et al., 2008; Gonzales et al., 2016) examined the impact of targeted interventions on the QOL of Hispanic/Latino immigrant cancer survivors.

*Quality of Life*

The QOL among Latina immigrant breast cancer survivors was explored by Lopez-Class et al. (2011) in their qualitative study that involved 28 women who were from the Latin American Cancer Research Coalition, an NCI-funded network. All but one of the women originated from Mexico and various countries in Central ($n$ = 11) and South America; most (68%) had been living in the United States for a decade or more. Their perspectives were captured using interviews conducted in Spanish followed by focus groups. Findings revealed that language and inexperience in navigating the healthcare system were hurdles for these women. Most importantly, the women's experiences as cancer survivors were strongly influenced by cultural beliefs specific to the Latina culture and their lives as immigrants; these nuances included being secretive and feeling shame about having breast cancer, familism (value of family), less personalismo (fewer social relationships in the United States), and machismo (challenges in male partner support; pp. 727–730). While many women expressed how their relationship with God and their overall spirituality had helped them deal with the challenge of living with cancer, others now questioned their prior faith after receiving a cancer diagnosis. In addition, many women talked about being more self-reliant after receiving a cancer diagnosis. The authors recommend various strategies to improve the QOL of Hispanic/Latino immigrant cancer survivors, such as using interpreters to minimize any language barriers, conducting psychosocial needs assessments, and providing culturally appropriate navigation support.

Taking QOL a step further, Costas-Muniz et al. (2015) determined the relationship between QOL and depression symptoms (somatic/nonsomatic) with self-reported appointment keeping in immigrant cancer survivors ($N$ = 622) who accessed healthcare services at Memorial Sloan Kettering's CPP. While all participants were immigrants, a little more than half of them (53.5%) were Hispanic/Latinos from Central and South American countries and the Hispanic Caribbean; nearly half of the study sample had lived in the United States for more than two decades. The sample was comprised of males (*n* = 229) and females (*n* = 393) with a mean age of 55.5 years and diagnosed mainly with breast, gastrointestinal, and prostate cancers. Data were collected using clinic-based needs assessment surveys and translated instruments that measured both QOL (Functional Assessment of Cancer Therapy [FACT-G]) and depression (European Quality of Life Five Dimensions). Results revealed that the immigrants' depression and poor physical and emotional well-being predicted missed appointments, treatment delays, or interrupted them (adherence). The authors identify the need to modify these factors in order to treat or improve patients' treatment adherence.

Finally, the relationship between cancer-related, contextual, and dispositional variables with QOL, depression, and affect was explored in Latina immigrants (*N* = 54) diagnosed with cervical cancer (D'Orazio et al., 2011). The women ranged in age from 30 to 75 years (mean 50.48 years), were born in Mexico, Central, or South America, and had lived in the United States for 5–38 years (mean 16.19 years). Data were collected from the women's clinic-based medical charts and through Spanish-translated instruments that measured several variables: acculturation (Acculturation Rating Scale for Mexican Americans-II Brief Version), depression (The Center for Epidemiologic Studies Depression Scale), affect (The Spanish Positive and Negative Affect Scale), QOL (Functional Assessment of Cancer Treatment–Cervical Cancer), coping (Brief Coping Orientation to Problems Experienced Scale), social support (Medical Outcomes Study Social Support Survey, life stress (Hispanic Stress Inventory—Immigrant Version), and adjustment (Life Orientation Test-Revised). Results revealed that the immigrant women had high levels of depression, negative affect, low levels of positive affect, and immigrant-related stress; however, they had sufficient social support. The authors recommend culturally appropriate interventions such as coping strategies and language-appropriate support services for Latina immigrant cancer survivors with cervical cancer.

*Depression*

Depression in cancer survivors was also the focus of a retrospective analysis reported by Costas and Gany (2013) who compared depressive symptoms (screening and diagnosis) between Latino (*n* = 145) and African Caribbean (*n* = 44) immigrants who were receiving cancer care through the Memorial Sloan Kettering's CPP. This sample of 189 immigrants were mostly women (*n* = 94, 68%), had a mean age of 54.19 years, and had been diagnosed with various types of cancers (breast, gastrointestinal, prostate, blood, and gynecological) at all stages, with breast cancer being the most common (38.6%). All participants had lived in the United States anywhere from fewer than 5 years to over 20 years; the Latinos were born in Latin American countries. Data were obtained from clinic-based needs assessment surveys along with measures to screen for depressive symptoms (Patient Health Questionnaire). While both groups of immigrants had positive depression screens, more Latino immigrants had a depressed mood, experienced more intense depressive and anxiety symptoms, and were diagnosed with depression. The authors advise using depression screening tools tailored to needs of immigrant cancer survivors from diverse cultures in order to implement timely interventions for the disease.

*Coping*

Coping was the primary focus of four studies that involved Latino immigrant cancer survivors. Most recently, Carrion et al. (2017) captured the perceptions of 60 Latino immigrants about coping with their cancer diagnosis. Participants were comprised of both males ($n$ = 15) and females ($n$ = 45) with a median age of 55 years and who had been diagnosed with various types of cancer (breast, prostate, ovarian, throat, stomach, skin, brain colorectal, and lung), with breast (80%) and prostate cancers (94%) being the most common diagnoses in respective genders. The Latinos originated from Columbia, Cuba, Mexico, Puerto Rico, and Venezuela and had lived in the United States anywhere from 1 to over 31 years, fairly evenly distributed across age years. Participants' perspectives were captured through semi-structured interviews that focused on coping with cancer. Findings revealed several themes that described their coping strategies, which involved support from their family and healthcare providers, the use of religion and spirituality, and their use of "positive reframing" (Carrion et al., 2017, p. 235). The authors urge practitioners to help support Latino immigrant cancer survivors so they are able to take part in meaning-based coping; they also advise researchers to study survivor coping by cancer type and at the end of life.

The association between cancer-specific coping, dispositional emotional expressivity, and distress was studied by Moreno et al. (2016) in their path model analysis involving 95 female Latina immigrants (93%) diagnosed with breast cancer and receiving care at a California-based safety net hospital. This study was part of a larger study that focused on QOL and adjustment in this population. Participants had a mean age of 52 years and, on average, lived in the United States for 24.13 years. While more than half (58.4%) of the immigrants were born in Mexico ($n$ = 52), others came from Central and South America. Data were collected using phone interviews scheduled at 18 months of diagnosis and later at 3 months. In addition to demographic and cancer-related data, multiple study variables and associated measures included (1) dispositional emotional expressivity (Berkeley Expressivity Questionnaire), (2) emotional approach coping (Emotional Approach Coping Scale), (3) avoidance coping subscales (COPE), (4) intrusive thoughts (Impact of Event Scale), and (5) depressive symptoms (CES-D). Results showed that immigrants, who had migrated to the United States more recently than others, possessed greater dispositional emotional expressivity (i.e., tendency to express emotions in a strong manner) and used greater avoidance and emotional approaches in coping with their cancer diagnosis. Participants' use of avoidance predicted an increase in their intrusive thoughts at 3 months after diagnosis. No depressive effects were noted in the sample. The authors recommend attention be paid to Latina breast cancer survivors who tend to experience and show their emotions in a strong way, as they may become overwhelmed by their cancer diagnosis, and subsequently, cope with it using avoidance tactics.

Congruent with coping strategies used by Latina immigrants in dealing with a cancer diagnosis, two studies tested their interventions on various QOL dimensions. Nearly a decade ago, Changrani et al. (2008) studied the benefits of an online support group (OSG) aimed to support Hispanic immigrants with breast cancer. A sample of 68 women who primarily spoke Spanish were divided into either an experimental group (EG; *n* = 48 divided into six groups) who engaged in the OSG or a control group (CG; *n* = 20) that received usual care. The women originated from Latin American countries, mainly the Dominican Republic (25.5%) and Columbia (18.2%), and on average, lived in the United States for 14 (EG) and 24.2 years (CG). Mean ages by group were 46.2 years (EG) and 50.8 years (CG). The EG met in the OSG for 90 minutes each week for 30 weeks; the OSG was facilitated by bilingual staff who focused on symptom management, treatment side effects, and the women's concerns. Various psychosocial variables and their measures were collected pre–post intervention such as (1) depression (CES-D), (2) personal growth (Posttraumatic Growth Inventory), (3) QOL (FACT-B), (4) pain (subscales measuring intensity, interference, and reactions), and (5) transcript interaction to measure components of speech (Linguistic Inquiry and Word Count). Although results failed to demonstrate a significant difference in outcomes between the two groups, the authors noted statistical trends toward positive outcomes (i.e., seeing new possibilities and increased feelings of strength). They concluded that the OSG was an acceptable and feasible mechanism for professionals to provide cancer support for immigrant women, despite language barriers.

More recently, Gonzales et al. (2016) tested the effect of coping strategies on emotional support, fatalism, acceptance, and emotional well-being QOL in

Latina immigrants ($N$ = 150) who were recently diagnosed with breast cancer (about 1 year prior to the study). The women's mean age was 50.1 years, they spoke only Spanish, and came from Mexico (67.33%), Central (23.33%), and South America (9.33%). Using a randomized control trial design, the researchers tested if coping strategies (fatalism or acceptance) mediated the effects of emotional support on the women's emotional well-being. Data were collected at baseline in person and later at 6 months via telephone and included several variables and their associated measures: (1) emotional support (Medical Outcomes Study Social Support Survey); (2) fatalism (Powe Fatalism Inventory); (3) acceptance (Benefit Finding Scale); (4) emotional well-being (Functional Assessment of Cancer Therapy QOL); and (5) acculturation. Results revealed that emotional support was negatively correlated with fatalism and positively associated with acceptance; emotional support and acceptance were positively associated with the women's emotional well-being; fatalism was negatively associated with emotional well-being; emotional support was associated with emotional well-being and continued when controlling for fatalism. The authors stress the impact that emotional support has on the well-being of Latina immigrant cancer survivors by reducing their fatalism.

*Social Support*

Finally, the social support needs of 22 immigrant Latina breast cancer survivors were explored by Galvan et al. (2009) using a qualitative approach. The immigrant sample had a mean age of 51 years and all ($n$ = 20) but two of the women were born in South America (41%), Central America (36%), and Mexico (14%). Data were collected via focus groups and interviews guided by demographic and interview guides. Data analysis revealed that the women who reported receiving various types of social support had lower levels of psychological distress and adjusted better to their cancer diagnosis; different points during survivorship journey (diagnosis, treatment, and posttreatment) warranted different types of social support. The women reported experiencing barriers related to their language, culture, and finances during their cancer survivorship. The authors offered five clinical recommendations aimed to improve the QOL among this immigrant population and tailored by the cancer survivors' diagnosis, treatment, and posttreatment periods.

## DISCUSSION

This scoping review study addressed the evidence that has been published over the past decade that focused on adult cancer survivors who were also Hispanic/Latino immigrants. In accordance with Arksey and O'Malley's scoping methodology (2005), this chapter provides readers with a "narrative account" (p. 27) of current evidence on the topic; no attempts were made to evaluate the quality of each study through a "weight" (p. 27), to synthesize this research evidence, or to aggregate the results of the 18 sample studies (Arksey & O'Malley, 2005, p. 27). To our best knowledge, this scoping study is the first report that offers an inclusive review of the research focused on Hispanic/Latino immigrants in the United States who are also cancer survivors.

**Demographics**

The demographic section of this scoping review provided readers with a "numerical analysis of the extent, nature, and distribution" of the 18 sample studies included in this scoping review (Arksey & O'Malley, 2005, p. 27). Interestingly, this demographic account illustrated a fairly even distribution of studies that have been published over the past decade about Hispanic/Latino immigrants as cancer survivors, with several studies authored by the same researchers who accessed data from national databases and/or medical records of underserved patients who received care at their health systems. Many studies were conducted in U.S. cities or states (i.e., New York City, Florida, California, Texas, and Arizona) that have experienced increased numbers of Hispanic/Latino immigrants. Given the day-to-day interactions that clinical nurses have with this population and the priority given to nursing research about minority and underserved populations and cancer survivors (LoBiondo-Wood et al., 2014), it was surprising that only one of the 18 sample studies was authored by nurse researchers and published in a journal dedicated to nursing (Campesino et al., 2009). In addition, further exploration is warranted regarding the cancer care needs of Hispanic/Latino immigrants residing in rural areas of the United States. Based on these findings, attention needs paid to disseminating research to nurses who can apply these study findings with their patients in clinical practice, mentor future nurses through their teaching, and effect change through advocacy and health policy changes. This need is especially important, given the current and projected growth of the Hispanic/Latino population in the United States, as previously discussed in this chapter (Colby & Ortman, 2014).

The majority ($n$ = 11) of the sample studies that utilized quantitative designs were mostly nonexperimental in nature, except for two studies that tested interventions aimed to help the immigrant cancer survivors manage their stress (Gonzales et al., 2016) or gain support (Changrani et al., 2008). The qualitative studies ($n$ = 7) give a "voice" to the sample population by allowing them to provide their personal perspectives about what life is like for them as Hispanic/Latino immigrants who are dealing with various types and stages of cancer. These latter studies provide valuable information that can be used to inform future research. Appropriately, all studies dealt with language barriers using bilingual researchers (Spanish–English) and/or used instruments that had been translated into Spanish (and back-translated).

Confirming studies that met our inclusion criteria was a challenge in this scoping review for several reasons. First, some retrieved studies used the terms "Latino" or "Hispanic" loosely or did not clarify the immigrants' country of birth. Similarly, other studies included only a small portion of Hispanics/Latinos in their ethnically diverse samples. In order to manage this challenge, we adopted a clear operational definition for "Hispanic/Latino" participants that was published by U.S. Census Bureau (see the "Methods" section). In an attempt to align with the original purpose of our scoping review, we limited our sample studies to those in which Hispanics/Latinos comprised over 50% of the sample. Similarly, many of the studies included immigrants who represented the multiple subgroups (birth countries) within the Latino/Hispanic domain; it is not clear if their diverse backgrounds posed different perspectives or experiences. This same concern aligns with that of D'Orazio et al. (2011) who recommended attention be given to the context in which immigrants live and cautions against mixing ethnicities for fear of missing relevant factors related to immigrants from diverse ethnic/racial backgrounds. Other researchers echo the need for researchers to realize that immigrants contained within the Hispanic culture may differ in their cancer survivor needs (Costas & Gany, 2013; Siegel et al., 2015). Because the various subgroups contained within the Hispanic culture have different lifestyle behaviors and cancer risks, Siegel et al. (2015) advise that aggregated statistics that describe cancer among Hispanics should be interpreted with caution. Finally, information about the immigrant status and length of time immigrants lived in the United States varied widely across sample studies and were tracked accordingly for this review.

A great deal of diversity existed among the sample studies. While several studies included mixed samples of males and females who were diagnosed with various types and stages of cancer, most studies focused on either women with breast cancer ($n$ = 15) or men with prostate cancer ($n$ = 6); also, most studies reported mean ages for samples around the 50 or mid-50 year age bracket. This emphasis on cancer type and age is quite appropriate, given the high mortality rates of these gender-associated cancers within the Hispanic/Latino population (Siegel et al., 2015) and the increased risk of developing cancer with advancing age (ACS, 2018). In fact, adults who are 50 years of age and over comprise 87% of all cancers diagnosed in the United States (ACS, 2018). As previously mentioned, the cancer survivorship period begins with diagnosis and ends at the end of life (ACS, 2016). Interestingly, only two of the 18 sample studies addressed the needs of cancer survivors over this entire cancer trajectory with only one study dedicated to ACP (Carrion, Nedjat-Haiem, Martinez-Tyson, & Castaneda, 2013). None of the sample studies addressed cancer screening, early detection, and/or vaccination initiatives among adult Hispanic/Latino immigrants who already were at an increased risk for cancer recurrence and the development of new secondary cancers, despite the screening priority for oncology nursing research (LoBiondo-Wood et al., 2014). Finally, no studies focused on identifying risk factors and/or existing comorbidities among Latino/Hispanic cancer survivors such as obesity, the use of tobacco and alcohol, and exposure to infectious agents (Siegel et al., 2015), despite the added risk that these factors place on a person's cancer risk and outcomes (National Center for Health Statistics, 2015).

## Themes

Our analysis provides readers with a scoping review of the current research evidence ($N = 18$) organized thematically by the following four topics as experienced by Hispanic/Latino immigrant cancer survivors living in the United States: (1) survival patterns, (2) barriers, (3) decision-making issues, and (4) QOL. These themes provide a foundation to guide future studies about this population for the ultimate purpose of developing evidence-based best practices and advancing population-based health promotion in this underserved and vulnerable population. However, it should be noted that the sample studies presented a great deal of diversity with foci that often overlapped across these four themes. The current researchers made every effort to capture the "essence" of each study as expressed by its title and purpose using a charting template (Table 4.2) and mapping techniques for consistency when comparing across sample studies.

Overall, the sample studies reflect the multitude of issues faced daily by individuals who are dealing with a cancer diagnosis, its associated surgical and medical treatments, and the vulnerability of being a cancer survivor. However, Hispanic/Latino cancer survivors in these studies also had to manage a multitude of barriers associated with, but not limited to, their cultural beliefs and customs, policies, limited/no English language, and limited/lack of health insurance and access to health care while living in the United States. Unfortunately, many of these burdens may worsen based on anticipated immigration legislation.

First, research on survival patterns illustrated the influence that one's nativity and neighborhood enclave had on cancer stage at diagnosis and survival outcomes. Interestingly, high-enclave neighborhoods provided a "protective" feature for Hispanic/Latino immigrants, despite the low socioeconomics in these communities. Unfortunately, acculturation may reduce this defense when immigrants adopt the U.S. lifestyle. As previously mentioned, it is important to interpret

Hispanic/Latino survival statistics with caution in light of multiple subgroups (Siegel et al., 2015) and the "salmon bias" or "reverse migration bias" (Gomez et al., 2015).

Second, previous research has revealed that cancer survivors who were born and living in the United States often encounter multiple challenges over their lifetimes due to their cancer diagnosis and treatment that can impact their overall QOL (ACS, 2016). However, being a Hispanic/Latino immigrant living in the United States and diagnosed with cancer adds an additional layer of burden to their experience as cancer survivors. For example, immigration legislation can prevent or halt their access to cancer care services; language barriers may hinder their understanding of the cancer diagnosis, desire for healthcare information, and treatment adherence; cultural beliefs combined with these previous barriers create a fearful cancer care experience. However, adopting unhealthy American lifestyles over their lifetimes may place these Hispanic/Latino immigrants at risk for developing additional cancers and/or associated comorbidities such as obesity (Siegel et al., 2015). Interestingly, Siegel et al. (2015) noted that first-generation Hispanic/Latino immigrants experienced lower rates of cancer than their offspring.

Third, what it is like to be a male or female Hispanic/Latino immigrant diagnosed with cancer and living in the United States was illustrated related to ACP and treatment decision-making (Carrion, Nedjat-Haiem, Martinez-Tyson, & Castaneda, 2013; Gany et al., 2011). These processes were influenced by factors such as a lack of knowledge (about ACP and/or a cancer diagnosis), limited/or lack of English proficiency that hindered communication, financial issues, and cultural changes related to family support and roles. Jaramillo and Hui (2016) cite that limited research exists regarding end-of-life care among undocumented immigrants in the United States that number over 11 million, of which the majority are Latinos. These authors provide a case study that describes the experience of a Latino undocumented immigrant who is dying from his cancer; they illustrate the unique challenges of this population such as ". . .a delayed diagnosis, limited social support, financial issues, fear of deportation, and language and cultural barriers" (Jaramillo & Hui, 2016, p. 784). Unfortunately, many of these issues were similar ones addressed in this scoping review.

Finally, most attention paid in this scoping review focused on QOL ($n$ = 9). Although many general QOL models exist in the literature, a model specific to cancer survivors that was developed by expert oncology researchers (Ferrell, Dow, & Grant, 2005) provides a meaningful context for understanding the QOL research included in this scoping review. More specifically, their model contains four dimensions of well-being (physical, psychosocial, social, and spiritual) with each containing multiple concepts. When viewed using this model, most of the sample studies about Hispanic/Latino immigrant cancer survivors focused on the psychosocial well-being dimension; two of the QOL studies addressed the sociological dimension (social support). No studies focused on their physical well-being (symptom management); one older study addressed/mentioned "pain" but within a coping perspective (i.e., coping with pain; Changrani et al., 2008). However, some of the qualitative studies in this review addressed the strength and importance of spiritual well-being heard through the voices of the study participants as they described their experiences as immigrant cancer survivors. Spirituality was not addressed as a primary study variable. Exploring physical and spiritual well-being dimensions of the cancer survivor experience may be an opportunity for future researchers.

Siegel et al. (2015) provide several recommendations for healthcare professionals to consider in an attempt to advance cancer control efforts such as "culturally appropriate lay-health advisors and patient navigators, targeted community-based interventions programs to increase screening and vaccination rates and encouraging healthy lifestyle behaviors" (p. 476). Based on the results of our scoping review, Hispanic/Latino immigrants would also benefit from these efforts as cancer survivors. Lastly, Siegel et al. (2015) also urge funders to support research focused on subgroups within the Hispanic population and focused on specific types of cancers.

## Limitations

Despite ongoing efforts taken by the current authors to collect, analyze, and report accurate evidence in this scoping review, four possible limitations may exist. However, the authors used a variety of approaches to promote accurate results, such as the use of web-based meetings scheduled every 2 weeks, constant comparisons and discussions, and cross-checking of retrieved data. Despite these efforts, we offer the following limitations.

First, results may be limited based on the search terms, databases, and 10-year limit previously described (see the "Methods" section); therefore, additional studies aligned with our inclusion criteria may exist that were not located through our search process. To minimize this limitation, we relied on our expertise as a health science librarian (D.A.N.) and experienced oncology nurse researchers (J.S.L. and M.G.O.).

Second, results are limited based on our strict inclusion criteria (see the "Methods" section), in particular, limiting our sample studies to those in which Hispanic/Latino immigrant cancer survivors comprised the majority of the total study sample (over 50%). We decided upon these criteria to ensure that our results would reflect the targeted population. While several reviewed studies included Hispanic/Latino immigrant cancer survivors in their sample populations, they either were combined with adults from other cultural groups and/or comprised a minority of the total study sample.

Third, we often encountered overlap between/among the sample studies during the thematic analysis process. Therefore, the authors carefully discussed the primary focus of these studies that straddled themes and subthemes until consensus was reached. A decision was made to assign each study to only one theme and subtheme.

Finally, our scoping review contained studies that utilized a wide range of terms to describe their study sample demographics. For example, participants were sometimes instructed to self-identify as being "Hispanic" or "Latino(a)," or report their birth country (i.e., Columbia, Cuba, Mexico, etc.). Some studies labeled the geographic continent/region of participants as only being North America, Central America, South America, and Spanish Caribbean. In order to describe the participants in our sample studies in an accurate fashion, we relied on the U.S. Census definition (2014) to categorize participants by their specific subculture

## CONCLUSION

This chapter describes the results of a scoping review of research published over the past decade and focused on cancer survivors who are adult immigrants of Hispanic/Latino ethnicity and living in the United States. This method provided a rigorous and transparent method for mapping published research and identifying existing gaps. Four major themes were identified through thematic analysis of 18 sample studies: survival patterns, barriers, decision-making, and QOL. Results offer evidence to guide informed, patient-centered care and culturally appropriate interventions tailored to the needs of Hispanic/Latino immigrants. Finally, results can be used by nurses to guide future oncology research about this vulnerable and underserved population of cancer survivors.

## REFERENCES

American Cancer Society. (2015). *Cancer facts and figures for Hispanics/Latinos 2015–2017*. Atlanta, GA: Author.

American Cancer Society. (2016). *Cancer treatment & survivorship: Facts and figures 2016–2017*. Atlanta, GA: Author.

American Cancer Society. (2018). *Facts and figures, 2018*. Atlanta, GA: Author.

Arksey, H., & O'Malley, L. (2005). Scoping studies: Towards a methodological framework. *International Journal of Social Research Methodology, 8*(1), 19–32. doi:10.1080/1364557032000119816

Bluethmann, S. M., Mariotto, A. B., & Rowland, J. H. (2016). Anticipating the "Silver Tsunami": Prevalence trajectories and comorbidity burden among older cancer survivors in the United

States. *Cancer Epidemiology Biomarkers and Prevention, 25,* 1029–1036. http://dx.doi.org/10.1158/1055-9965

Buki, L. P., Garces, D. M., Hinestrosa, M. C., Kogan, L., Carrillo, I. Y., & French, B. (2008). Latina breast cancer survivors' lived experiences: Diagnosis, treatment, and beyond. *Cultural Diversity and Ethnic Minority Psychology, 14*(2), 163–167.

Bustamante, A., Fang, H., Garza, J., Carter-Pokras, O., Wallace, S. P., Rizzo, J. A., et al. (2010). Variations in healthcare access and utilization among Mexican immigrants: The role of documentation status. *Journal of Immigration and Minority Health, 14,* 146. http://dx.doi.org/10.1007/s10903-10-9406-9

Campesino, M., Ruiz, E., Glover, J. U., & Koithan, M. (2009). Counternarratives of Mexican-Origin women with breast cancer. *Advances in Nursing Science, 32*(2), B57–B67.

Carrion, I. V., Nedjat-Haiem, F., Macip-Billbe, M., & Black, R. (2017). "I told myself to stay positive" - Perceptions of coping among Latinos with a cancer diagnosis living in the United States. *American Journal of Hospice & Palliative Medicine, 34*(3), 233–240. http://dx.doi.org/10.1177/1049909115625955

Carrion, I. V., Nedjat-Haiem, F. R., Martinez-Tyson, D. X. (2013). Examining cultural factors that influence treatment decisions: A pilot study of Latino men with cancer. *Journal of Cancer Education, 28*, 729–737. http://dx.doi.org/10.1007/s13187-013-0522-9

Carrion, I. V., Nedjat-Haiem, F. R., Martinez-Tyson, D., & Castaneda, H. (2013). Advance care planning among Columbian, Mexican, and Puerto Rican women with a cancer diagnosis. *Supportive Care Cancer, 21,* 1233–1239. http://dx.doi.org/10.1007/s00520-012-1652-z

Castro-Echeverry, E., Kao, L. S., Robinson, E. K., Silberfein, E. J., Ko, T. C., & Wray, C. J. (2013). Relationship between documentation status and survival for medically underserved Hispanic breast cancer patients. *Journal of Surgical Research, 180,* 284–289. http://dx.doi.org/10.1016.j.jss2012.04.072

Centers for Disease Control and the Lance Armstrong Foundation. (2004). *A national action plan for cancer survivorship: Advancing public health strategies.* Washington, DC: U.S. Department of Health and Human Services.

Changrani, J., Lieberman, M., Golant, M., Rios, P., Damman, J., & Gany, F. (2008). Online cancer support groups: Experiences with underserved immigrant Latinas. *Primary Psychiatry, 15*(1), 55–62. Retrieved from http://primarypsychiatry.com/online-cancer-support-groups-experiences-with-underserved-immigrant-latinas

Colby, S. L., & Ortman, J. M. (2014). *Projections of the size and composition of the U.S. population: 2014 to 2060*. Washington, D.C.: US Census Bureau.

Costas, R., & Gany, F. (2013). Depressive symptoms in a sample of Afro-Caribbean and Latino Immigrant cancer patients: A comparative analysis. *Supportive Cancer Care, 21*, 2461–2468. http://dx.doi.org/10.1007/s00520-013-1813-8

Costas-Muniz, R., Leng, J., Diamond, L., Aragones, A., Ramirez, J., & Gany, F. (2015). Psychosocial correlates of appointment keeping in immigrant cancer patients. *Journal of Psychosocial Oncology, 33*(2), 107–123. http://dx.doi.org/10.1080/07347332.2014.992084

Costas-Muniz, R., Sen, R., Leng, J., Aragones, A., Ramirez, J., & Gany, F.(2013). Cancer stage Knowledge and desire for information: Mismatch in Latino cancer patients. *Journal of Cancer Education, 28,* 458–465. http://dx.doi.org/10.1007/s13187-013-0487-8

D'Orazio, L. M., Meyerowitz, B. E., Stone, P. J., Felix, J., & Muderspach, L. I. (2011) Psychosocial adjustment among low-income Latina cervical cancer patients. *Journal of Psychosocial Oncology, 29*, 515–533. http://dx.doi.org/10.1080/07347332.2011.599363

Delgado, R., & Stefancic, J. (2001). *Critical race theory: An introduction*. New York, NY: University Press.

Du, X. L., Fang, S., Coker, A. L., Sanderson, M., Aragaki, C., Cormier, J. N., et al. (2006). Racial disparity and socioeconomic status in association with survival in older men with local/regional stage prostate carcinoma: Findings from a large community-based cohort. *Cancer, 106*(6), 1276–1285.

Esbach, K., Stimpson, J. P., Kuo, Y., & Gooewin, J. S. (2007). Mortality of foreign-born and US-born Hispanic adults at younger ages: A reexamination of recent patterns. *American Journal of Public Health, 97*, 1297–1304. http://dx.doi.org/10.2105/AJPH.2006.094193

Ferrell, B. R., Dow, K. H., & Grant, M. (2005). Measurement of the quality of life in cancer survivors. *Quality of Life Research, 4*, 523–531.

Galvan, N., Buki, L. P., & Garces, D. M. (2009). Suddenly, a carriage appears: Social support needs of Latina breast cancer survivors. *Journal of Psychosocial Oncology, 27*(3), 361–382. http://dx.doi.org/10.1080/07347330902979283

Gany, F., Ramirez, J., Nierodzick, M. L., McNish, T., Lobach, I., & Leng, J..(2011). Cancer portal project: A multidisciplinary approach to cancer care among Hispanic patients. *American Society of Clinical Oncology, 7*(1), 31–38. http://dx.doi.org/10.1200/JOP.2010.000036

Gany, F., Yogendran, L., Massic, D., Ramirez, J., Lee, T., Winkel, G., et al. (2013). "Doctor, what do I have?" Knowledge of cancer diagnosis among immigrant/migrant minorities. *Journal of Cancer Education, 28*, 165–170. http://dx.doi.org/10.1007/s13187-012-0429-x

Gomez, N., Guendelman, S., Harley, K. G., & Gomez, S. L. (2015). Nativity and neighborhood characteristics and cervical cancer at diagnosis and survival outcomes among Hispanic women in California. *American Journal of Public Health, 105*(3), 538–545. http://dx.doi.org/10.2105/AJPH.2014.302261

Gonzales, F. A., Hurtado-de-Mendoza, A, Santoyo-Olsson, J., & Napoles, A. M. (2016). Do coping strategies mediate the effects of emotional support on emotional well-being among Spanish-speaking Latina breast cancer survivors? *Psycho-Oncology, 25*, 1286–1292. http://dx.doi.org/10.1002/pon.3953

Grant, S. R., Walker, G. V., Guadagnolo, B. A., Koshy, M., Allen, P. K., & Mahmood, U. (2015). Variation in insurance status by patient demographics and tumor site among nonelderly adult patients with cancer. *Cancer, 121*, 2020–2028. http://dx.doi.org/10.1002/cncr.29120

Hewitt, M., Greenfield, S., & Stovall, E. (Eds.) (2005). *From cancer patient to cancer survivor: Lost in transition*. Washington, D.C.: The National Academies Press.

Hoffmann, R. M., Gilliland, F. D., Eley, J. W., Harlan, L. C., Stephenson, R. A., Stanford, J. L., et al. (2001). Racial and ethnic differences in advanced-stage prostate cancer: the Prostate Cancer Outcomes Study. *JNCI: Journal of the National Cancer Institute, 93*(5), 388–395. http://dx.doi.org/10.1093/jnci/93.5.388

Hsu, C. E., Mas, F. S., Miller, J. A., & Nkhoma, E. T. (2007). A spatial-temporal approach to surveillance of prostate cancer disparities in population subgroups. *Journal of the National Medical Association, 99*, 72–87.

Institute of Medicine. (1999). *The unequal burden of cancer.* Washington, DC: National Academy Press.

Jaramillo, S., & Hui, D. (2016). End-of-life care for undocumented immigrants with advanced cancer: Documenting the undocumented. *Journal of Pain and Symptom Management, 51*(4), 784–788. http://dx.doi.org/10.1016/j.jpainsymman.2015.11.009

Kagawa-Singer, M., Dadia, A. V., Yu, M. C., & Surbone, A. (2010). Cancer, culture, and health disparities: Time to chart a new course? *CA: A Cancer Journal for Clinicians, 60*, 12–39. http://dx.doi.org/10.3322/caac.20051

Kennedy, S., Kidd, M. P., McDonald, J. T., & Biddle, N. (2015). The healthy immigrant effect: Patterns and evidence from four countries. *International Journal of Migration and Immigration, 16*, 317–332. http://dx.doi.org/10.1007/s12134-014-0340-x

Krogstad, J. M., Passel, J. S., & Cohn, D. (2018). 5 Facts about illegal immigration in the U.S. Pew Research Center. Retrieved from http://www.pewresearch.org/fact-tank/2017/04/27/5-facts-about-illegal-immigration-in-the-u-s

Latini, D. M., Elkin, E. P., Cooperberg, M. R., Sadetsky, N., Duchane, J., & Carroll, P. R. (2006). Differences in clinical characteristics and disease-free survival for Latino, African American, and non-Latino white men with localized prostate cancer: Data from CaPSURE. *Cancer, 106*(4), 789–795.

LoBiondo-Wood, G., Brown, C. G., Knobf, M. T., Lyon, D., Mallory, G., Mitchell, S. A., et al. (2014). Priorities for oncology nursing research: The 2013 national survey. *Oncology Nursing Forum, 42*(1), 67–76. http://dx.doi.org/10.1188/14.onf.67-76

Lopez-Class, M., Perret-Gentil, M., Kreling, B., Caicedo, L., Mandelblatt, J., & Graves, K. D. (2011). Quality of life among immigrant Latina breast cancer survivors: Realities of culture and enhancing cancer care. *Journal of Cancer Education, 26,* 724–733.

Moher, D., Liberati, A., Tetzlaff, J., & Altman, D. G. (2009). Preferred reporting items for systematic reviews and meta-analyses: the PRISMA statement. *PLoS Medicine, 6*(7), e1000097. http://dx.doi.org/10.1371/journal.pmed.1000097

Moreno, P. I., Bauer, M. R., Yanez, B., Jorge, A., Maggard-Gibbons, M., & Stanton, A. L. (2016). Dispositional emotional expressivity, cancer-specific coping, and distress in socioeconomically-disadvantaged Latinas. *Health Psychology, 35*(6), 584–593. http://dx.doi.org/10.1037/hea0000319

National Center for Health Statistics. (2015). *Health, United States, 2014: With special feature on adults aged 55-64.* Hyattsville, MD: Author.

Pinheiro, P., Callahan, K., Jin, H., & Morris, C. (2016). Rethinking the Hispanic advantage in cancer outcomes: Influence of birthplace. *Journal of Clinical Oncology, 34*(15_suppl), 1575. http://dx.doi.org/10.1200/jco.2016.34.15_suppl.1575

Schupp, C. W., Press, D. J., & Gomez, S. L. (2014). Immigration factors and prostate cancer survival among Hispanic men in California. *Cancer, 120*(9), 1401–1408. http://dx.doi.org/10.1002/cncr.28587

Siegel, R. L., Fedewa, S. A., Miller, K. D., Goding-Sauer, A., Pinheiro, P. S., Martinez-Tyson, D., et al. (2015). Cancer statistics for Hispanics/Latinos, 2015. *CA: A Cancer Journal for Clinicians, 65*, 457–480. http://dx.doi.org/10.3322/caac.21314

Siegel, R. L., Miller, K. D., & Jemal, A. (2018). Cancer statistics, 2018. *CA: A Cancer Journal for Clinicians, 68*, 7–30. http://dx.doi.org/10.3322/caac.21442

Singh, G. K. & Hiatt, R. A. (2006). Trends and disparities in socioeconomic and behavioural characteristics, life expectancy, and cause-specific mortality of native-born and foreign-born populations in the United States, 1979-2003. *International Journal of Epidemiology, 35,* 903–919. http://dx.doi.org/10.1093/ije/dyl089

Singh, G. S., & Siahpush, M. (2001). All-cause mortality and cause-specific mortality of immigrants and native born in the United States. *American Journal of Public Health, 91,* 393–399. http://dx.doi.org/10.2105/AJPH.91.3.392

Smith, B. D., Smith, G. I., Hurria, A., Hortobagyi, G. N., & Buchholz, T. A. (2009). Future of cancer incidence in the United States: Burdens upon an aging, changing nation. *Journal of Clinical Oncology, 27,* 2881–2885. http://dx.doi.org/10.1200/JCO.2008.20.8983

Stern, M. C., Fejerman, L., Das, R., Setiawan, V. W., Cruz-Correa, M. R., Perez-Stable, E. J., et al. (2016). Variability in cancer risk and outcomes within US Latinos by national origin and genetic ancestry. *Current Epidemiology Reports, 3,* 181–190. http://dx.doi.org/10.1007/s40471-016-0083-7

Turra, C. M., & Elo, I. T. (2008). The impact of Salmon Bias on the Hispanic mortality advantage. *Population Research Policy Review, 27*(5), 515–530. http://dx.doi.org/10.1007/s11113-008-9087-4

US Census Bureau. (2005). *Texas becomes nation's "Majority-Minority" state.* Washington, DC: US Census Bureau.

US Census Bureau. (2014). *2011-2013 American community survey 3-year estimates*. Washington, DC: US Census Bureau. MGO

U.S. Census Bureau. (2018, March 7). Hispanic origin: About. Retrieved from https://www.census.gov/topics/population/hispanic-origin/about.html

White, A., Coker, A. L., Du, X. L., Eggleston, K. S., & Williams, M. (2011). Racial/ethnic disparities in survival among men diagnosed with prostate cancer in Texas. *Cancer, 117*, 1080–1088. http://dx.doi.org/10.1002/cncr.25671

CHAPTER 5

# Prevention and Treatment of Overweight and Obesity Among African Immigrant Populations

## *A Systematic Review of the Literature*

Melanie T. Turk, Melissa A. Kalarchian, David A. Nolfi, and Abimbola Fapohunda

ABSTRACT

Obesity increases with duration of residence in the United States, and confers risk for cardiovascular disease, type 2 diabetes mellitus and other chronic illnesses. Therefore, this review focused on the topic of prevention and treatment of overweight and obesity among immigrants and refugees from Africa. In a systematic review of the literature, five articles published after 2000 were identified that address this topic, including reports on intervention development and intervention delivery. We describe these reports with a focus on cultural implications. Research on this topic supports the importance of engaging community partners, delivering interventions in community settings, and using the parent as an agent for family behavior change. We note the limitations of this small body of work, and present recommendations for developing and evaluating future programs. As healthcare professionals with knowledge of and connections to immigrant communities, nurses can play a key role in the delivery of culturally congruent interventions to reduce obesity-related health disparities in this growing population.


http://dx.doi.org/10.1891/0739-6686.37.161

## INTRODUCTION

Obesity has tripled worldwide since 1975 and is currently recognized as an epidemic in the United States and globally (World Health Organization, 2017). According to the latest data from the 2015–2016 U.S. National Health and Nutrition Examination Survey (NHANES), designed to assess the health and nutrition of the nation, 39.8% were obese in 2015–2016, defined as a body mass index (BMI) of ≥ 30 kg/m$^2$ (Hales, Carroll, Fryar, & Ogden, 2017). If current trends continue, most U.S. adults are projected to become obese by 2030 (Guh et al., 2009; Hales et al., 2017; Trust for America's Health, 2013). Serious health consequences of obesity include type 2 diabetes mellitus, cardiovascular disease, and certain types of cancer (Jensen et al., 2014).

National U.S. data also indicated that some groups are more vulnerable to obesity than others (Ogden, Carroll, Kit, & Flegal, 2014). For example, non-Hispanic Black adults have the highest age-adjusted rates of obesity (48.1%), followed by Hispanic (42.5%), non-Hispanic White (34.5%), and non-Hispanic Asian (11.7%) adults. Rates of obesity are also higher among middle-age adults 40–59 years (40.2%) and older adults > 60 years (37.0%) as compared to adults aged 20–39 years (32.3%). Of note, irrespective of the country of origin, adult immigrants to the United States have a lower prevalence of overweight and obesity than their racial/ethnic counterparts born in the United States (Tovar, Renzaho, Guerrero, Mena, & Ayala, 2014). Obesity is also associated with gender and socioeconomic status (Ogden et al., 2014). For example, women with higher incomes are less likely to be obese than those with lower incomes. Conversely, among non-Hispanic Black and Mexican American men, those with higher incomes have a higher prevalence of obesity as compared to men with lower incomes. Among women (but not men), there is a trend toward college graduates being less likely to be obese than those who have not received a college degree. Thus, disparities in obesity in the United States exist not only with respect to race and ethnicity, but also immigration status, as well as gender, age, education and income.

Nurses and other healthcare professionals need to be prepared to prevent and treat obesity in an increasingly diverse population. This systematic review will focus on African immigrants and refugees, a growing group. In the United States, the African immigrant population has doubled every decade since 1970, totaling 2.1 million in 2015 (Anderson, 2017). Individuals who immigrate to the United States are expected to comprise approximately 20% of the population by the year 2060 (Colby & Ortman, 2014). Thus, these demographic trends indicate that addressing the health needs of immigrants is essential.

## OBESITY AND IMMIGRATION

Immigration is typically defined as permanently relocating from one's country of origin to another country (Parry, 2007), whereas migration typically refers to movement more generally. Data from the 2010–2014 National Health Interview Survey indicates that the prevalence of overweight/obesity is highest among immigrants to the United States from Africa, Russia, and Mexico (61%, 61%, and 71%, respectively) as compared to other regions (Commodore-Mensah et al., 2016). Data suggest that risk for obesity and type 2 diabetes may be related to increased urbanization and socioeconomic status, as reflected in a stepwise increase in the prevalence of obesity following a common path of migration of Black individuals from Africa to the United States centuries ago, from 5% in Nigeria, to 23% in Jamaica, and 39% in the United States (Misra & Ganda, 2007).

Diseases associated with a sedentary lifestyle and poor diet, such as overweight/obesity, hypertension, diabetes mellitus, and hyperlipidemia, are of specific concern among immigrant groups (Commodore-Mensah et al., 2016), and achieving and maintaining a healthy body weight is key to cardiovascular risk reduction among immigrants. Most adult immigrants to the United States arrive with a lower BMI than individuals born in the United States (Murphy, Robertson, & Oyebode, 2017). However, the prevalence of overweight and obesity among migrant groups increases the longer they reside in the United States (Goel, McCarthy, Phillips, & Wee, 2004; Koya & Egede, 2007; Singh, Siahpush, Hiatt, & Timsina, 2011). Furthermore, within 10–15 years post-migration, rates of overweight and obesity are comparable to or surpass rates of native U.S. residents (Delavari, Sonderlund, Swinburn, Mellor, & Renzaho, 2013; Hao & Kim, 2009). Analysis of nearly 55,000 immigrants (Commodore-Mensah et al., 2016) revealed that immigrants who resided in the United States for more than 10 years were significantly more likely to be overweight/obese (adjusted odds ratio [AOR] = 1.19, 95% Confidence Interval [CI] = 1.10–1.29), have hypertension (AOR = 1.18, 95% CI = 1.05–1.32), and have diabetes mellitus (AOR = 1.43, 95% CI = 1.17–1.73) than those living in the United States for less than 10 years. The prevalence of hypertension was highest among Russian immigrants (25%) followed closely by immigrants from Southeast Asia (22%), and Africa (22%); the prevalence of diabetes mellitus and hyperlipidemia was highest among Mexican, European and Southeast Asian immigrants, respectively (10% for all).

### Acculturation

Acculturation may be defined as the individual processes by which immigrants attain the attitudes, values, and behaviors of the receiving country (Lopez-Class, Castro, & Ramirez, 2011). Various proxy variables are used to measure acculturation, such as birth place, age at migration, length of residence in the host country, citizenship status, and primary language spoken, and these factors are often associated with worsening health outcomes (Viruell-Fuentes, Miranda, & Abdulrahim, 2012). For example, a systematic review on the relationship between immigrant duration of residence in the United States and BMI documented that obesity is associated with longer duration in the mainland United States and other measures of acculturation among women from Puerto Rico, such as birth place and self-evaluation of English language proficiency; women who self-rated their English fluency as very good or fluent had significantly higher BMIs than those whose English was not-so-good or good (Himmelgreen et al., 2004). However, the most appropriate ways to measure acculturation, and how acculturation affects obesity independently of race and ethnicity, are not well understood (Di Noia, Furst, Park, & Byrd-Bredbenner, 2013; Salant & Lauderdale, 2003). Along with acculturation, variables posited to be associated with weight gain among immigrant populations include epi-genetic and genetic factors; diet and physical activity behaviors; preference for body size; exposure to stress; and socioeconomic status (Murphy et al., 2017).

## Lifestyle Behaviors

Migration from one's country of origin to a receiving country presents new challenges with respect to diet and physical activity. Access to native foods may be limited. Changes in eating after migration are often referred to as dietary acculturation (Terragni, Garnweidner, Pettersen, & Mosdol, 2014), or the process by which immigrants adopt the food selections and eating behaviors of the new setting (Satia-Abouta, 2003). As part of this process, immigrants may keep and discover new methods of using native foods, exclude some traditional foods, and/or begin to eat unfamiliar foods (Satia, 2010). Adapting to a different food environment may be particularly challenging for immigrants from countries with a lower income and level of education (Gilbert & Khokhar, 2008; Satia-Abouta, 2003); if native foods are available in the new environment, they are likely to be higher in cost (Satia, 2010). Limited knowledge of how to source ingredients to cook traditional dishes, along with significant lifestyle and employment changes in a new country, may result in dietary changes that negatively affect health and food security among migrants (Hadley, Patil, & Nahayo, 2010; Saleh, Amanatidis, & Samman, 2002).

Physical activity also plays an important role in weight control (Jensen et al., 2014; United States Department of Health and Human Services, 2008), and activity behaviors are likely to be negatively affected by migration (Gadd, Sundquist, Johansson, & Wandell, 2005; Sternfeld, Ainsworth, & Quesenberry, 1999). For example, Nigerian immigrants have reported higher levels of lifestyle activity while living in their native country as compared to living in the United States

(Turk, Fapohunda, & Zoucha, 2015). Other barriers to engaging in healthy levels of physical activity include time constraints from work/family commitments; cost of belonging to an exercise facility; cultural and religious beliefs that influence exercise participation; routine use of vehicles for transportation; and the hectic pace of immigrants' new lifestyles (Caperchione, Kolt, & Mummery, 2009; Ibe-Lamberts, Tshiswaka, Onyenekwu, Schwingel, & Iwelunmor, 2018; Mohamed, Hassan, Weis, Sia, & Wieland, 2014; Turk et al., 2015).

## TREATMENT OF OBESITY

Obesity is a chronic condition, and treatments include behavioral therapy, pharmacotherapy, and bariatric surgery. Lifestyle intervention, or standard behavioral therapy rooted in Social Cognitive Theory (Bandura, 2004), is the first line of treatment, consisting of diet, exercise, and behavior modification (Jensen et al., 2014; United States Department of Health and Human Services, 2008). Fundamental behavioral change strategies include self-monitoring of dietary intake and physical activity, goal setting, enhancing self-efficacy, cognitive restructuring and social support; feedback on progress toward goals is often provided by behavioral counselors or interventionists (Burke & Turk, 2014). Modest weight losses approximating 8%–10% of initial weight typically result over 6 months followed by a pattern of gradual weight regain (Jensen et al., 2014).

Pharmacotherapy is a second level of treatment used together with lifestyle intervention. Pharmacotherapy is considered for persons with a BMI > 30 kg/m$^2$ and no contraindications to the medication, or those with a BMI of > 27 kg/m$^2$ and significant comorbidities, such as type 2 diabetes mellitus or hypertension (Srivastava & Apovian, 2018). Some medications, for example, bupropion, work centrally to promote appetite suppression and satiety, whereas orlistat is designed to prevent the absorption of 25%–30% of calories from fat (Srivastava & Apovian, 2018). Compared to placebo, medications for weight loss are associated with at least a 5% weight loss at 1 year (Khera et al., 2016). However, weight loss medications also have side effects, and persons must continue lifestyle changes to maintain weight loss.

Bariatric surgery can lead to substantial and sustained weight loss for individuals with higher levels of obesity (Ricci et al., 2015). The eligibility criteria for surgical intervention includes Class 3 obesity [BMI ≥ 40 kg/m$^2$] or Class 2 obesity [BMI 35–39.9 kg/m$^2$] with obesity-related comorbidities, as well as failure to attain a sustained weight loss with previous weight loss attempts (American Society for Metabolic and Bariatric Surgery, 2016). Although post-surgery weight loss is substantial, weight regain has been noted as early as 6 months postoperatively (Courcoulas et al., 2013). Weight recidivism has been linked to health-related behaviors such as diet, metabolic factors, and type of surgical procedure (Karmali et al., 2013).

Evidence suggests that nurses and other healthcare professionals may need additional training in weight management and obesity care to participate in interdisciplinary management models (Bleich, Bandara, Bennett, Cooper, & Gudzune, 2015; Lazarou & Kouta, 2010; National Clinical Guideline Centre, 2014). A compilation of education, assessment, and treatment tools, as well as links to current clinical practice guidelines are available through the American Association of Nurse Practitioners (AANP) (American Association of Nurse Practitioners, 2018). Furthermore, the American Academy of Physician Assistants (AAPA) has announced a collaboration with the AANP and the Obesity Medicine Association (OMA) to develop an educational program that will award a Certificate in Primary Care Obesity Management to Physicians' Assistants and Nurse Practitioners who are interested in expanding care to patients with obesity (American Academy of Physician Assistants, 2018).

## Cultural Considerations

Although frameworks have been proposed for adapting behavioral interventions for weight management to specific racial and ethnic groups (Kong, Tussing-Humphreys, Odoms-Young, Stolley, & Fitzgibbon, 2014; Perez et al., 2013), there has been relatively less attention in the literature paid to immigrant populations specifically. For example, a cross-sectional study in Israel investigated factors associated with childhood overweight and obesity among acculturated and new immigrants. Investigators found that acculturation, perception of child's weight status, and parental smoking were associated with overweight/obesity (Kaufman-Shriqui et al., 2013) and recommend that immigration should be considered when implementing programs to prevent obesity. A team in Australia used the Analysis Grid for Elements Linked to Obesity (ANGELO) framework to understand perspectives related to obesity prevention in the African community in Melbourne; the aim was to elicit priorities and suggestions of culturally centered methods for implementation (Halliday et al., 2014), which included a need for culturally and age-appropriate interventions while reducing intergenerational and gender role conflicts. Studies on predictors of obesity in specific immigrant populations may also suggest targets for culturally tailored interventions. For example, an association between weekly consumption of alcohol and obesity, rather than traditional predictors from the general population, suggests that specifically targeted obesity screening and obesity prevention intervention programs may benefit Nigerian immigrants to the United States (Obisesan et al., 2017). Previous reviews of obesity prevention interventions among immigrants and refugee populations suggest that they are limited by methodological weaknesses, and most have targeted Latinos (Kong et al., 2014; Perez et al., 2013; Renzaho, Mellor, Boulton, & Swinburn, 2010; Tovar et al., 2014).

## PREVENTION AND TREATMENT OF OVERWEIGHT AND OBESITY AMONG AFRICAN IMMIGRANTS

There has been scant literature on interventions for African immigrants and refugees. The Research on Obesity and Diabetes among African Migrants (RODAM) study is a multicenter cross-sectional study of individuals from Ghana, living in rural and urban Ghana, the Netherlands, England, and Germany. RODAM is designed to elucidate the mechanisms underlying the high prevalence of obesity and diabetes in African populations residing in Europe (Addo et al., 2017). Results suggest a complex interplay of sociodemographic factors that may have direct implications for prevention in different locations. For example, Ghanaian women living in Europe who had a higher education level (tertiary) had a lower prevalence of diabetes (prevalence ratio [PR]: 0.65; 95% CI 0.45 to 0.93) compared to women with elementary level education; yet, this relationship was not accounted for by dietary intake, physical activity or BMI. Indeed, studies on predictors in specific African immigrant populations may suggest points of emphasis for interventions. As noted above, obesity screening and prevention programs targeting alcohol consumption may benefit Nigerian immigrants to the United States (Obisesan et al., 2017). Overall, however, there is a dearth of research to guide the development of theory-driven, culturally tailored, evidence-based prevention and treatment programs. Thus, we conducted a systematic review of interventions that focused on the prevention and treatment of overweight and obesity for African immigrants and refugees.

## METHODS

One author (DN) conducted searches systematically in PubMed, CINAHL, Scopus, and PsycINFO using combinations of keywords and subject terms for African immigrants, overweight or obesity, and prevention or treatment strategies. Although Scopus lacks its own subject terms, it includes searchable subject terms from other databases. The authors used keyword truncation and subject explosions where appropriate. Based on two authors' (MK and MT) previous experience with obesity research, the authors expected they would find relatively few intervention studies for obesity treatment or prevention in African immigrants. After confirming this expectation, the authors decided to use OR to combine the problem terms (obesity, overweight) with the intervention and prevention terms (diet, weight management, etc.). The authors incorporated intervention terms used in a previous systematic review (Bryant et al., 2014) and obtained full search strategies from the authors (J. Wright, personal communication, January 22, 2018). Search terms are included in Table 5.1 (except for the lengthy list of names of African countries and their residents). To obtain a full list of search terms and search strategies, contact the corresponding author. All searches were run on January 27, 2018. After completing the initial inclusion process, the authors performed ancestry searches of the references for the included articles and looked for the publication of trial results from articles that reported the study design only; one additional article was identified. The authors used EndNote to store search results and locate full text. Covidence review management software was used to screen studies independently and compare evaluations.

### Inclusion/Exclusion Criteria

Study inclusion was based on the following criteria: African immigrants or refugees (living in the United States or other countries), overweight or obese, interventions (prevention or treatment), and family-based, children, or adults. Exclusion criteria included outcomes that did not incorporate prevention or

**TABLE 5.1**
*Search Terms*

| Keywords | Subject Headings |
|---|---|
| Africa/Africans<br>Names of all African countries/residents | Africa<br>African Continental Ancestry Group<br>African Cultural Groups |
| Adiposity<br>BMI<br>Body Mass Index<br>Body Weight<br>Diet<br>Obese/Obesity<br>Overeating<br>Overweight<br>Weight Control<br>Weight Gain<br>Weight Loss<br>Weight Management | Body Mass Index<br>Body Weight<br>Diet<br>Obesity<br>Overweight<br>Weight Control<br>Weight Loss |
| Aliens<br>Asylum seekers<br>Emigres<br>Immigrants<br>Refugees | Emigrants and Immigrants<br>Emigration and Immigration<br>Human Migration<br>Immigrants<br>Refugees |

treatment of overweight or obesity, languages other than English, duplicate studies, and published before 2000. This date cutoff was intended to capture both current state of the science in prevention and treatment, as well as current demographics of immigrants and refugees from Africa. Two authors (MT and MK) independently reviewed the titles, abstracts, and full text to apply the inclusion and exclusion criteria. Figure 5.1 reports the major steps of the study selection process using the Preferred Reporting Items for Systematic Reviews and Meta-Analyses (PRISMA) guidelines (Moher, Liberati, Tetzlaff, Altman, & Group, 2009). This process yielded a final result of five articles, which the researchers analyzed and used to extract the data presented in Table 5.2 including Study, Purpose, Sample/Setting, Intervention, Results, and Cultural Implications. These elements were chosen to characterize efforts at developing and evaluating obesity prevention and/or treatment interventions for immigrants from Africa, with a focus on how interventions have been adapted for this population.

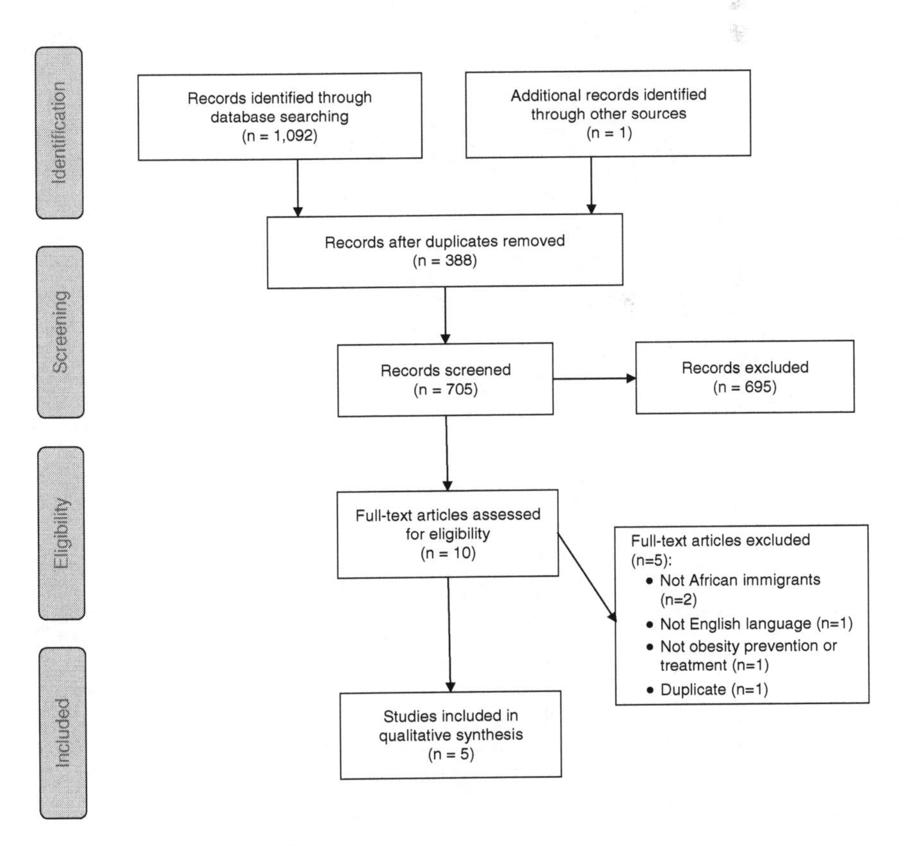


**FIGURE 5.1** PRISMA 2009 flow diagram.

**TABLE 5.2**
*Summary of Studies Reviewed*

| Study | Purpose | Sample/Setting | Intervention | Results | Cultural Implications |
|---|---|---|---|---|---|
| Renzaho, Halliday, Mellor, and Green (2015) | To report on development of a culturally competent obesity prevention program for sub-Saharan African families using a community-partnered participatory approach | Targeting families in Melbourne, Australia, with children between the ages of 12 and 17 | Healthy Migrant Families Initiative: Challenges and Choices program developed in 3 phases:<br>(1) Focus groups, interviews, workshops, and surveys of African teens, parents, community members, and health care providers identified the main drivers of obesity among children<br>(2) Survey of 208 participants indicated the types of strategies that might be helpful<br>(3) Development of a 9-session program informed by 10 cultural competence strategies:<br>"Healthy lifestyles in a new culture" module consists of 5, 90-minute group sessions about healthy eating and body weight, physical activity<br>"Healthy families in a new culture" module consists of 4, 90-minute group sessions on family communication, parenting and problem solving | Resources developed to promote consistent program delivery including Power Point slides, learning materials, program implementation manual, facilitator manual, and group session guide<br>Program has not yet been implemented. | Group sessions should be run by health professionals who are bilingual and have experience working with African migrant families.<br>Interventions need to consider the acculturation gap between different generations within migrant families to maximize involvement of parents and to promote community ownership of the program.<br>Interventions should consider cultural foods and practices by working with individuals to identify methods of modifying traditional foods so that they are healthier. |

| | | | | | |
|---|---|---|---|---|---|
| Wieland et al. (2012) | To systematically develop and evaluate a physical activity and nutrition program for immigrant and refugee women using a community-based participatory approach | Immigrant and refugee women in Rochester, MN<br>*N* = 29 women for retreat with focus groups to develop socioculturally appropriate fitness program<br>*N* = 45 women for pilot study (18 Hispanic, 14 Somali, 10 Sudanese, & 3 non-immigrant African American), mean age 40 years (range 22–68) | Two, 90-minute classes per week for 6 weeks conducted at YMCA<br>60 minutes of exercise (aerobic dance and strength training with resistance bands)<br>30 minutes of nutrition education (used food props and lay interpreters)<br>Child care or child recreation, taxi vouchers, and light snacks provided | Acceptability of classes rated highly (4.85/5.0)<br>29% reported regular physical activity before the intervention vs. 82% after, $p \leq .001$<br>Trends for weight loss (–3.6 kg, $p$ =.65), waist circumference –4.1 cm, $p$ = .35), and blood pressure (125/80 vs. 122/76 mm/Hg; $p$ = .27)<br>Significant improvements in quality of life and self-efficacy for diet and exercise | Exercise should begin slowly and increase incrementally in intensity, in a women-only space.<br>Family-focused nutrition education should highlight proper portion sizes and recommend modifications to traditional dishes.<br>Childcare and activities for children are advantageous as children pressure parents to attend.<br>Ethnic heterogeneity is beneficial for exercise but detrimental for nutrition component due to language barriers. |

(*Continued*)

**TABLE 5.2**
*Summary of Studies Reviewed (Continued)*

| Study | Purpose | Sample/Setting | Intervention | Results | Cultural Implications |
|---|---|---|---|---|---|
| Wieland et al. (2016) | To describe participatory development and baseline characteristics of a physical activity and nutrition program for immigrant and refugee families | 144 families (151 individuals) in Rochester, MN<br>Family eligibility criteria: household with at least 1 adult and 1 adolescent age 10–18 years | Work group meetings for 6 months with 16 community/academic partners to develop and refine intervention<br>based on preliminary research<br>Manual with 12 content modules based in Social Cognitive Theory including self-efficacy, social support, outcome expectations, social reinforcement<br>Face-to-face and word-of mouth recruitment entirely by community partners in each of three ethnic communities (Hispanic, Somali, Sudanese)<br>Study staff member who was language-congruent called family to screen for eligibility | Baseline characteristics of the sample (81 adolescents, 40 adults; 44 families) indicated adolescents and adults spent 64.7 (302.) and 43.1 (35.4) minutes per day in moderate-to-vigorous physical activity<br>45.7% of adolescents and 80% of adults were overweight or obese<br>Both groups had moderate dietary quality<br>Moderate levels of self-efficacy and social support reported for activity and nutrition | Co-creation with immigrant communities of a multi-component physical activity and nutrition intervention is feasible using community based participatory approach.<br>Recruitment using community partners can significantly help efforts to recruit diverse immigrant groups to participate. |

| | | | | | |
|---|---|---|---|---|---|
| Wieland et al. (2018) | Randomized, controlled trial to evaluate a healthy eating and physical activity intervention for immigrant families | 25 families randomized to intervention and 19 families to control<br>81 Adolescents, 51% female (45.7% Hispanic, 49.4% Somali, 4.9% Sudanese), mean age 13.5 ± 2.5 years<br>70 Adults, 71% female (61.5% Hispanic, 34.3% Somali, 4.3% Sudanese), mean age 39.1 ± 10.9 years | Healthy Immigrant Families intervention consisting of 12 home visits over 6 months (60–90 minutes) then phone calls every 2 weeks during the next 6 months (maximum of 12 calls)<br>12 learning modules (6 on healthy eating, 4 on physical activity, and 2 to reinforce content)<br>Home visits included assessment of knowledge and current behaviors for each topic, information delivery, interactive learning activities, discussion of barriers to and facilitators of healthful behaviors, family goal setting<br>Intervention delivered by bilingual family health promoters with 250 hours of training<br>Assessments at 6, 12, and 24 months | No significant differences in outcomes between the 3 racial/ethnic groups<br>Improvements in adults (but not adolescents) in intervention compared to control as measured by Healthy Eating Index at 12 months (+8.6 vs. −4.4, $p < .01$) and 24 months (+7.4, $p < .01$)<br>Effect mediated by reductions in empty calories, increases in vegetable and bean intake and decreases in refined carbohydrates<br>No improvements in physical activity (measured by accelerometer), Body Mass Index, waist circumference, blood pressure, or quality of life domains for adults or adolescents compared to controls at 12 or 24 months | High baseline activity and family priority of nutrition over activity may account for lack of improvements baseline levels of physical activity.<br>Consistent participation by the adolescents is challenging due to after-school activities.<br>Specific engagement of adolescents in planning phase needed.<br>Social networks of immigrant families can lead to diffusion of the intervention to the control group. |

*(Continued)*

**TABLE 5.2**
*Summary of Studies Reviewed (Continued)*

| Study | Purpose | Sample/Setting | Intervention | Results | Cultural Implications |
|---|---|---|---|---|---|
| Wilson & Elgoghail (2016) | To implement a health education program for West African immigrants to the United States to address health risks associated with the modern diet | Bronx, NY, medical clinic that serves primarily West African patients<br>Young to older-adult clinic patients<br>English not the primary language for most | 3-month program including:<br>1) Group education sessions based on a "Healthy Choices" program (healthy diet, exercise, and lifestyle behaviors) in waiting room of clinic offered twice a week<br>2) Individual, one-on-one education sessions in a private exam room to address individual patient health issues and reinforce group topics<br>3) Health education pamphlets in English, French, and Spanish about services for obtaining inexpensive produce and healthier foods, management of hypertension and prevention of diabetes, changing one's diet for weight loss | Project was successfully implemented<br>Patients engaged in discussions about health issues and what they could do to lower their risks<br>Data on intervention effectiveness not collected | A targeted health education program can address health risk related to diet.<br>Language barriers can persist despite the use of translation services because of the number of different languages spoken in one clinic.<br>Educational materials should be offered in a variety of languages.<br>Consider using a health educator with knowledge of the culture and language of the immigrant population. |

### Study Evaluation

The five studies in this review were assessed for quality using the Quality Assessment Tool for Quantitative Studies, developed by the Effective Public Health Practice Project as a specific part of a systematic review process, (Armijo-Olivo, Stiles, Hagen, Biondo, & Cummings, 2012; Thomas, Ciliska, Dobbins, & Micucci, 2004), and the tool has established validity and reliability (Thomas et al., 2004). This tool was used to assess the studies according to sample selection bias; study design; recognition and treatment of confounders; blinding; data collection methods; withdrawals/dropouts; intervention integrity; and analysis. The studies were given a rating for each component, and then a global rating was assigned as strong, moderate, or weak (Thomas et al., 2004).

## RESULTS

Of the five articles that met the eligibility criteria, two describe the development of interventions for obesity prevention and health promotion via physical activity and nutrition (Renzaho et al., 2015; Wieland et al., 2016), two present the outcomes of interventions (Wieland et al., 2018; Wieland et al., 2012), and one describes a program for which outcomes were not collected (Wilson & Elgoghail, 2016). Three of these five reports were from one research group (Wieland et al., 2018; Wieland et al., 2016; Wieland et al., 2012). Participants included sub-Saharan African immigrant families in Melbourne, Australia (Renzaho et al., 2015); Hispanic, Somali, and Sudanese partners and participants in Rochester, Minnesota (Wieland et al., 2016); (Wieland et al., 2018); immigrant and refugee women of Hispanic, Somali, and Cambodian descent (Wieland et al., 2012); and West African immigrants in the Bronx, New York (Wilson & Elgoghail, 2016). Three of the five articles were rated as weak quality studies (Renzaho et al., 2015; Wieland et al., 2012; Wilson & Elgoghail, 2016), and two articles that pertained to the same study (development and baseline characteristics then intervention testing) were rated as strong (Wieland et al., 2018; Wieland et al., 2016). Findings are discussed in the context of intervention development and intervention delivery.

### Reports on Intervention Development

Researchers from Australia (Renzaho et al., 2015) and from Minnesota (Wieland et al., 2016) described the development of culturally appropriate physical activity and nutrition interventions for African immigrants using community-engaged and community-based participatory research approaches (see Table 5.2). Renzaho and colleagues describe the use of a cultural competence theoretical framework to inform the development of their intervention. Plans for creating the program included theoretically based strategies such as forming community partnerships, continuously collaborating with the target population, defining research questions reflecting a genuine knowledge of the culture, and displaying sensitivity to cultural considerations when developing and implementing the methods. Specifically, members of the African immigrant community were solicited and educated to engage in all aspects of the project's development; an African Review Panel served as a steering committee for the study within the community. The Healthy Migrant Families: Challenges and Choices intervention was developed in three phases with focus groups, interviews, workshops, and surveys with African teens, parents, community members, and health care providers to address obesity-related lifestyle behaviors in families. Focusing on the acculturation gap between parents and adolescents, the intervention aims to address two main aspects of being a healthy family in a new country—living a healthy lifestyle and having positive family relationships. The nine sessions of the intervention centered on topics such as how living in a different culture impacts health, improving communication among family members, making healthy food choices when eating at home and away, and promoting physical activity as part of one's ordinary routine. The importance of the family among migrants from sub-Saharan African in Australia seemed to be an essential cultural consideration with program development.

A community-based participatory research (CBPR) collaboration between the Mayo Clinic and the immigrant and refugee communities of Rochester, Minnesota, originally began in 2004 and was used to develop a culturally appropriate physical activity and nutrition intervention for immigrants and refugees from the Hispanic, Somali, and Sudanese neighborhoods in the area (Wieland et al., 2016). Initial pilot work using focus groups revealed common barriers and facilitators of physical activity and proper nutrition among the three immigrant groups that suggested similar experiences from immigration. These similarities included socioeconomic and language issues affecting participation in physical activity, and dietary intake being influenced by the context and cultural meanings of food within a new environment. The theoretical basis for the intervention was Social Cognitive Theory (Bandura, 2004) with key concepts thought to be relevant to vulnerable populations (Eyler et al., 1999), for example, social support through family and self-efficacy. In order to prepare for a grant submission, a 16-member work group with members from each immigrant sector and the academic medical center collaboratively developed the intervention over 6 months during weekly meetings. After the grant was received, 8 work groups of 8-14 members met to refine aspects of the intervention including physical activity content, dietary content, measurement tool translation and modification, interventionist training and sustainability. Interventionists, bilingual community members called "family health promoters" (FHP) (p. 24), were recruited and trained to deliver the intervention to individuals from their same immigrant community. FHPs received 250 hours of training, visited every participant family in their home prior to intervention delivery, and were employed and compensated via grant monies. Outcomes of interest—objective measurement of physical activity, 24-hour dietary recall data, BMI, blood pressure, waist circumference, and waist-to-hip ratio—are described in the recent report of the randomized controlled trial discussed next (Wieland et al., 2018).

### Reports on Intervention Delivery

As noted in Table 5.2, outcomes of the randomized controlled trial of the intervention developed by the Mayo Clinic group were published in 2018 (Wieland et al., 2018). Randomization occurred at the family level, and eligibility criteria indicated the household needed to have a minimum of one adult and one adolescent between the ages of 10 and 18 years; adolescents were a focus rather than younger children because of an identified need in the community. The 12-month Healthy Immigrant Family intervention was delivered via the FHPs during 12 home visits over 6 months and biweekly phone calls over 6 months with 6, 4, and 2 content modules focused on healthy eating, physical activity and reinforcement of content, respectively. FHPs used theory-based methods, such as feedback on behavior and social support, to promote self-efficacy for behavior change. FHPs also worked individually with families to tailor strategies for each family. Despite the rigorous development and intensity of the intervention, intervention fidelity between 82-89%, and objective measurement of most outcomes, results at 6, 12, and 24 months were modest with similar results among the three ethnic groups. The only outcome that improved significantly in the intervention compared to the control group was self-reported overall diet quality at 12 months for adults, which was sustained at 24 months (see Table 5.2). No significant changes were noted among adolescents. The authors noted that, because most families had more than one adolescent, engagement in the intervention components was inconsistent among the adolescent participants compared to the adults, which might have affected adolescent outcomes.

An earlier intervention study for immigrant and refugee women was designed and implemented using CBPR by the same Mayo Clinic research group (Wieland et al., 2012). After development with women from the community, the 6-week exercise and nutrition intervention was piloted at a local Young Men's Christian Association (YMCA) among 45 immigrant and refugee women, 24 of whom were from Somalia and Sudan. On average, 25 women attended the Tuesday evening session, and 22 attended the Saturday morning session, with a retention rate of 71%. The focus on dance as a means of exercise was highly endorsed by all ethnic groups, and the overall acceptability of the intervention was excellent. Regarding the nutrition education component, participants recommended using visual food props due to potential language barriers, emphasizing healthy family nutrition and suggesting adaptations to culturally based foods to enhance nutritional value. Significantly more women reported engaging in regular physical activity after the intervention, and psychosocial outcomes improved as well (Table 5.2), although the quality of life tool had not been validated among Cambodian or Somali populations. Non-statistically significant, but potentially clinically significant, decreases were noted for weight, waist circumference and blood pressure; as this was a pilot study, it might have been underpowered to detect significant changes (Wieland et al., 2012).

A 3-month intervention for West African immigrants implemented in the Bronx, New York, aimed to address health issues, such as obesity, diabetes, and coronary heart disease, associated with poor dietary intake (Wilson & Elgoghail, 2016). The intervention was delivered at a community-based health clinic serving mainly West African patients who were Medicare or Medicaid recipients with low health literacy and for whom English was a second language. Twenty-minute, nutrition education sessions took place twice weekly within the waiting room area of the clinic with groups of 12-15 patients. Content focused on lifestyle behaviors that could help manage chronic diseases, such as following a healthy diet and exercising, with time devoted to actively engaging patients to ask questions and discuss their ideas about how they could improve their health. Individual private sessions focused on patient-specific health concerns and interests. Educational handouts were also distributed to raise awareness of services available in the Bronx area to promote healthy lifestyle choices and weight loss as well as to prevent or manage chronic illnesses. The authors report that the health education intervention was successfully implemented among West African immigrants in the clinic setting, but no outcome data were collected because, although patients provided consent to participate, Institutional Review Board approval was not obtained for the project.

## DISCUSSION

The African immigrant population in the U.S. continues to climb (Anderson, 2017), and rates of obesity have been found to increase with duration of residence in the United States (Goel et al., 2004; Oza-Frank & Cunningham, 2010). Despite calls for preventing obesity among immigrants to the United States (Oza-Frank & Cunningham, 2010), there is a dearth of research on prevention programs for obesity and chronic diseases among immigrants to developed countries (Renzaho et al., 2010). To inform future intervention efforts, we conducted a systematic review with a focus on prevention and treatment of overweight and obesity among African immigrants and refugees. A total of five studies from three research teams were identified (Renzaho et al., 2015; Wieland et al., 2018; Wieland et al., 2016; Wieland et al., 2012; Wilson & Elgoghail, 2016), which offer several pearls of wisdom for developing culturally appropriate programming.

This review highlights the importance of engaging community members and key stakeholders such as patients, families, gatekeepers and health care providers. CBPR is uniquely suited to engaging immigrants, from identifying program priorities through dissemination of findings, and carries benefits for both researchers (e.g., relevant questions, more reliable data, and better dissemination) and immigrant communities (e.g., raised awareness and leadership opportunities) (Vaughn, Jacquez, Lindquist-Grantz, Parsons, & Melink, 2017). CBPR methods have been successfully used to improve the health of Asian immigrants (Joo, 2014; Katigbak, Foley, Robert, & Hutchinson, 2016), as well as Hispanic (Shelton, 2008; Tapp, White, Steuerwald, & Dulin, 2013) communities. In this review, two of the three teams adopted a CBPR approach. The Healthy Immigrant Families study was a product of the Rochester (Minnesota) Healthy Community Partnership (RHCP) (Wieland et al., 2018). The RHCP contributed to the organization, implementation, and dissemination of the work, including recruiting participants from the Hispanic, Somali, and Sudanese communities with promising results. The Healthy Migrant Families: Challenges and Choices Program was developed in partnership with communities in Melbourne, Australia, as well as health care providers working with African communities and an African Review Panel (Renzaho et al., 2015). Future research on prevention and treatment of overweight or obesity for immigrants and refugees from Africa will require community collaborations that take months or years to develop. To that end, it is encouraging that promoting community-engaged research methodologies and collaborations for early phase translational research are priorities at the National Institute of Nursing Research (NINR), especially among individuals who experience disparate health outcomes (NINR, 2016, 2018).

Results of this review also suggest the importance of delivering programs in community sites in order to reach African immigrant and refugee participants (Wieland et al., 2018; Wieland et al., 2016; Wieland et al., 2012; Wilson & Elgoghail, 2016). Indeed, community-based healthy living initiatives have been found to be highly effective in delivering a range of programs, education, and support to the general population with the goal of reducing cardiovascular disease risk factors and improving outcomes (Berra, Franklin, & Jennings, 2017). The Bronx Health Education Project for West African Immigrants was delivered at a community medical clinic (Wilson & Elgoghail, 2016), and the Healthy Immigrant Families program was delivered at the YMCA, with evidence of significant improvements in healthy eating sustained through 2 years (Wieland et al., 2018). It is noteworthy that the YMCA has also been a successful site for translating the Diabetes Prevention Program into the general population, with weight loss maintained through 1 year (Ackermann, Finch, Brizendine, Zhou, & Marrero, 2008). Further exploration of community settings for intervention delivery to diverse groups is warranted (Ackermann et al., 2008). Faith-based organizations such as churches may also serve as sites for obesity prevention and treatment programs (Lancaster, Carter-Edwards, Grilo, Shen, & Schoenthaler, 2014; Maynard, 2017), but have not been evaluated specially for immigrants and refugees from Africa.

Studies identified and described here also underscore the importance of engaging the entire family in obesity prevention efforts. Only one report included family outcomes, showing sustained improvements in diet quality among adults, but not adolescents, who were randomized to intervention as compared to control (Wieland et al., 2018). This study included Hispanic, Somali, and Sudanese refugees, which can present challenges for working with participants to modify traditional foods that vary for different ethnic groups (Wieland et al., 2012). Although this study indicates additional efforts are needed to reach adolescents, working with adults who prepare food and influence the family lifestyle may be an important conduit for promoting child weight control. Evidence suggests parent-only interventions for childhood overweight may be an effective treatment option (Loveman et al., 2015), but data are not available specifically for parents who have immigrated from Africa. The Healthy Migrant Families initiative will address this gap in the literature by working with parents from Sub-Saharan families to target a primary outcome of child BMI (Renzaho et al., 2015), but this intervention has not yet been implemented and evaluated.

This systematic review also reveals some limitations in the literature. The one randomized controlled trial included a sample that was approximately half Hispanic (Wieland et al., 2018), which was not our population focus. Two papers focused exclusively on immigrants from Africa, but one program has not yet been implemented (Renzaho et al., 2015), and the other was a clinic sample that did not have approval to report outcomes (Wilson & Elgoghail, 2016). Three of the five studies were rated as weak quality. Additionally, while all interventions included weight loss as at least a secondary outcome, only one intervention had an explicit primary focus on obesity (Renzaho et al., 2015); the others focused more on healthy eating and physical activity without specific strategies for weight loss (Wieland et al., 2018; Wilson & Elgoghail, 2016). Two studies were conducted in the United States (Wieland et al., 2018; Wilson & Elgoghail, 2016) and one was designed for implementation in Australia (Renzaho et al., 2015). It is likely that acculturation and the environment of the receiving country is relevant to tailoring effective prevention and treatment programs.

It is also important to consider African immigrants' or refugees' specific country of origin when creating a culturally appropriate program. Immigrants from different regions may have varied views on healthy eating and physical activity. For example, some immigrants may be comfortable participating in certain physical activities, such as traditional dance, but may prefer gender-exclusive settings for women only, for example (Wieland et al., 2012). With respect to diet, one must consider that a significant number of immigrants and refugees continue to eat their native foods, which may include highly palatable foods prepared using traditional oils, for example, palm oil (Turk et al., 2015), that they have consumed since childhood. Interventionists should be very familiar with these foods and methods of cooking, as well as frequency of consumption, in order to suggest potential dietary modifications to prevent and treat obesity.

Moving forward, more methodologically rigorous, theory-driven research testing interventions for the prevention and treatment of overweight and obesity among African immigrants is needed. Full-scale clinical trials with more potent, multi-level interventions and longer-term follow-up are essential. Future research should aim to elucidate the mechanisms for intervention effects and include active comparison groups. In order to increase the public health impact, different approaches may be needed for prevention versus treatment. It may also be necessary to target overweight and obesity specifically, rather than overall health more broadly. In addition to utilizing community settings, incorporating technology (telephone coaching, text messaging, video conferencing) and expanding home visits may increase reach and scalability (Berra et al., 2017), but these have not been evaluated with African immigrant populations. Nurse scientists can play an important role in leading research teams in the development and delivery of novel obesity interventions and their translation into real world settings, in order to reduce health disparities for underserved groups such as immigrants.

In conclusion, the overall body of literature on weight gain prevention and treatment lacks adequate representation of racial and ethnic minority populations, which limits generalizability (Haughton et al., 2018). We found this to be particularly true for African immigrant populations. The five studies identified in this review may have implications for how to develop culturally appropriate obesity prevention and treatment for immigrants and refugees from Africa. Pearls of wisdom from teams working in this area include developing community partnerships, delivering programs in community settings, and engaging the parent as an agent for family lifestyle change.

## REFERENCES

Ackermann, R. T., Finch, E. A., Brizendine, E., Zhou, H., & Marrero, D. G. (2008). Translating the Diabetes Prevention Program into the community. The DEPLOY Pilot Study. *American Journal of Preventive Medicine, 35*(4), 357–363. http://dx.doi.org/10.1016/j.amepre.2008.06.035

Addo, J., Agyemang, C., de-Graft Aikins, A., Beune, E., Schulze, M. B., Danquah, I., et al. (2017). Association between socioeconomic position and the prevalence of type 2 diabetes in

Ghanaians in different geographic locations: the RODAM study. *Journal of Epidemiology and Community Health, 71*(7), 633–639. http://dx.doi.org/10.1136/jech-2016-208322

American Academy of Physician Assistants. (2018). New Certificate in Obesity Management to be Available to PAs and NPs. Retrieved from https://www.aapa.org/news-central/2018/01/new-certificate-obesity-management-available-pas-nps

American Association of Nurse Practitioners. (2018). Education tools - Obesity. Retrieved from https://www.aanp.org/education/education-toolkits/obesity#clinician-resource

American Society for Metabolic and Bariatric Surgery. (2016). Who is a candidate for Bariatric Surgery? Retrieved from https://asmbs.org/patients/who-is-a-candidate-for-bariatric-surgery

Anderson, M. (2017). *African immigrant population in U.S. steadily climbs*. Retrieved from http://www.pewresearch.org/fact-tank/2017/02/14/african-immigrant-population-in-u-s-steadily-climbs

Armijo-Olivo, S., Stiles, C. R., Hagen, N. A., Biondo, P. D., & Cummings, G. G. (2012). Assessment of study quality for systematic reviews: a comparison of the Cochrane Collaboration Risk of Bias Tool and the Effective Public Health Practice Project Quality Assessment Tool: methodological research. *Journal of Evaluation in Clinical Practice, 18*(1), 12–18. http://dx.doi.org/10.1111/j.1365-2753.2010.01516.x

Bandura, A. (2004). Health promotion by social cognitive means. *Health Education & Behavior, 31*(2), 143–164. http://dx.doi.org/10.1177/1090198104263660

Berra, K., Franklin, B., & Jennings, C. (2017). Community-Based Healthy Living Interventions. *Progress in Cardiovascular Diseases, 59*(5), 430–439. http://dx.doi.org/10.1016/j.pcad.2017.01.002

Bleich, S. N., Bandara, S., Bennett, W. L., Cooper, L. A., & Gudzune, K. A. (2015). U.S. health professionals' views on obesity care, training, and self-efficacy. *American Journal of Preventive Medicine, 48*(4), 411–418. http://dx.doi.org/10.1016/j.amepre.2014.11.002

Bryant, M., Ashton, L., Brown, J., Jebb, S., Wright, J., Roberts, K., et al. (2014). Systematic review to identify and appraise outcome measures used to evaluate childhood obesity treatment interventions (CoOR): evidence of purpose, application, validity, reliability and sensitivity. *Health Technology Assessment, 18*(51), 1–380. http://dx.doi.org/10.3310/hta18510

Burke, L. E., & Turk, M. W. (2014). Obesity. In K. A. Reikert, J. K. Ockene, & L. Pbert (Eds.), *Handbook of Health Behavior Change* (4th ed., pp. 363–378). New York, NY: Springer Publishing.

Caperchione, C. M., Kolt, G. S., & Mummery, W. K. (2009). Physical activity in culturally and linguistically diverse migrant groups to Western society: a review of barriers, enablers and experiences. *Sports Medicine, 39*(3), 167–177. http://dx.doi.org/10.2165/00007256-200939030-00001

Colby, S. L., & Ortman, J. M. (2014). *Projections of the Size and Composition of the U.S. Population: 2014 to 2060* (p. 25–1143). Washington, DC: Current Population Reports. Retrieved from https://census.gov/content/dam/Census/library/publications/2015/demo/p25-1143.pdf

Commodore-Mensah, Y., Ukonu, N., Obisesan, O., Aboagye, J. K., Agyemang, C., Reilly, C. M., et al. (2016). Length of Residence in the United States is Associated With a Higher Prevalence of Cardiometabolic Risk Factors in Immigrants: A Contemporary Analysis of the National Health Interview Survey. *Journal of the American Heart Association, 5*(11). http://dx.doi.org/10.1161/JAHA.116.004059

Courcoulas, A. P., Christian, N. J., Belle, S. H., Berk, P. D., Flum, D. R., Garcia, L., et al. (2013). Weight change and health outcomes at 3 years after bariatric surgery among individuals with severe obesity. *The Journal of the American Medical Association, 310*(22), 2416–2425. http://dx.doi.org/10.1001/jama.2013.280928

Delavari, M., Sonderlund, A. L., Swinburn, B., Mellor, D., & Renzaho, A. (2013). Acculturation and obesity among migrant populations in high income countries--a systematic review. *BMC Public Health, 13*, 458. http://dx.doi.org/10.1186/1471-2458-13-458

Di Noia, J., Furst, G., Park, K., & Byrd-Bredbenner, C. (2013). Designing culturally sensitive dietary interventions for African Americans: review and recommendations. *Nutrition Reviews, 71*(4), 224–238. http://dx.doi.org/10.1111/nure.12009

Eyler, A. A., Brownson, R. C., Donatelle, R. J., King, A. C., Brown, D., & Sallis, J. F. (1999). Physical activity social support and middle- and older-aged minority women: results from a US survey. *Social Science & Medicine, 49*(6), 781–789.

Gadd, M., Sundquist, J., Johansson, S. E., & Wandell, P. (2005). Do immigrants have an increased prevalence of unhealthy behaviours and risk factors for coronary heart disease? *European Journal of Cardiovascular Prevention and Rehabilitation, 12*(6), 535–541.

Gilbert, P. A., & Khokhar, S. (2008). Changing dietary habits of ethnic groups in Europe and implications for health. *Nutrition Reviews, 66*(4), 203–215. http://dx.doi.org/10.1111/j.1753-4887.2008.00025.x

Goel, M. S., McCarthy, E. P., Phillips, R. S., & Wee, C. C. (2004). Obesity among US immigrant subgroups by duration of residence. *The Journal of the American Medical Association, 292*(23), 2860–2867. http://dx.doi.org/10.1001/jama.292.23.2860

Guh, D. P., Zhang, W., Bansback, N., Amarsi, Z., Birmingham, C. L., & Anis, A. H. (2009). The incidence of co-morbidities related to obesity and overweight: a systematic review and meta-analysis. *BMC Public Health, 9*, 88. http://dx.doi.org/10.1186/1471-2458-9-88

Hadley, C., Patil, C. L., & Nahayo, D. (2010). Difficulty in the food environment and the experience of food insecurity among refugees resettled in the United States. *Ecology of Food and Nutrition, 49*(5), 390–407. http://dx.doi.org/10.1080/03670244.2010.507440

Hales, C. M., Carroll, M. D., Fryar, C. D., & Ogden, C. L. (2017). Prevalence of Obesity Among Adults and Youth: United States, 2015-2016. *NCHS Data Brief* (288), 1–8. Retrieved from https://www.cdc.gov/nchs/products/databriefs/db288.htm

Halliday, J. A., Green, J., Mellor, D., Mutowo, M. P., de Courten, M., & Renzaho, A. M. (2014). Developing programs for African families, by African families: engaging African migrant families in Melbourne in health promotion interventions. *Family & Community Health, 37*(1), 60–73. http://dx.doi.org/10.1097/FCH.0000000000000011

Hao, L., & Kim, J. J. (2009). Immigration and the American Obesity Epidemic. *International Migration Review, 43*(2), 237–262. http://dx.doi.org/10.1111/j.1747-7379.2009.00764.x

Haughton, C. F., Silfee, V. J., Wang, M. L., Lopez-Cepero, A. C., Estabrook, D. P., Frisard, C., et al. (2018). Racial/ethnic representation in lifestyle weight loss intervention studies in the United States: A systematic review. *Preventive Medicine Reports, 9*, 131–137. http://dx.doi.org/10.1016/j.pmedr.2018.01.012

Himmelgreen, D. A., Pérez-Escamilla, R., Martinez, D., Bretnall, A., Eells, B., Peng, Y., et al. (2004). The longer you stay, the bigger you get: Length of time and language use in the U.S. are associated with obesity in Puerto Rican women. *American Journal of Physical Anthropology, 125*(1), 90–96. http://dx.doi.org/10.1002/ajpa.10367

Ibe-Lamberts, K., Tshiswaka, D. I., Onyenekwu, I., Schwingel, A., & Iwelunmor, J. (2018). Dance and Hometown Associations are Promising Strategies to Improve Physical Activity Participation Among US Nigerian Transnational Immigrants. *Journal of Racial and Ethnic Health Disparities, 5*(2), 253–260. http://dx.doi.org/10.1007/s40615-017-0365-x

Jensen, M. D., Ryan, D. H., Apovian, C. M., Ard, J. D., Comuzzie, A. G., Donato, K. A., et al. (2014). 2013 AHA/ACC/TOS guideline for the management of overweight and obesity in adults: a report of the American College of Cardiology/American Heart Association Task Force on Practice Guidelines and The Obesity Society. *Circulation, 129*(25 Suppl 2), S102–S138. http://dx.doi.org/10.1161/01.cir.0000437739.71477.ee

Joo, J. Y. (2014). Effectiveness of culturally tailored diabetes interventions for Asian immigrants to the United States: a systematic review. *The Diabetes Educator, 40*(5), 605–615. http://dx.doi.org/10.1177/0145721714534994

Karmali, S., Brar, B., Shi, X., Sharma, A. M., de Gara, C., & Birch, D. W. (2013). Weight recidivism post-bariatric surgery: a systematic review. *Obesity Surgery, 23*(11), 1922–1933. http://dx.doi.org/10.1007/s11695-013-1070-4

Katigbak, C., Foley, M., Robert, L., & Hutchinson, M. K. (2016). Experiences and Lessons Learned in Using Community-Based Participatory Research to Recruit Asian American Immigrant Research Participants. *Journal of Nursing Scholarship, 48*(2), 210–218. http://dx.doi.org/10.1111/jnu.12194

Kaufman-Shriqui, V., Fraser, D., Friger, M., Bilenko, N., Vardi, H., Abu-Saad, K., et al. (2013). Factors associated with childhood overweight and obesity among acculturated and new immigrants. *Ethnicity & Disease, 23*(3), 329–335. Retrieved from https://www.ethndis.org/edonline/index.php/ethndis/article/view/344

Khera, R., Murad, M. H., Chandar, A. K., Dulai, P. S., Wang, Z., Prokop, L. J., et al. (2016). Association of Pharmacological Treatments for Obesity With Weight Loss and Adverse Events: A Systematic Review and Meta-analysis. *The Journal of the American Medical Association, 315*(22), 2424–2434. http://dx.doi.org/10.1001/jama.2016.7602

Kong, A., Tussing-Humphreys, L. M., Odoms-Young, A. M., Stolley, M. R., & Fitzgibbon, M. L. (2014). Systematic review of behavioral interventions with culturally-adapted strategies to improve diet and weight outcomes in African-American women. *Obesity Reviews, 15*, 62–92. http://dx.doi.org/10.1111/obr.12203

Koya, D. L., & Egede, L. E. (2007). Association between length of residence and cardiovascular disease risk factors among an ethnically diverse group of United States immigrants. *Journal of General Internal Medicine, 22*(6), 841–846. http://dx.doi.org/10.1007/s11606-007-0163-y

Lancaster, K. J., Carter-Edwards, L., Grilo, S., Shen, C., & Schoenthaler, A. M. (2014). Obesity interventions in African American faith-based organizations: a systematic review. *Obesity Reviews, 15 Suppl 4*, 159–176. http://dx.doi.org/10.1111/obr.12207

Lazarou, C., & Kouta, C. (2010). The role of nurses in the prevention and management of obesity. *British Journal of Nursing, 19*(10), 641–647. http://dx.doi.org/10.12968/bjon.2010.19.10.48203

Lopez-Class, M., Castro, F. G., & Ramirez, A. G. (2011). Conceptions of acculturation: a review and statement of critical issues. *Social Science & Medicine, 72*(9), 1555–1562. http://dx.doi.org/10.1016/j.socscimed.2011.03.011

Loveman, E., Al-Khudairy, L., Johnson, R. E., Robertson, W., Colquitt, J. L., Mead, E. L., et al. (2015). Parent-only interventions for childhood overweight or obesity in children aged 5 to 11 years. *The Cochrane Database of Systematic Reviews* (12), CD012008. http://dx.doi.org/10.1002/14651858.CD012008

Maynard, M. J. (2017). Faith-based institutions as venues for obesity prevention. *Current Obesity Reports, 6*(2), 148–154. http://dx.doi.org/10.1007/s13679-017-0257-8

Misra, A., & Ganda, O. P. (2007). Migration and its impact on adiposity and type 2 diabetes. *Nutrition, 23*(9), 696–708. https://doi.org/10.1016/j.nut.2007.06.008

Mohamed, A. A., Hassan, A. M., Weis, J. A., Sia, I. G., & Wieland, M. L. (2014). Physical activity among Somali men in Minnesota: barriers, facilitators, and recommendations. *American Journal of Men's Health, 8*(1), 35–44. http://dx.doi.org/10.1177/1557988313489132

Moher, D., Liberati, A., Tetzlaff, J., Altman, D. G., & Group, P. (2009). Preferred reporting items for systematic reviews and meta-analyses: the PRISMA statement. *PLoS Medicine, 6*(7), e1000097. http://dx.doi.org/10.1371/journal.pmed.1000097

Murphy, M., Robertson, W., & Oyebode, O. (2017). Obesity in International Migrant Populations. *Current Obesity Reports, 6*(3), 314–323. http://dx.doi.org/10.1007/s13679-017-0274-7

National Clinical Guideline Centre. (2014). *Obesity: Identification, assessment and management of overweight and obesity in children, young people and adults: partial update of CG43*. London. Retrieved from https://www.ncbi.nlm.nih.gov/pubmed/25535639

National Institute of Nursing Research. (2016). *The NINR strategic plan: Advancing science, improving lives*. (Publication No. 16-NR-7783). Bethesda, MD. Retrieved from https://www.ninr.nih.gov/sites/files/docs/NINR_StratPlan2016_reduced.pdf

National Institute of Nursing Research. (2018). *Director's message: Enhancing the impact of nursing research through community-based participatory research*. Bethesda, MD. Retrieved from National Institute of Nursing Research, National Institutes of Health website: https://www.ninr.nih.gov/aboutninr/directors-message/enhancing-impact-of-nursing-research

Obisesan, O., Kuo, W. H., Brunet, M., Obisesan, A., Akinola, O., & Commodore-Mensah, Y. (2017). Predictors of Obesity Among Nigerian Immigrants in the United States. *Journal of Immigrant and Minority Health, 19*(2), 328–332. http://dx.doi.org/10.1007/s10903-016-0404-4

Ogden, C. L., Carroll, M. D., Kit, B. K., & Flegal, K. M. (2014). Prevalence of childhood and adult obesity in the United States, 2011-2012. *The Journal of the American Medical Association, 311*(8), 806–814. http://dx.doi.org/10.1001/jama.2014.732

Oza-Frank, R., & Cunningham, S. A. (2010). The weight of US residence among immigrants: a systematic review. *Obesity Reviews, 11*(4), 271–280. http://dx.doi.org/10.1111/j.1467-789X.2009.00610.x

Parry, S. (2007). Immigration. In M. Bevir (Ed.), *Encyclopedia of governance* (Vol. 1, pp. 438–436). Thousand Oaks, CA: SAGE.

Perez, L. G., Arredondo, E. M., Elder, J. P., Barquera, S., Nagle, B., & Holub, C. K. (2013). Evidence-based obesity treatment interventions for Latino adults in the U.S.: a systematic review. *American Journal of Preventive Medicine, 44*(5), 550–560. http://dx.doi.org/10.1016/j.amepre.2013.01.016

Renzaho, A. M., Halliday, J. A., Mellor, D., & Green, J. (2015). The Healthy Migrant Families Initiative: development of a culturally competent obesity prevention intervention for African migrants. *BMC Public Health, 15*, 272. http://dx.doi.org/10.1186/s12889-015-1628-2

Renzaho, A. M., Mellor, D., Boulton, K., & Swinburn, B. (2010). Effectiveness of prevention programmes for obesity and chronic diseases among immigrants to developed countries - a systematic review. *Public Health Nutrition, 13*(3), 438–450. http://dx.doi.org/10.1017/S136898000999111X

Ricci, C., Gaeta, M., Rausa, E., Asti, E., Bandera, F., & Bonavina, L. (2015). Long-term effects of bariatric surgery on type II diabetes, hypertension and hyperlipidemia: a meta-analysis and meta-regression study with 5-year follow-up. *Obesity Surgery, 25*(3), 397–405. http://dx.doi.org/10.1007/s11695-014-1442-4

Salant, T., & Lauderdale, D. S. (2003). Measuring culture: a critical review of acculturation and health in Asian immigrant populations. *Social Sciences & Medicine, 57*(1), 71–90.

Saleh, A., Amanatidis, S., & Samman, S. (2002). The effect of migration on dietary intake, type 2 diabetes and obesity: The Ghanaian health and nutrition analysis in Sydney, Australia (Ghanaisa). *Ecology of Food and Nutrition, 41*(3), 255–270.

Satia, J. A. (2010). Dietary acculturation and the nutrition transition: an overview. *Applied Physiology, Nutrition, and Metabolism, 35*(2), 219–223. http://dx.doi.org/10.1139/H10-007

Satia-Abouta, J. (2003). Dietary acculturation: Definition, process, assessment, and implications. *International Journal of Human Ecology, 4*(1), 71–86.

Shelton, D. (2008). Establishing the public's trust through community-based participatory research: a case example to improve health care for a rural Hispanic community. *Annual Review of Nursing Research, 26*, 237–259.

Singh, G. K., Siahpush, M., Hiatt, R. A., & Timsina, L. R. (2011). Dramatic increases in obesity and overweight prevalence and body mass index among ethnic-immigrant and social class groups in the United States, 1976-2008. *Journal of Community Health, 36*(1), 94–110. http://dx.doi.org/10.1007/s10900-010-9287-9

Srivastava, G., & Apovian, C. (2018). Future pharmacotherapy for obesity: New anti-obesity drugs on the horizon. *Current Obesity Reports, 7*(2), 147–161. http://dx.doi.org/10.1007/s13679-018-0300-4

Sternfeld, B., Ainsworth, B. E., & Quesenberry, C. P. (1999). Physical activity patterns in a diverse population of women. *Preventive Medicine, 28*(3), 313–323. http://dx.doi.org/10.1006/pmed.1998.0470

Tapp, H., White, L., Steuerwald, M., & Dulin, M. (2013). Use of community-based participatory research in primary care to improve healthcare outcomes and disparities in care. *Journal of Comparative Effectiveness Research, 2*(4), 405–419. http://dx.doi.org/10.2217/cer.13.45

Terragni, L., Garnweidner, L. M., Pettersen, K. S., & Mosdol, A. (2014). Migration as a turning point in food habits: the early phase of dietary acculturation among women from South Asian, African, and Middle Eastern Countries living in Norway. *Ecology of Food and Nutrition, 53*(3), 273–291. http://dx.doi.org/10.1080/03670244.2013.817402

Thomas, B. H., Ciliska, D., Dobbins, M., & Micucci, S. (2004). A process for systematically reviewing the literature: providing the research evidence for public health nursing interventions. *Worldviews on Evidence-Based Nursing, 1*(3), 176–184. http://dx.doi.org/10.1111/j.1524-475X.2004.04006.x

Tovar, A., Renzaho, A. M., Guerrero, A. D., Mena, N., & Ayala, G. X. (2014). A Systematic Review of Obesity Prevention Intervention Studies among Immigrant Populations in the US. *Current Obesity Reports, 3*, 206–222. http://dx.doi.org/10.1007/s13679-014-0101-3

Trust for America's Health. (2013). *F as in fat: How obesity threatens America's future issue [Report]*. Retrieved from https://www.rwjf.org/content/dam/farm/reports/reports/2013/rwjf407528

Turk, M. T., Fapohunda, A., & Zoucha, R. (2015). Using photovoice to explore Nigerian immigrants' eating and physical activity in the United States. *Journal of Nursing Scholarship, 47*(1), 16–24. http://dx.doi.org/10.1111/jnu.12105

United States Department of Health and Human Services. (2008). *2008 Physical Activity Guidelines for Americans*. (ODPHP Publication No. U0036). Retrieved from https://health.gov/paguidelines/pdf/paguide.pdf

Vaughn, L. M., Jacquez, F., Lindquist-Grantz, R., Parsons, A., & Melink, K. (2017). Immigrants as Research Partners: A Review of Immigrants in Community-Based Participatory Research (CBPR). *Journal of Immigrant and Minority Health, 19*(6), 1457–1468. http://dx.doi.org/10.1007/s10903-016-0474-3

Viruell-Fuentes, E. A., Miranda, P. Y., & Abdulrahim, S. (2012). More than culture: structural racism, intersectionality theory, and immigrant health. *Social Science & Medicine, 75*(12), 2099–2106. http://dx.doi.org/10.1016/j.socscimed.2011.12.037

Wieland, M. L., Hanza, M. M. M., Weis, J. A., Meiers, S. J., Patten, C. A., Clark, M. M., et al. (2018). Healthy Immigrant Families: Randomized Controlled Trial of a Family-Based Nutrition and Physical Activity Intervention. *American Journal of Health Promotion, 32*(2), 473–484. http://dx.doi.org/10.1177/0890117117733342

Wieland, M. L., Weis, J. A., Hanza, M. M., Meiers, S. J., Patten, C. A., Clark, M. M., et al. (2016). Healthy immigrant families: Participatory development and baseline characteristics of a community-based physical activity and nutrition intervention. *Contemporary Clinical Trials, 47*, 22–31. http://dx.doi.org/10.1016/j.cct.2015.12.004

Wieland, M. L., Weis, J. A., Palmer, T., Goodson, M., Loth, S., Omer, F., et al. (2012). Physical activity and nutrition among immigrant and refugee women: a community-based participatory research approach. *Women's Health Issues, 22*(2), e225–e232. http://dx.doi.org/10.1016/j.whi.2011.10.002

Wilson, R. D., & Elgoghail, N. (2016). Bronx Health Education Project for West African Immigrants. *Journal of Cultural Diversity, 23*(1), 34–36.

World Health Organization. (2017). Obesity and overweight. Retrieved from http://www.who.int/mediacentre/factsheets/fs311/en

CHAPTER 6

# The Impact of the Political and Policy Cultures of Washington, DC, on the Affordable Care Act

Sr. Rosemary Donley and Carmen Kiraly


## ABSTRACT

The Patient Protection and Affordable Care Act of 2010 (PPACA) is the health policy framework to discuss the contemporary culture and political landscape of Washington, DC. Since its implementation, PPACA has directly engaged the White House, Executive agencies, the Congress, the Circuit and Supreme Courts, governors, state legislators, health insurers, the pharmaceutical industry, health lobbyists, the media and the press. What makes the Patient Protection and Affordable Care Act so provocative? Passed as the centerpiece of the legislative legacy of President Barack Obama, PPACA was designed to provide under- and uninsured American citizens access to continuous affordable health insurance. During Congressional debates, objections to PPACA were based on its cost and its impact on enhancing the role of the federal government in the design and financing of public and private health insurance plans. The bill passed Congress with a narrow margin of Democratic votes. After PPACA was enacted, specific objections focused on its mandates: the Individual, the Provider, and the Employer mandates, and the expansion of Medicaid. In the 2015–16 Presidential campaign, Repealing "Obama Care," another name for PPACA, was a centerpiece of Donald J. Trump's presidential campaign platform. When all electoral votes



http://dx.doi.org/10.1891/0739-6686.37.187

were counted, Donald J. Trump became the 45th President of the United States and both branches of Congress were under the control of the Republican Party. Repeal of PPACA was back on the Presidential and Congressional agenda.

## INTRODUCTION

This chapter examines government culture in Washington, DC, during and after the passage of the Patient Protection and Affordable Care Act (ACA) of 2010 (PPACA, 2010). Why was the time surrounding the passage of the ACA, as the Patient Protection and ACA is now called, selected to exemplify the political and cultural environment of the federal government? The ACA, the signature piece of legislation of the 111th Congress, passed by a party-oriented vote during the presidency of Barack Obama (2009–2017) (Beaussier, 2012). The ACA is important; it is the first major health law enacted since Medicare and Medicaid in 1965. Its passage was a major policy accomplishment because the ACA has the potential to radically transform the healthcare delivery environment (Skinner & Amitabh, 2016), healthcare financing (Hall & McCue, 2016), and the work of health professionals (Anderson, 2014).

The ACA was designed to reduce the number of under- and uninsured Americans, the only developed country that links access to health insurance to employment status, age, poverty, or disability rather than to citizenship (Vladeck, 2003). Although the ACA is not a comprehensive national health insurance plan, 23 million of the previously uninsured 37 million citizens had obtained affordable health insurance by 2016 (The Commonwealth Fund, 2016).

The ACA also engages the federal government more intimately in healthcare financing and in the design of mandated health benefits (Hill, 2012). These initiatives were expressed in key components of the law: the Individual, Employer, and Provider mandates, and the Medicaid Expansion program (Quadagno, 2014).

The ACA has ardent supporters and vigorous opponents within and outside of Washington, DC. Repealing ACA, pejoratively called "Obamacare," was a campaign issue during the 2015–16 presidential election and dominated the congressional agenda during the fall of 2017 (Oberlander, 2014). Near the end of 2017, Congress passed a tax bill. An amendment to repeal the ACA's Individual Mandate was appended to the tax bill (Wagner, 2017). Although the ACA was not on the public agenda in the spring or summer of 2018, federal agencies used their regulatory power to impede its implementation (Cunningham, 2018). The 2019 budget also proposed cuts to Medicare and Medicaid. While these proposed budget changes are directed at the two largest entitlement programs, Medicare and Medicaid, they also represent an effort to strip away some of the benefits to the elderly, disabled, and poor Americans that were enacted in the ACA (Bunis, 2018b).

## WASHINGTON, DC, IS A SMALL SOUTHERN TOWN

Americans and others, whose careers, incomes, and world views center on government, live in the capital city of the free world. These citizens of the Beltway, a name used to describe residents of the District of Columbia and daily commuters from nearby Maryland and Virginia, are ambassadors and embassy staff, judges of the Supreme Court, members of Congress, Cabinet members, members of the military, and staff who work at all levels of government. They may be lobbyists, scholars, or staff members at universities and think tanks, or employees at local hotels and restaurants. They are members of the media and the press or workers in service and transportation industries. Another group, former government employees who live inside the Beltway, is composed of private sector contractors who perform work previously done by federal workers in security, military operations, and aerospace activities around the world. Blackwater, perhaps the most recognized of this group, was hired during the Bush administration to offer security services during the Iraq war. The engagement of Blackwater's employees in a deadly gun battle in Baghdad raised questions about the legal status of private sector contractors and the management and oversight of their work (Singer, 2007).

In addition to the Beltway residents, visitors come to Washington, DC, from all parts of the United States and around the world. Tourists marvel at the symbols of governmental culture: the White House, the Houses of Congress, and the Supreme Court, while others seek to influence the work of government.

Career pathways and upward mobility exist inside the Beltway. Some political appointees leave town when the persons or party that brought them to Washington loses a position or political influence; others succumb to "Potomac Fever," developing a deep attachment to the alluring capital city. The political and policy environments in Washington energize them; they relish that national news is local news. Inside the Beltway, you do not need to move to another part of the country when seeking a new job. Washingtonians frequently change jobs within governmental agencies and supporting structures and industries. For example, during their careers, many former members of Congress and their staffs work in executive agencies and think tanks, teach at local universities, or join private contractors or lobbying firms (Center for Responsive Politics, n.d.; Rennie, n.d.). These transitions commonly occur after elections, when the President or Members of Congress change. Social introductions in the capital city usually include brief bios of career pathways.

## THE CULTURE IN WASHINGTON, DC

The government shapes the culture of Washington, DC. Although most residents of the Beltway work for the government directly or indirectly, many were not born in Washington, DC. They came or were assigned for academic or employment reasons. The climate of the area, the many beautiful buildings, museums, libraries, concert halls, theaters, restaurants, and social events make it a desirable and ideal place to live (Weiner, n.d.). In DC, it is possible to live in a single house, an apartment in a condominium, or on a houseboat on the Potomac. The citizenry spans many age groups and is ethnically and racially diverse (Stein, 2015). Consequently, Washington is more than a stop of "must see cities," described in tour books or restaurant guides. It is a mecca that attracts people not only from the United States, but from around the world.

Anthropologists have struggled for years to define culture. A common theme in most definitions is that culture and its knowledge, beliefs, morals, laws and customs are shared among individuals in a society (Tyler, 1871). If you look at the cultures that drive and inspire the American government, you realize that the American government has many cultures. The cultures of the White House and the executive agencies differ from the cultures of the House of Representatives or the Senate. Cultures vary within and among the estimated 480 Federal departments, agencies, executive agencies, and units (Crews, 2015). The houses of Congress express their own cultural norms and practices. There are significant cultural differences within and between the House and the Senate. The culture of the Supreme Court is unique because its members hold life time terms of office (Taylor, 2005).

## THE CULTURE OF THE WHITE HOUSE

Spencer-Oatey (2008) described culture as "shared basic assumptions and values, ways of living, belief systems, policies, procedures and behavioral conventions that influence how a person behaves and how he/she interprets the behavior of others" (p. 3). The culture of the White House revolves around the personality and value system of the President and the people whom he selects as his closest advisors and staff members. It is also affected by national and world events. Gone are the days when the President could walk across the street from the White House to enjoy a glass of brandy and a cigar in the lobby of the Willard Hotel ("Where does the term," n.d.) Because terrorism has become commonplace around the world, the President is a protected and isolated person. Surrounded by live-in bodyguards, members of the Secret Service guard the President and his family. They are driven in convoys of armored vehicles, transported in military airplanes, and generally kept away from ordinary citizens. The White House, a "no fly zone," is enclosed within high fences and under continuous human and electronic surveillance. The private residence of the President and his family is not accessible. No one can drop in and visit the White House (Walsh, 2013). Tours are scheduled and guests and visitors are carefully screened. When the current President goes to one of his golf resorts or to his home in Palm Beach, Florida, trees, artificial barriers, and electronic and personal security systems protect him and his family. Security is a little more difficult in New York City because Trump Tower is a public building with offices, stores, restaurants, and private apartments (Watson, 2017).

Ordinary people see and hear the President during television appearances, news conferences, or when he welcomes and honors Americans and visiting international dignitaries in the Rose Garden. President Trump has increased his access to the public through his use of social media such as Twitter. He also holds campaign style rallies around the United States and visits states and districts to support Republican candidates. Although President Trump limits interviews and news conferences, his spokespeople are interviewed on most of the Sunday TV talk shows. Several DC-based news services, notably the Cable News Network (CNN), Consumer News and Business Channel (CNBC), and Fox News focus the majority of their coverage on the White House and the President. Although Donald Trump was not named *Time* magazine's 2017 Man of the Year, he dominates the news cycle.

President Trump has an ambitious global and domestic policy agenda. Although, some items on his agenda were campaign promises, other issues have risen or gained primacy during his first year and one half in office. Globally, there is concern with the Islamic State of Iraq and Syria (ISIS), refugees, climate change, and trade. This agenda engages many countries: Russia, North Korea, South Korea, Turkey, China, Iran, Mexico, and the European Union (Goldberg, 2017). President Trump's domestic agenda include: repealing the ACA, middle class tax cuts, controlling immigration, building a wall between the United States and Mexico, improving the infrastructure in the United States, and reviewing safety net programs such as food stamps, housing, and Medicaid (Berenson, 2018).

## THE CULTURE OF THE EXECUTIVE AGENCIES

Each agency has its own culture and ethos. Although the leadership team in the executive agencies is appointed and serves at the will of the President, the agencies are staffed by professional career employees who are experts in their fields. Although most agency employees have political preferences, over their careers they work in bi-partisan environments with Republican and Democratic administrations.

Bureaucracy is the term used to characterize the structure and decision-making processes used by governmental agencies. Sociologist Max Weber (1978) identified two essential elements of successful bureaucracies: hierarchical structures and rational–legal decision-making rules. He argued that bureaucracies eliminate favoritism, maximize efficiency, and maintain order (Phillips, n.d.). In well-developed bureaucracies, work products and recommendations may originate at the lower rungs of the organization. These recommendations wind their way through a serpentine process that ends at the top of the hierarchical pyramid. The outcome of the decision is then filtered down to the group that prepared the documents for consideration and will be responsible for their implementation. In most bureaucracies, the process is reversed; what is to be done comes "top down" (Sisney, 2016). The President or the Secretary of the Agency tells its staff what programs to emphasize or ignore. For example, during the Trump administration, the Secretary of the Environmental Protection Agency (EPA) has targeted 67 regulations that he plans to eliminate (Popovich, Albeck-Ripka, & Pierre-Louis, 2018).

Sharing information within large bureaucratic structures is a slow process. In the days when communication was a flow of paper, important documents were hidden in stacks of paper. Failure to move the paper up or down the hierarchical lattices delayed decision making and program implementation. In a computerized world, data files contain and store the work of government and the outcomes of decision making processes. Computerized data can become buried in file systems or placed in wrong files. Potter (2016) offers an explanation that goes beyond losing track of papers or computerized files. She argues that agencies can speed up or slow down the regulation development process to avoid Presidential or Congressional oversight.

A newer concern with electronic data storage systems is their vulnerability to being tampered with or erased by others who are not authorized to use or know the content of these files. Many individuals, even those who are not computer literate, are familiar with break-ins, leaked emails, secret servers, and unsecured cell phones (Storm, 2017). Although government agencies and offices have security systems to protect their data, hacking remains an international threat. As WikiLeaks (n.d.) aptly demonstrated, it is possible to hack and then leak or publish confidential files.

While some people fault bureaucratic processes as slow and top heavy, they are the mode of operations in federal agencies. The chain of command is clear, and rules are to be followed.

The Agencies in the Executive branch of government have a reciprocal relationship and influence with the President and the Congress (University of Minnesota, n.d.).

The culture of each agency is shaped by its mission and history. For example, the mission of the State Department requires its political appointees, career bureaucrats, and foreign service employees to work domestically and globally. Employees of the State Department travel frequently and often live for years in different countries (United States Department of State, n.d.). The culture in the Department of Health and Human Services reflects the diverse mission of its departments. Regulatory agencies, such as the Food and Drug Administration (FDA) that work with pharmaceutical industries, farmers, and lobbyists, have a different culture than the National Institutes of Health whose constituencies are faculty and researchers in academic health centers across the United States (DHHS, n.d.).

The Department of Justice emphasizes compliance and accountability. While the impetus of this guidance around compliance may have come from efforts to investigate fraud, the call for accountability addresses the Justice Department's code of silence (Robertson, 2017). This code of silence or secrecy reflects a protective instinct of the Department and its tendency to resist change or new ideas. The Agency's tendencies to work alone and limit the sharing of intelligence with other governmental agencies or local justice and police authorities were called into question after 9/11 (September 11, 2001) when 19 Islamic terrorists hijacked four plans and attempted to destroy significant American buildings in New York and Washington, DC ("9/11 attacks," 2001). It became apparent that federal agencies entrusted with security were not sharing information with each other. While Washington is a city where information is leaked, some agencies espouse the policy that information obtained by their agents or informants stays within their agency. The Justice Department is an Agency that is known for keeping its business out of the public view (Smith, 2017). However, during the presidencies of President Obama and Trump, the Justice department was instructed to investigate the use of excessive force by police departments in various cities and states (Editorial Board, 2017). The interested citizens that evoked this public response were not world leaders or powerful lobbies. Those most concerned about this issue were families, neighbors, and citizens who believed that they and their neighbors and family members deserved to be treated with dignity and justice. This directive to the Justice department to investigate police brutality brought Justice Department employees into neighborhoods and communities and gave them direct contact with local police and security forces (Hersher, 2017). Contemporary culture makes it difficult to conduct secret investigations because ordinary citizens have smart cell phones and recording devices; situations being investigated can be seen on social media long before official reports are written or made.

The Department of Justice is frequently in the news. During the presidencies of President Clinton and President Trump, the Justice Department appointed special prosecutors to examine behaviors and activities that negatively impacted the President and the White House (Isaac, 2017). Currently the investigation into Russian interference in the 2016 election is wide reaching, and of serious concern to the Congress, the Justice Department and the White House. President Trump frequently refers to this investigation as a "witch hunt" designed to cast doubt on the validity of his election (Scott & Burton, 2018). Others argue that foreign government's interference in American elections is a threat to democracy that merits investigation (Zarate, 2017).

In our global world, withholding information from other intelligence agencies or from the public is no longer the preferred practice. Yet, it is hard to change practices that are deeply rooted in workplaces cultures where people stay for many years. Deputy Assistant Attorney General Snyder spoke to this phenomenon in the paper he presented to the International Chamber of Commerce, *Compliance is part of the culture, not just a policy* (Snyder, 2014).

## THE CULTURE OF THE CONGRESS

The Congress is accessible to ordinary people. Although persons without badges must go through security screening processes similar to those found in airports, ordinary citizens can visit Congressional offices and meet with their Congressman's personal and legislative staffs. If the Congressmen or Congresswomen are available, they can speak directly with them. The Congress is composed of two bodies: House of Representatives and the Senate. Although each body shares legislative responsibility, each makes its unique contributions to governmental and legislative endeavors. The culture of the House of Representatives, the lower House, was modeled on the House of Commons in the British Parliament. In the United States, the House of Representatives' accountability is to its constituents in their Districts, specific geographical areas within each state. The total number of members in the House of Representative is 435, a number determined by each state's population (United States House of Representatives, n.d.). In large states like Pennsylvania, the majority of Representatives cluster in the state's populous areas. To assure their responsiveness to constituents, Representatives serve 2-year terms. The length of their terms and their close association with their constituents influence the culture of the House of Representatives. Representatives make frequent trips to their Districts, monitor local news and print media, and speak and vote for issues in committees, conferences and on the floor of the

House that affect the economic and personal well-being of their constituents (New York Times, 2013).

Two Senators who serve 6-year terms represent each state. The Senate of the United States was modeled on the British Parliament's House of Lords. Senators are not as accessible to ordinary citizens as are members of the House. Senators focus on statewide corporate issues and the economy of their states. While it is possible for an ordinary person to meet with a Senator, it is more likely that he or she will talk with a member of the Senator's personal, legislative or committee staffs. Senators have unique responsibilities, often explained by the phrase, the Senate's role is to advise and consent. These duties are reflected in the Committee structure in the Senate that differs from that of the House. Only the Senate can approve major Presidential appointments to the Cabinet and Executive branch of government, ratify treaties, and preside over Presidential impeachment trials (United States Senate, n.d.a). However, the power to introduce tax bills is reserved for members of the House of Representatives.

In the past, it was possible to compare the credentials and experiential background of Senators with members of the House. These comparisons addressed education, professional training, previous governmental experience, personal or family wealth, party identification and ideological positions. Today, there are fewer differences among Senators and Representatives. More members of Congress possessed some governmental experience, often in their state assemblies, before they ran for Congress. Some Senators were once members of the House of Representatives. Many members of Congress are lawyers; some have been federal prosecutors. Social status and personal wealth no longer distinguish members of the Senate from their colleagues in the House of Representatives (United States Senate, n.d.b).

One factor that has not disappeared with time is the desire to remain in Congress. No one becomes a committee chair, a ranking member, or a political leader by serving one term in office. Members of Congress are always working to stay in office. Representatives begin to campaign during their first year of their first 2-year term. Campaigning means returning to the District frequently and keeping in contact with constituents and what they want. It means keeping promises, mailing newsletters, accepting invitations to District or state events, actively pursuing campaign promises, seeking endorsements from influential organizations and individuals in the state or District, and introducing new legislation, and/or voting in favor of bills that are important to constituents and financial supporters (Lewis & Arkedis, 2014). Some members of Congress represent "safe districts" or hold "safe seats." However, even in safe Districts, members of Congress in their first terms and those who have served in Congress for many years are vulnerable at election time. Another factor that influences election outcomes is the political and ideological composition of the district. When the composition of a district changes, the incumbent must forge new relationships and build new coalitions (Levitt, n.d.). Although party identification was once very important in elections, support from the party and its leaders does not always assure election.

Partisan politics remain a major determinant of Congressional culture, expressed through party identification and a shared political ideology. Even though party loyalty is a major theme, it is too simple to say that one is a Republican, a Democrat, or an Independent. There is a continuum of political and policy ideologies within each major party (Khan Academy, n.d.). Historically, Republicans valued free trade, low taxes, and less government regulation of the economy or interference in business or persons' lives. Republicans support the second amendment and vehemently oppose gun control. They endorse a strong military, family values, and private schools. They are conservative on many social issues, women's and gay rights, and abortion ("Democrat vs. Republican," n.d.). Today, there are identifiable groups within the Republican Party: the Tea Party, Libertarians, Freedom Caucus, Alt Right and Moderates; each group or members within each group emphasize one or more traditional Republican values. It is difficult to gain consensus among the Republicans.

The Party of Jefferson takes a more liberal stand on policy issues. Democrats believe that government should be engaged in the lives of Americans, especially those in need. They oppose policies and laws that benefit the rich, especially when the poor are most affected by these decisions. They endorse organized labor, women's rights, social welfare programs, Medicaid, the entitlement programs, and public schools. They believe in equality. Politicians identify with typical Democratic values along a continuum of moderate, liberal, and far left perspectives ("Democrat vs. Republican," n.d.). Political ideology influences what issues come before the Congress and what bills become Public Laws. When one party holds the White House and the majority of seats in both Houses, they are able to advance their agenda if they can get agreement among members of their party. In 2016, Republicans won the majority of seats in the Congress and elected a Republican as the 45th President (Berky & Kazda, 2018).

As noted earlier in this chapter, repeal of the ACA was one of the major themes in the presidential campaign of Donald Trump (Blendon & Benson, 2014). After the 2016 election, the Republicans had enough votes to pass any bill that they introduced. However, even with a majority in both Houses, Republicans found that constituents and party members valued and supported some of the programs in the ACA. For example, under the ACA, young adults can be insured under their parents' health plans until they are 26 years of age. People with existing illnesses, heart disease, cancer, or other chronic diseases, cannot be denied access to health insurance plans or be forced to pay expensive premiums to maintain their health insurance coverage (Blumenthal & Collins, 2014). Faced with constituent objections to repeal the ACA, the Republican leaders developed new language to express their intent: Repeal became Repeal and Replace (Lambrew, 2017).

On the President's 105th day in office, the Republican members of the House of Representatives passed their effort to replace rather than repeal the ACA. The American HealthCare Reform Act of 2017 (HCRA) (HR 277, 2017) was passed in the House and sent to the Senate (Kaplan & Pear, 2017). However, HCRA faced a different fate in the Senate. In the end, it failed to obtain the necessary number of votes; the deciding vote that defeated HCRA was cast by Senator John McCain (Pear & Kaplan, 2017). Republicans in both houses went back to the drawing board. The Senate produced what was called the "Skinny bill," a proposal to repeal the Individual and the Employer mandates and defund Planned Parenthood (Luhby, 2017; Sullivan, 2017). The Skinny bill was also defeated (Pear & Kaplan, 2017). The Majority leader in the Senate, Mitch McConnell, said that it was time to move on (LoGiurato, 2017).

Near the end of 2017, the Republican Congress found another vehicle to lessen the impact of the ACA. During his campaign, Donald Trump promised to lower taxes for the middle class. As the tax bill was debated, an amendment to repeal the Individual Mandate, one of the pillars of the ACA, was introduced, debated, passed, and appended to the tax bill ("The GOP tax bill," 2017).

The Individual Mandate was not the most popular component of the ACA (Traser, 2017). Designed to reduce the cost of increasing access to health insurance for the under- and uninsured, the ACA required that everyone ineligible for employer-based, the healthcare program of the U.S. Department of Defense (TRI-CARE) or other federal health insurance programs must obtain an approved healthcare plan from the ACA Exchange or pay for it from his or her own resources. All approved insurance plans specified a preventative health benefit. Objections to the Individual Mandate came from many constituents and members of Congress. Concern was expressed that mandating preventative health benefits increased the cost of the health insurance plan and contained health services that were not needed by everyone such as prenatal care. Other criticisms centered on the limited number of providers included within some provider networks. Others found that the plan that they selected required them to change physicians or hospitals and pay more for their new insurance coverage (Hardcastle, Record, Jacobson, & Gostin, 2011). However, the most vocal objections to the Individual Mandate came from many members of congress, their constituents, and church groups who objected to the health promotion section of the ACA. They argued that the requirement to purchase health plans that included contraception and abortion violated their religious beliefs (Bill of Rights Institute, n.d.).

The tax bill proved to be a good vehicle to repeal the Individual Mandate. The tax bill was attractive to many Americans; the Individual mandate was not. After much debate, an amended tax bill was passed in the House and Senate. The tax bill and the amendment to repeal the Individual Mandate was signed into law by President Trump (Paletta & Stein, 2017). The Individual Mandate is no longer a component of the ACA.

Since this repeal, no new Congressional efforts to replace or repeal the ACA have been undertaken. However, there is concern that the House plans to reform Medicare and reexamine Medicaid Expansion (Rosenbaum, 2012). The outcome of the Republican leaders' plan to use savings from cuts to Medicare and Medicaid to pay for the tax cuts contained in the recent tax bill will be determined by the 2018 Congressional elections (Bunis, 2018b).

Because of the deep divisions within and between the Houses of Congress, legislative activity has lessened. Congress is investigating Russian involvement in the election of 2016 and visiting shelters for children that have been separated from their families who came across U.S. borders without proper documents (Delk, 2018; Weigel, 2018). While there is rhetoric and growing public concern around gun control, fueled by the young people who attended schools where gun violence has occurred, there has been no executive or legislative efforts to mandate background checks on gun buyers, regulate gun sales, especially at gun shows or online websites, or ban the sale of assault-type weapons. Evidence shows that after a mass shooting, gun sales increase. Commentators speculate that gun owners know that President Trump will not support gun control legislation (Locker, 2017).

## THE CULTURE OF THE SUPREME COURT

The culture in the Supreme Court differs from that of the White House, the Executive Agencies, and the Congress as is evident when the President selects a Justice for the High Court. After the President interviews and then nominates a candidate for the Supreme Court, the candidate is interviewed by the Judiciary Committee of the Senate. After this interview process is completed, the members of the Judiciary Committee vote on whether the nomination of the candidate should go forward to the Senate. When the name of the candidate is forwarded to the Senate, the process continues. If a simple majority of the Senate affirms the candidate, the name of the candidate is forwarded to the President. If this candidate remains the President's choice, he or she is appointed to the Supreme Court (Morrison, 2016). Supreme Court judges have life-long terms to preserve their integrity and keep them somewhat separated from influence by the political side of

Washington. Presidents and members of their parties are very pleased when they have the opportunity to appoint a Supreme Court Justice because it is believed that these appointees will reflect and sustain their party's ideologies and values well past the terms of those who appointed them (Hirschfeld Davis & Landler, 2017).

Over the past 20 years, six justices have been appointed to the nine-member High Court. Ronald Regan (1998), George H. W. Busch (1991), and Donald Trump (2017) appointed one justice during their terms of office. Presidents Clinton (1993, 1994) and George Bush, and Barack Obama (2009, 2010) and Donald Trump (2017, 2018) appointed two Justices (Hirschfeld Davis & Landler, 2017; Tilllmann, n.d.). Given the importance of their work and the length of their tenure, it is not surprising that a highly charged political climate surrounds confirmation hearings to fill vacancies on the Court. Confirmations can be lengthy and tedious. Justice Clarence Thomas was nominated on 1 July 1991; his hearings began on 10 September 1991, and he was confirmed on 15 October 2016 after hours of questioning by the Senate Judiciary Committee (Truffaut-Wong, 2016).

The Supreme Court has exclusive jurisdiction over civil actions and appellate jurisdiction over decisions made by state and federal circuit courts (Sousa, 2017). Another interesting component of the High Court is that its Justices decide which of the cases referred by lower courts within their jurisdiction will be heard (FindLaw, n.d.). *Certiorari* (cert) is the term used when the Supreme Court decides to review the judgment of a lower court (Legal Information Institute, n.d.). Given the focus of this chapter, it is appropriated to ask how did the Justices respond to lower court challenges to the ACA?

The ACA, signed into law by President Obama on March 23, 2010, extended health insurance benefits to all American citizens. Twenty-six states, along with several private parties, challenged the ACA in several federal circuit courts. The Supreme Court granted cert and, during March 2012, heard oral arguments regarding the ACA's constitutionality. The Court released its opinion on June 28, 2012 regarding challenges to two key provisions of the ACA: Medicaid Expansion and the Individual Mandate. In discussing Medicaid Expansion, the Court ruled that expanding Medicaid to cover all individuals living at or under 133% of the federal poverty level (FPL) exceeded the federal government's power to require states to comply with federal regulations (Kaiser Family Foundation [KFF], 2012).

Chief Justice Roberts, the writer of the Majority opinion, said that the Medicaid Expansion is constitutional if applied only to new Medicaid funds. The ruling also concluded that the Medicaid Expansion is unconstitutional if it allows the Secretary of Health and Human Services (HHS) to withdraw all Medicaid funding from states that do not comply with the expansion. If, the Secretary's power only applies to new Medicaid funding, the expansion is constitutional.

In the case of the Individual Mandate, the Court ruled that the requirement to maintain minimum essential coverage is unconstitutional if it is dependent upon Congress's Commerce power, but is Constitutional as a tax under Congress's taxing power. Commenting further, Justice Roberts wrote that The Anti-Injunction Act (AIA) does not bar suits challenging the individual mandate. He argued that although the mandate is a tax under Article 1 of the Constitution, Congress labeled the tax a "penalty," indicating that it did not intend the AIA to apply. He also opined that the requirement that nonexempt individuals obtain health insurance is constitutional under Congress' authority to tax and spend (Center for Health Law and Policy Innovation, 2012).

## THE CULTURE OF THE WHITE HOUSE REVISITED

Many politicians come to Washington, DC, promising to change its culture. While President Trump may be the latest person to announce his intention to "drain the swamp," he is not the only President or newly elected politician to run on an agenda of change (Overby, 2017). Once politicians arrive on Capitol Hill, they learn that cultural change is a lengthy process and is not the real business of government. Culture is expressed through customs about behaviors not outcomes. Successful politicians adapt and learn to manipulate cultural obstacles and maneuver through Washington, DC, and the halls of the White House, the Congress, and the Supreme Court. Congressional newcomers to Washington learn the culture in their new home town from experienced law makers and their political advisors, "old Washington hands," and staff members who work with them in Washington and in their district offices ("Capitol Hill Definitions and Congressional Staff Positions," n.d.). They are given opportunities for formal orientations and guidance on setting up an office and an office budget (Bowman, 2014). Initial and frequent briefing sessions conducted by both parties' leadership teams and political caucuses explain the current legislative agenda and how the various branches of government work. Staying in contact with their district offices and their constituents reminds members of Congress of their campaign promises and the concerns of the persons who elected them. Newcomers learn to look at each bill through the eyes of their constituents and the needs of their districts. Some newly elected Presidents or members of Congress bring their campaign staffs/advisors with them to Washington. However, being in the White House or serving in Congress is very different than running a successful political campaign (Tenpas, 2018).

Political appointees to the many federal agencies learn the rules of the various bureaucracies from the professional careerists in their agencies. The process of going from the private sector into the federal bureaucracy has been studied by the Brookings Institute, a respected think tank in Washington, DC (Cohen, 1995). Cabinet members have major responsibilities and budgets. Although their number is small when compared to the career bureaucrats, there is a predictable rhythm to the legislative cycle and the work of the Supreme Court, the President and the White House influence the Congressional agenda. President Trump is not as predictable as his predecessors. He has the ability to confuse and sometimes contradict his staff, Cabinet secretaries and Congressional leaders.

A glimpse into Donald Trump's style of decision-making is revealed in his 1987 book, *The Art of the Deal* (Trump & Schwartz, 1987). Early in the book, Donald Trump describes an average week in his life. His report of conversations and meetings provide details of planned real estate ventures and discussions about the pros and cons of real estate that he wants to purchase or sell. The reader also learns about his litigation history with contractors and others. Many of his reported phone calls are with attorneys. His self-report describes a hard-working man who admires people who give terse reports and conduct business quickly. His account of a typical week suggests that he knows influential people who will take his calls. When the book was published, Donald Trump was a 40-year-old man with a young family. He had many deals going on simultaneously. Reading the book in 2018, you can hear President Trump speaking as if he were at his town meetings. You also get an insight into how he thinks and acts. In the real estate business, he relied on his instincts as much as he listened to the words of his advisors, even those whom he considered smart and competent. He has been socialized to win and to make money. He seems to be comfortable with ambiguity and uncertainty. His previous world did not involve separation of powers or bureaucratic hierarchies. He wants things done quickly and in his way. He is used to being boss and the person in charge. He values success and the respect that comes with it. He speaks freely and does not seem to be restrained by facts or the presentation of evidence. He creates his own world. He obviously wants to be the most successful President in the history of the United States. It is hard to know if Donald Trump's style will permanently influence the culture or the politics of Washington, DC.

## THE CULTURE OF NURSING

What impact does knowledge of the culture and politics of Washington, DC, have on the nursing community. The Kaiser Family Foundation (KFF, 2018) reports there are 3,386,668 professionally active registered nurses in the United States. Everyone knows a nurse; many politicians have nurses in their families and in their neighborhoods. Nurses should have influence on health policy because of their knowledge, their practices, their numbers, and their geographic dispersion (Burke, 2016). Yet in the opinion of this author, nurses are noticeable absent at policy tables, possibly because their leadership has failed to resolve its classic policy disagreement about the level of education that nurses should have before they enter professional practice. Recently, 53 years since the ANA's position paper on entry into practice, two major organizations, the American Association of Colleges of Nursing and the National League for Nursing (NLN) issued draft documents that re-affirmed their traditional positions on entry into practice (NLN Communications, 2018). While these documents are still under development, they provide evidence that the lack of consensus on the initial educational preparation of new nurses persists.

## REFERENCES


Anderson, A. (2014). The impact of the Affordable Care Act on the health care workforce. Retrieved from http://www.heritage.org/healthcare-reform/report/the-impact-the-affordable-care-act-the-healthcare-workforce

Beaussier, A. (2012). The patient protection and Affordable Care Act: The victory of unorthodox lawmaking. *Journal of Health Politics, Policy and Law*, *37*(5), 741–778.

Berenson, T. (2018). 4 things President Trump wants to accomplish in 2018. Retrieved from http://time.com/5084907/donald-trump-2018-calendar

Berky, B., & Kazda, A. (2018). Here's what Congress will try to accomplish in 2018 and the likelihood of it happening. Retrieved from https://www.ourpursuit.com/congress-accomplish-2018/?gclid=EAIaIQobChMI08ifiYHj3AIVjuDICh27uwF8EAAYASAAEgKIb_D_BwE

Bill of Rights Institute. (n.d.). Religious freedom and Affordable Care Act. Retrieved from https://billofrightsinstitute.org/educate/educator-resources/lessons-plans/current-events/religious-freedom-and-the-affordable-care-act

Blendon, R. J., & Benson, J. M. (2014). Votes and the Affordable Care Act in 2014 election. *New England Journal of Medicine*, *371*, E31(1)–E31(7).

Blumenthal, D., & Collins, S. R. (2014). Healthcare coverage under the Affordable Care Act-A progress report. *New England Journal of Medicine*, *371*, 275–281.

Bowman, B. (2014). New member orientation welcomes new class of lawmakers. Retrieved from https://www.rollcall.com/news/new-member-orientation-welcomes-new-class-of-lawmakers

Bunis, D. (2018a). Will the next Congress cut Medicaid? AARP Bulletin. Retrieved from https://www.aarp.org/politics-society/government-elections/info-2018/medicare-midterm-elections.html

Bunis, D. (2018b). President's budget targets Medicare, Medicaid and food stamps. Retrieved from https://www.aarp.org/politics-society/government-elections/info-2018/trump-budgetaffects-seniors-fd.html

Burke, S (2016). Influence through policy: Nurses have a unique role. *Reflection on Nursing Leadership (RNL)*. Indianapolis, IN: Sigma Theta Tau Int.

Capitol Hill Definitions and Congressional Staff Positions. (n.d.). Retrieved from https://www.ncoa.org/public-policy-action/advocacy-toolkit/understanding-congress/capitol-hill-terms

Center for Health Law and Policy Innovation. (2012). Summary of the decision of the U.S. Supreme Court on the Patient Protection and Affordable Care Act. Retrieved from https://www.chlpi.org/wp-content/uploads/2013/12/SCOTUS_ACA_Summary_6-29-12.pdf

Center for Responsive Politics. (n.d.). Influence and lobbying. Retrieved from https://www.google.com/search?source=hp&ei=FG1oW4yFMoG4ggeF-42wBA&q=opensecrets.org&oq=opensecrets.org&gs_l=psy-ab.3..0l10.27206.33668.0.35203.15.9.0.6.6.0.72.540.9.9.0....0...1c.1.64.psy-ab..0.15.568...0i131k1j0i10k1.0.Y3oOkoMftVg

Cohen, D. M. (1995). Amateur government: When political appointees manage the federal bureaucracy. Retrieved from https://www.brookings.edu/wp-content/uploads/2016/06/amateur.pdf

The Commonwealth Fund Biennial Health Insurance Survey. (2016). How the Affordable Care Act has improved Americans' ability to buy health insurance on their own. Retrieved from http://www.commonwealthfund.org/publications/issue-briefs/2017/feb/how-the-aca-has-improved-ability-to-buy-insurance

Crews, C. W. (2015). Nobody knows how many Federal Agencies exist. Competitive Enterprise Institute. Retrieved from https://cei.org/blog/nobody-knows-how-many-federal-agencies-exist

Cunningham, P. W. (2018). The Health 202: Trump health officials rewrite big Obamacare rules. PowerPost. Retrieved from https://www.washingtonpost.com/news/powerpost/paloma/the-health-202/2018/04/10/the-health-202-trump-health-officials-rewrite-big-obamacare-rules/5acbc54c30fb0406a5a122cd/?utm_term=.09b01b3aca34

Delk, J. (2018). Giuliani calls Mueller probe 'tremendous' distraction, 'totally unjustified.' The Hill. Retrieved from https://thehill.com/blogs/blog-briefing-room/386388-giuliani-calls-mueller-probe-tremendous-distraction-and-totally

Democrat vs. Republican. (n.d.). Diffen. Retrieved from https://www.diffen.com/difference/Democrat_vs_Republican

Department of Health and Human Service. (n.d.). About HHS. Retrieved from https://www.hhs.gov

Editorial Board. (2017). Bringing a culture of accountability to CPD: Begin by breaking the code of silence. Chicago Tribune. Retrieved from http://www.chicagotribune.com/news/opinion/editorials/ct-cops-chicago-justice-department-police-0122-md-20170120-story.html

FindLaw. (n.d.). How does the U.S. Supreme Court decide whether to hear a case? Retrieved from https://litigation.findlaw.com/legal-system/how-does-the-u-s-supreme-court-decide-whether-to-hear-a-case.html

Goldberg, M. L. (2017). 9 stories that will drive the global agenda. Retrieved from https://www.undispatch.com/9-stories-will-drive-global-agenda-2018

The GOP tax bill kills Obamacare's Individual Mandate: Here's what that means? (2017). Retrieved from http://time.com/money/5067044/gop-tax-plan-individual-mandate-obamacare

Hall, M. A., & McCue, M. J. (2016). How has the Affordable Care Act affected health insurers' financial performance? *The Commonwealth Fund*, *18*, 1–14.

Hardcastle, L. E., Record, K. L., Jacobson, P. D., & Gostin, K. L. (2011). Improving the population's health: The Affordable Care Act and the importance of integration. *Journal of Law, Medicine and Ethics*, *39*, 317–327.

Hersher, R. (2017). DOJ 'severely deficient training' has led to patterns of abuse by Chicago police. Retrieved from https://www.npr.org/sections/thetwo-way/2017/01/13/509646186/doj-severely-deficient-training-has-led-to-pattern-of-abuse-by-chicago-police

Hill, B. J. (2012). What is the meaning of health? Constitutional implications of defining "medical necessity" and "essential health benefits" under the Affordable Care Act. *American Journal of Health and Medicine*, *38*, 445–470.

Hirschfeld Davis, J., & Landler, M. (2017). Trump nominates Neil Gorsuch to the Supreme Court. *New York Times*. Retrieved from https://www.nytimes.com/2017/01/31/us/politics/supreme-court-nominee-trump.html

HR 277. (2017). The American HealthCare Reform Act. Retrieved from https://www.govtrack.us/congress/bills/115/hr277

Isaac, J. (2017). Possible $10.4 million money funnel from Putin Associates to GOP uncovered. Bipartisan Reports. Retrieved from https://www.google.com/search?ei=1-4SW866Ko_r5gK85Z-YDw&q=Isaac+2017+%2410+million+dollars++funnel+from+Putin+asssociates&oq=Isaac+2017+%2410+million+dollars++funnel+from+Putin+asssociates&gs_l=psy-ab.12...16403.39916.0.42436.30.30.0.0.0.0.230.3755.0j27j1.28.0....0...1.1.64.psy-ab..2.1.155...33i21k1.0.IdQ--LfgXBA

Khan Academy. (n.d.). Ideologies of political parties: Lesson overview. Retrieved from https://www.khanacademy.org/humanities/ap-us-government-and-politics/american-political-beliefs-and-behaviors/ideologies-of-political-parties/a/lesson-summary-ideologies-of-political-parties

Kaiser Family Foundation (KFF). (2012). A guide to the Supreme Court's decision on the ACA's Medicaid expansion. Retrieved from https://kaiserfamilyfoundation.files.wordpress.com/2013/01/8347.pdf

The Kaiser Family Foundation. (2018). Total number of professionally active nurses. Retrieved from https://www.kff.org/other/state-indicator/total-registered-nurses/?currentTimeframe=0&sortModel=%7B%22colId%22:%22Location%22,%22sort%22:%22asc%22%7D

Kaplan, T., & Pear, R. (2017). House passes measure to repeal and replace The Affordable Care Act. Retrieved from https://www.nytimes.com/2017/05/04/us/politics/healthcare-bill-vote.html

Lambrew, J. (2017). Trump's ACA Executive Order: Will it reduce "burden," or shift it to patients? Retrieved from https://www.ourpursuit.com/congress-accomplish-2018/?gclid=EAIaIQobChMI08ifiYHj3AIVjuDICh27uwF8EAAYASAAEgKIb_D_BwE

Legal Information Institute. (n.d.). Cornell University Law School. Certiorari. Retrieved from https://www.law.cornell.edu/wex/certiorari

Levitt, J. (n.d.). All about redistricting. Los Angeles, CA: Loyola Law School. Retrieved from http://redistricting.lls.edu/why.php

Lewis, L. M., & Arkedis, J. (2014). So you've won a seat in Congress—Now what? The Atlantic. Retrieved from https://www.theatlantic.com/politics/archive/2014/11/so-youve-won-election-to-congressnow-what/382421

Locker, M. (2017). Here is the depressing reason why gun stocks go up after mass shootings. Retrieved from https://www.fastcompany.com/40475808/why-gun-stocks-always-go-up-after-an-attack

LoGiurato, B. (2017). Trump fumes at McConnell says it's time to move on after healthcare collapse. Retrieved from https://www.businessinsider.com/mcconnell-healthcare-vote-failure-2017-7

Luhby, T. (2017). What was in the failed Senate 'skinny repeal' healthcare bill? Retrieved from https://www.ourpursuit.com/congress-accomplish-2018/?gclid=EAIaIQobChMI08ifiYHj3AIVjuDICh27uwF8EAAYASAAEgKIb_D_BwE

Morrison, C. (2016). Four steps to appointing a Supreme Court justice. Retrieved from https://theconversation.com/four-steps-to-appointing-a-supreme-court-justice-54715

National League for Nursing (NLN) Communications. (2018). National League for Nursing responds to AACN draft vision statement for the future of nursing education. Retrieved from https://outlook.office.com/owa/projection.aspx

New York Times. (2013). How lawmakers can stay connected to their constituents. Retrieved from https://www.nytimes.com/roomfordebate/2013/08/13/how-lawmakers-can-stay-connected-to-constituents

9/11 attacks—facts & summary. (2001). Retrieved from https://www.history.com/topics/9-11-attacks

Oberlander, J. (2014). Unraveling Obamacare-Can Congress and the Supreme Court undo health-care reform. *New England Journal of Medicine*, *371*, 2445–2447.

Overby, P. (2017). Trump's efforts to 'drain the swamp' lagging behind his campaign rhetoric. Retrieved from https://www.npr.org/2017/04/26/525551816/trumps-efforts-to-drain-the-swamp-lagging-behind-his-campaign-rhetoric

Paletta, D., & Stein, J. (2017). Sweeping tax overhaul clears Congress. *The Washington Post*. Retrieved from https://www.washingtonpost.com/business/economy/gop-tax-bill-passes-congress-as-trump-prepares-to-sign-it-into-law/2017/12/20/0ba2fd98-e597-11e7-9ec2-518810e7d44d_story.html?noredirect=on&utm_term=.e7b6ae882a29

Patient Protection and Affordable Care Act, 42 U.S.C. § 18001 (2010).

Pear, R., & Kaplan, T. (2017). Senate rejects slimmed down Obamacare Repeal as McCain votes no. New York Times. Retrieved from https://www.nytimes.com/2017/07/27/us/politics/obamacare-partial-repeal-senate-republicans-revolt.html

Phillips, J. L. (n.d.). "What Is the bureaucratic model?" Small Business - Chron.com, Retrieved from http://smallbusiness.chron.com/bureaucratic-model-66119.html

Popovich, N., Albeck-Ripka, L., & Pierre-Louis, K. (2018). 76 environmental rules on the way out under trump. Retrieved from https://www.nytimes.com/interactive/2017/10/05/climate/trump-environment-rules-reversed.html

Potter, R. A. (2016). Slow rolling and fast pacing and the pace of bureaucratic decisions in rule-making. Retrieved from https://www.princeton.edu/csdp/events/Potter%2004142016/Potter-04142016-RAP.slowroll.CSDP.pdf

Quadagno, J. (2014). Right-Wing conspiracy? Socialist plot? The origins of the Patient Protection and Affordable Care Act. *Journal of Health Politics, Policy and Law*, *39*(1), 35–56.

Rennie, G. (n.d.). The revolving door: Why politicians become lobbyists and lobbyists become politicians. Retrieved from http://theconversation.com/the-revolving-door-why-politicians-become-lobbyists-and-lobbyists-become-politicians-64237

Robertson, T. (2017). United States Department of Justice promotes the need for a culture of compliance. Retrieved from https://blogs.thomsonreuters.com/financial-risk/risk-management-compliance/u-s-doj-promotes-the-need-for-a-culture-of-compliance

Rosenbaum, S. (2012). Threading the needle-Medicaid and the 113th Congress. *New England Journal of Medicine*, *367*(25), 2368–2369.

Scott, D., & Burton, T. I. (2018). "Witch hunts" explained, from Salem to Donald Trump. Vox. Retrieved from https://www.vox.com/policy-and-politics/2018/4/17/17235546/witch-hunt-mueller-donald-trump-tweet-eric-greitens

Singer, P. W. (2007). The dark truth about Blackwater. Washington, DC: The Brookings Institute. Retrieved from https://www.brookings.edu/articles/the-dark-truth-about-blackwater

Sisney, L. (2016). Top-down vs. bottom up hierarchy: Or, how to design a self- managed organization. Retrieved from https://organizationalphysics.com/2016/10/13/top-down-vs-bottom-up-hierarchy-or-how-to-build-a-self-managed-organization

Skinner, J., & Amitabh, C. (2016). The past and future of the Affordable Care Act. *The Journal of the American Medical Association*, *316*(5), 497–499.

Smith, B. (2017). DOJ acts to curb the overuse of secrecy orders: Now it's Congress' turn. Retrieved from https://blogs.microsoft.com/on-the-issues/2017/10/23/doj-acts-curb-overuse-secrecy-orders-now-congress-turn/

Sousa, G. (2017). How are U.S. Supreme Court Justices appointed? Retrieved from https://www.worldatlas.com/articles/how-are-u-s-supreme-court-justices-appointed.html

Stein, P. (2015). Why do people move out of DC? Housing. Retrieved from https://www.google.com/search?source=hp&ei=ColoW8b-Bsy3ggel7rjwAg&q=stein++why+do+people+move+out+of

Snyder, B. (2014). Compliance is a culture, not just a policy. Retrieved from https://www.justice.gov/atr/file/517796/download

Spencer-Oatey, H. (2008). *Culturally speaking: Culture, communication, and politeness theory* (2nd ed.). London, UK: Continuum.

Storm, D. (2017). Hackers breached 63 universities and governmental agencies. Retrieved from https://www.computerworld.com/article/3170724/security/hacker-breached-63-universities-and-government-agencies.html

Sullivan, P. (2017). Senate GOP floats scaled down healthcare bill. The Hill. http://thehill.com/policy/healthcare/343611-senate-gop-floats-scaled-down-healthcare-bill

Taylor, S. (2005). Life tenure is too long for Supreme Court Justices. Retrieved from https://www.theatlantic.com/magazine/archive/2005/06/life-tenure-is-too-long-for-supreme-court-justices/304134/

Tenpas, K. D. (2018). Why is Trump's staff turnover higher than the 5 most recent presidents? Retrieved from https://www.brookings.edu/research/why-is-trumps-staff-turnover-higher-than-the-5-most-recent-presidents/

Tillman, Z (n.d.). Trump has a good year getting judges confirmed, but he's still a long way from reshaping the courts. BuzzFeedNews. Retrieved from: https://www.buzzfeednews.com/article/zoetillman/trump-had-a-good-year-getting-judges-confirmed-but-hes

Traser, Z. (2017). Axing the Individual Mandate, Obama's hated heart: Quick take. Washington Post. Retrieved from http://time.com/money/5067044/gop-tax-plan-individual-mandate-obamacare/

Truffaut-Wong, O. (2016). How long were Clarence Thomas' confirmation hearings? The HBO film version only highlights the Anita Hill testimony. Retrieved from https://www.bustle.com/articles/154791-how-long-were-clarence-thomas-confirmation-hearings-the-hbo-film-version-only-highlights-the-anita-hill

Trump, D. J., & Schwartz, J. (1987). *The art of the deal*. New York, NY: Random House.

Tyler, E. B. (1871). How culture works. Retrieved from https://ocw.mit.edu/courses/anthropology/21a-01-how-culture-works-fall-2012/readings/MIT21A_01F12_Sir_Edwrd_cul.pdf

United States Department of State. (n.d.). Retrieved from https://www.state.gov/r/pa/ei/rls/dos/436.htm

United States House of Representatives. (n.d.). The House explained. Retrieved from https://www.house.gov/the-house-explained

United States Senate. (n.d.a). The role and duties of the Senate. Retrieved from https://www.history.com/topics/history-of-the-us-senate

United States Senate. (n.d.b). Retrieved from https://www.senate.gov

University of Minnesota. (n.d.). Policymaking, power, and accountability in the bureaucracy. Retrieved from http://open.lib.umn.edu/americangovernment/chapter/14-2-policymaking-power-and-accountability-in-the-bureaucracy

Vladeck, B. (2003). Universal health insurance in the United States: Reflections on the past, the present and the future. *American Journal of Public Health*, *93*(1), 16–19.

Wagner, J. (2017). Trump begins sweeping tax bill into law. The Washington Post. Retrieved from https://www.washingtonpost.com/news/post-politics/wp/2017/12/22/trump-signs-sweeping-tax-bill-into-law/?utm_term=.796b9360e41d

Walsh, K. T. (2013). Isolation a threat to modern presidency. U.S. News. Retrieved from https://www.usnews.com/news/blogs/ken-walshs-washington/2013/05/10/isolation-a-threat-to-modern-presidency

Watson, K. (2017). Trump's security costs for one day in NYC equivalent to entire summer in Bedminister, N.J. Retrieved from https://www.cbsnews.com/news/trumps-security-price-tag-for-one-day-in-nyc-same-as-bedminster-n-j-all-summer

Weber, M. (1978). *Economy and society: An outline of interpretive sociology*. Berkeley, CA: University of California Press.

Weiner, M. (n.d.). What's it like to live in Washington, DC? Retrieved from https://realestate.usnews.com/places/district-of-columbia/washington

Weigel, D. (2018). Democrats visit detention centers to attack 'zero tolerance' immigration policies. The Washington Post. Retrieved from https://www.washingtonpost.com/news/powerpost/wp/2018/06/23/democrats-visit-detention-centers-to-attack-zero-tolerance-immigration-policy/?utm_term=.bdac10241e35

Where does the term "lobbyist" come from? (n.d.). Retrieved from http://political-lobbying.co.uk/where-does-the-term-lobbyist-come-from

WikiLeaks. (n.d.). Retrieved from https://wikileaks.org/ciav7p1

Zarate, J. V. (2017). The cyber-attacks on democracy. Retrieved from http://www.bushcenter.org/catalyst/democracy/zarate-cyber-attacks-on-democracy.html

CHAPTER 7

# The Current State of Transcultural Mental Health Nursing

## *A Synthesis of the Literature*

Kimberly M. Wolf, Katelin N. Umland, and Chai Lo

**ABSTRACT**

Objectives: The purpose of this chapter is to discuss the current state of transcultural mental health nursing and the work that has been done by nursing in this area. This chapter aims to discuss the current available literature that documents nurses' work toward addressing barriers and ensuring nondominant culture clients receive reliable and appropriate mental health care. Data Sources: A search of the published literature in English language using PubMed, MEDLINE, CINAHL, and the Cochrane databases over the past 10 years using the search words "transcultural nursing" and related terms and "mental health" and related terms was conducted by each author. Mental health nursing organizational websites that the authors are members of were also searched for information related to transcultural mental health nursing, as well as organizational websites the authors have known to have content related to mental health and immigrant health in the United States. Conclusion: Cultural care knowledge has grown due to the work of transcultural nurses. Mental health transcultural care knowledge, with its unique challenges, is especially in need of attention and advancement. Implications for Nursing Research: Mental health researchers, educators, and nurses are encouraged to identify, investigate, and


http://dx.doi.org/10.1891/0739-6686.37.209

disseminate mental health cultural knowledge learned, to continue to grow transcultural mental health nursing, and to promote culturally competent mental health care.

## INTRODUCTION

As inpatient psychiatric providers for a large metropolitan county hospital that serves and cares for a culturally diverse population with a culturally diverse multidisciplinary staff, engaging in developing treatment plans with consideration for culturally appropriate interventions is a daily practice for these authors. Despite the fact that the providers have access to culturally diverse staff members in a variety of disciplines, as well as interpreters who go above and beyond at times to explain the cultural relevance of answers provided by patients, challenges to understanding the whole situation and problem solving with cultural competence is also present on a daily basis. The purpose of this chapter is to discuss the current state of transcultural mental health nursing and the work that has been done by nursing in this area. Transcultural nursing was developed by Dr. Madeleine Leininger with the purpose of providing guidance for nursing care actions and decisions that include a client's cultural beliefs, practices, and values as nurse and client creatively and productively work together to design a care plan for a lifestyle of health and well-being (Leininger & McFarland, 2006). The transcultural nursing theory remains an essential part of nursing practice in this country's current climate of conflict, uncertainty, and change, especially including the changes in leadership and immigration laws. Furthermore, the addition of Standard 8 in 2015 to the American Nurses Association's (ANA's) standards of practice declares the necessity of the inclusion of culturally congruent practice "during a time of social change and an increase of culturally and ethnically diverse consumers" (Marion et al., 2017, p.1). Of concern is that there are discussions in the public healthcare systems, including the healthcare system that these authors work in, that the fear that is growing in the immigrant and nondominant cultures in this country regarding deportation is decreasing utilization of healthcare services, including for immigrants who are in this country legally.

Lack of access to, and underutilization of, mental health services is also of national concern. Over 40 million Americans live with a mental health condition and the numbers of youth who suffer from mental health conditions is growing. The Mental Health America (formerly known as the National Mental Health Association) 2018 report asserts that 56% of American adults with a mental illness do not receive treatment (Nguyen, Hellebuyck, Halpern, & Fritze, 2017). This same report asserts that youth mental health is worsening with rates of youth who suffer from severe depression increasing from 5.9% in 2012 to 8.2% in 2015. Sadly, this report indicates that even when youth suffer with severe depression, 76% either are not treated at all or receive insufficient treatment. Zoucha and Wolf (2018) maintain that nondominant cultures are also subject to a variety of experiences that challenge their mental health in ways that members of the dominant culture are not, including, but not limited to, the experience of being an immigrant with the associated loss and changes as well as socioeconomic disadvantages. According to Scuglik, Alarcón, Lapeyre, Williams, and Logan (2007), even if the immigration process follows the usual course, it is complicated by the impact of premigration losses and other traumatic events. Kahn (2017) also discusses the challenges of adjustment and acculturation on mental health in her publication on mass migration. Also of note is that the Substance Abuse and Mental Health Services Administration (SAMHSA) report (SAMHSA, 2015) indicates one of our national problems is the discrepancy in the use of mental health services among racial and ethnic groups. The American Psychiatric Nurses Association (APNA) president Linda Beeber, PhD, PMHCNS-BC, FAAN, asserts that this nation needs to prioritize mental health and substance use to at least the same level as other healthcare essentials and ensure that all groups receive equal access to care to promote whole health and full lives for all (Beeber, 2018).

The low percentage of people who are accessing mental health treatment in general, the assertion that nondominant cultures are even less likely to seek mental health treatment, the extra challenges that nondominant cultures face that may negatively affect their mental health, and the fear that is growing in the nondominant culture regarding deportation, combined with Standard 8, provide evidence that mental health nurses need to continue to work toward ensuring that transcultural nursing and culturally congruent practice is active and growing. Given the many barriers already described that are preventing nondominant culture clients from approaching the healthcare facilities for the mental health care they need, having the tools and skills necessary to build trust and provide culturally congruent care for those who do visit is crucial for mental health nurses. This chapter aims to discuss the current available literature that documents nurses' work toward addressing barriers and ensuring nondominant culture clients receive reliable and appropriate mental health care.

## LITERATURE REVIEW

A search of the published literature in English language using PubMed, MEDLINE, CINAHL, and the Cochrane databases over the past 10 years using the search words "transcultural nursing" and related terms and "mental health" and related terms was conducted by each author. Mental health nursing organizational websites that the authors are members of were also searched for information related to transcultural mental health nursing as well as organizational websites the authors have known to have content related to mental health and immigrant health in the United States.

## Conceptualization of Transcultural Mental Health Nursing

Dr. Madeleine M. Leininger founded the discipline of transcultural nursing and changed the way that nurses and other healthcare professionals care for culturally diverse populations around the world (Ray, 2012). Andrews (2017) indicates that a benefit of transcultural nursing is the fact that it helps us focus on what unites us as human beings. This author also indicates that this is especially important during these challenging times filled with adversity and unrest that currently exist in our country. Leininger developed the theory of Culture Care Diversity and Universality (Leininger & McFarland, 2006). This theory provides guidance for nursing interventions and decisions to incorporate each consumer's cultural values, cultural beliefs, and cultural practices. Leininger also crafted the qualitative research methodology of ethnonursing, the first research methodology developed by a nurse for use in research subjects relevant to nurses (Andrews & Boyle, 2016). Leininger also developed the Sunrise Enabler tool to assist these qualitative researchers to gather culture care phenomena from a holistic perspective, including a variety of factors that have the potential to influence a person's well-being (Leininger & McFarland, 2006). Andrews and Boyle (2016) assert that the ethnonursing research methodology has been used in hundreds of studies since its development. The Transcultural Nursing Society (TCNS) was also founded by Dr. Leininger with the identified mission "to enhance the quality of culturally congruent, competent, and equitable care that results in improved health and well-being for people worldwide" (TCNS, 2018).

Several researchers have found that Leininger's theory and methodology were ideal for studies that they conducted that were focused on a specific culture's mental healthcare beliefs, needs, and practices. Dieujuste (2016) studied mental health care among Haitian Americans utilizing the Sunrise Enabler to find characteristics of stigma, identified as "labelling, stereotypes, negative attitudes, emotional responses and discrimination" (p. 203) as hindrances to seeking effective mental health care. Doornbos, Zandee, and DeGroot (2014) found that women of diverse ethnics with mental health conditions in urban underserved areas had commonalities in their communication and interaction patterns, which can guide culturally sensitive nursing care in mental health. Millender's (2012) study used Leininger's framework to assess the indigenous Mayans' adjustment to life in the United States and expound their uniqueness from other immigrant groups due to displacement decades after civil discord, calling for further effort to meet the needs of those from another culture. An ethnonursing study conducted by Wolf et al. (2014) that utilized Leininger's theory and methodology to study Somali immigrants' perceptions of mental health and illness revealed how religion significantly influences this culture's mental health as well as how tribe connectedness, cultural history, and khat usage are significant in mental health.

## Related Theories, Tools, and Research

Other theories and their associated tools are also available to transcultural nurses and researchers. These are not specific to mental health but offer assistance to mental health nurses facing challenges when working with people of diverse cultural backgrounds. Andrews/Boyle Transcultural Interprofessional Practice (TIP) Model, with a five-step problem-solving process, was developed to provide nurses with a theoretically sound and evidence-based framework to guide them in their development of culturally congruent care plans and interventions (Andrews & Boyle, 2016). This model acknowledges the communication challenges that exist in contexts with diversity of languages, values, beliefs, and practices and offers instructive assistance to nursing facing these challenges. Mental health issues often pose extra challenges in the communication process, and this theory and its associated tool offer specifics on communicating with people who speak a different language and utilizing interpreters. The Process of Cultural Competence in the Delivery of Healthcare Services (PCCDHS) model was developed by Campinha-Bacote and requires the health-care professional to accept the concept of continual growth in becoming (as opposed to being) culturally competent with the integration of cultural desire, cultural awareness, cultural knowledge, cultural skill, and cultural encounters (Campinha-Bacote, 2011). This model's associated tool, Inventory For Assessing The Process of Cultural Competence Among Healthcare Professionals—Revised (IAPCC-R), also developed by Campinha-Bacote, produced research that prompted change in the model as it revealed the key construct in the process of becoming culturally competent is cultural encounters (Campinha-Bacote, 2011). This model and tool provide guidance that mental health nurses working with a culturally diverse population may easily utilize as they encourage mindful interactions with patients and adoption of an available and open presence, actions already known quite well to mental health nurses.

Other transcultural frameworks that can be utilized in mental health clinical environments and research studies have also changed and expanded with advancements in available knowledge. Jeffreys's Cultural Competence and Confidence (CCC) Model, along with the associated questionnaires and assessment tools, provides a framework for understanding the process of teaching and learning "optimal" cultural competence (Jeffreys, 2016). The model provides a guide for planning, implementing, and evaluating cultural competence education programs. Jeffreys acknowledges the increasing complexities, barriers, as well as the ethical and legal implications, in providing culturally competent care with increasing global migration and changes in demographic patterns. Jeffreys's model and concepts can easily be adapted to mental health nursing as well as mental health nursing research. The ethnonursing dissertation study conducted by Wolf utilized constructs adapted from the constructs in Jeffreys's model to study Somali immigrants' perceptions of mental health and illness. This research study was published to disseminate the valuable knowledge learned about this culture's mental health beliefs and practices (Wolf et al., 2014). Purnell's Model of Cultural Competence, along with the associated 12 domains of culture, also provides a framework to learn about the concepts and characteristics of culture (Purnell, 2013). Purnell (2013) asserts that cultural competence "has become one of the most important initiatives in health care in the United States and throughout most of the world" (p. 3). Mental health professionals related to his identification of the importance of relationships and communication in the model. The Giger and Davidhizar Transcultural Assessment was developed to meet the need for an assessment tool that could be easily utilized to gather information about cultural variables and the effects these variables have on a population's health and illness behaviors (Giger, 2017). The model identifies six cultural phenomena that are evident in all cultural groups and must be acknowledged by health-care professionals providing transcultural health care. SAMHSA (2003) adapted concepts from this model for the publication *Developing Cultural Competence in Disaster Mental Health Programs: Guiding Principles and Recommendations*.

The aforementioned models have been incorporated into studies. A study utilizing Purnell's Model of Cultural Competence studied cultural and spirituality in the palliative care setting (Long, 2011). Although not directly in reference to Purnell's model, a separate study referenced a case of self-mutilation in which the authors sought cultural sensitivity with concepts from Purnell and Paulanka's approach to transcultural health care (Williams & Hamilton, 2009). Singleton and Krause (2009) assessed health literacy in those nondominant cultures, referring to concepts of culture by Leininger, Campinha-Bacote, and Giger and Davidhizar. Harding (2017) used Giger and Davidhizar's model as a framework for assessing veterans' self-stigma as a hindrance to receiving mental health care. Assessment tools to measure cultural competence were used in a study to assess competence among nursing students. Mesler (2014) used Campinha-Bacote's IAPCC-R to valuate nursing students' confidence in cultural competence and Jeffreys's Transcultural Self-efficacy Tool to measure ascertain self-efficacy or confidence.

The Circular Model of Cultural Tailoring (CMCT) was developed to address substance use among Native American Indians (Patchell, Robbins, Lowe, & Hoke, 2012). The model consists of four elements: self, time, relationships, and tribes (Patchell, Robbins, Lowe, & Hoke, 2012). It also identifies three patterns of knowing: expressed experience of culture, lived experience of culture, and flashpoint (Patchell, Robbins, Lowe, & Hoke, 2012). Patchell, Robbins, Lowe, and Hoke (2015) used the CMCT model for treating substance abuse in Native American adolescents. The researchers also incorporated the traditional method of a talking circle within the schools to provide substance abuse prevention topics to high school students to show improvement in reported self-reliance and self-report substance use/abuse (Patchell et al., 2015). Adaptation of the CMCT to substance use among Native American Indian adolescents brings about likeliness that it can be modified and applied to other geographic areas with multiple cultures such as many different parts of Africa with the numerous tribes within a country. Other researchers recommend allowing the client to define health and heeding the client's social environment and traditional practices to increase adherence and success and allow each individual to be heard without conviction or assumptions (Yurkovich & Lattergrass, 2008). The researchers worked with Native American Indians with mental illnesses to define their perspective of health and unhealthiness and identify their sense of spirituality to invoke a sense of culturally competent care (Yurkovich & Lattergrass, 2008).

Warren (2007) addressed cultural implications specifically treating bipolar disorder. Bipolar disorder is a complex mental illness to diagnose and treat. Individuals with bipolar disorder may experience symptoms within their cultural beliefs, values, and norms. It is important psychiatric nurses understand the role that culture plays in mental health. Not understanding the role of culture in clients' lives can make caring for those with this disorder quite challenging. It can lead to misinterpretation of symptoms, which could in turn lead to misdiagnosis or reduction of the importance of symptoms. It is also important to consider pharmacological differences. Pharmacological research has been indicating that metabolic processes are different for racially and ethnically diverse groups than for those from groups that are not racially and ethnically diverse. This calls for dosages to be adjusted appropriately due to these genetic metabolic processes (Warren, 2007).

## Progress With Challenges

A descriptive study by Wilson (2010) explored the views of clients with mental illness regarding the overall effectiveness of psychiatric care in meeting their cultural needs and psychiatric nurses' own views of how and to what extent they were able to provide culturally competent psychiatric mental health nursing care to diverse populations. Clients described being encouraged and reassured, being spoken up for, and praying as essential to their care. Nurses participating in the study believed themselves to provide competent psychiatric nursing care but had actually lacked specific knowledge and the skills to do so effectively. To eliminate the gap between knowledge and practice, psychiatric nurses need to receive specific education focusing on cultural assessment, cultural communication, and other mental health nursing skills (Wilson, 2010). In working with patients who are refugees, providers should be mindful of intergenerational influences experienced on an individual basis and socially through one's own trauma and grief and through one's parental experience that has been transmitted over time (Hudson, Adams, & Lauderdale, 2016). Singleton and Krause (2009) provided similar suggestions but also included recommendation that nurses do a self-assessment of personal assumptions and biases; assessment of the patient's health literacy; professional education on culture; interdisciplinary collaboration; patient advocacy; establishment of an educational setting for patients, providers, and students; and interpreters or cultural brokers to bridge language and cultural barriers.

The *Diagnostic and Statistical Manual of Mental Disorders* has progressed in its addition of cultural considerations. Progress had previously been made with the addition of culturally bound syndromes in the *Diagnostic and Statistical Manual of Mental Disorders* (4th ed.; *DSM-IV*; American Psychiatric Association [APA], 1994). Although this edition did not contain every culturally bound syndrome, it did encourage clinicians to include a cultural assessment in their diagnostic formulation. The *DSM-IV* recommended that diagnostic impressions be formulated by considering the cultural identity of the person, cultural explanations for the illness, cultural factors related to the psychosocial environment and levels of functioning, as well as cultural elements of the relationship between the individual and the clinician in the development of diagnosis (O'Brien, 2006). The *DSM-IV* (APA, 2000) defined cultural formulation and included the culture-bound syndrome glossary, which further explicated the need for practitioners to further assess symptoms within the context of cultural and social influences and the patient's distress (Warren, 2013). The importance of the influence of culture on diagnosis is further recognized in the *Diagnostic and Statistical Manual of Mental Disorders* (5th ed.; *DSM-5*; APA, 2013). Instead of listing culture-bound syndromes, the *DSM-5* updates criteria throughout to address cross-cultural variations in presentations, gives further detailed information regarding cultural concepts of distress, and includes a clinical tool to facilitate more comprehensive, person-centered assessments (Warren, 2013). Different cultures may exhibit mental health symptoms in dissimilar ways. Crying and headaches may be symptoms of a panic attack in one culture, while shortness of breath may be a symptom in another culture. To address these cross-cultural variations, specific diagnostic criteria were changed to appropriately apply to a nondominant culture. An example is how the diagnosis of social anxiety disorder now includes the fear of offending others to reflect a Japanese concept where avoiding harm to others is emphasized rather than avoiding harm to oneself. Cultural concepts of distress are described through cultural syndromes, idioms of distress, and explanations that can help assist clinicians in recognizing how different cultures think and talk about psychological problems. The *DSM-5* also contains a cultural formulation interview guide to assist clinicians in assessing cultural factors influencing patients' perspectives of their symptoms and treatment options, giving the clinician a more comprehensive foundation on which to base both diagnosis and care (APA, 2013).

## RESEARCH PRIORITIES

Registered nurses from all areas of nursing have the ability to identify research questions that can be used in culturally congruent practice research with the goal "to eliminate racial and ethnic health disparities among all populations" (Marion et al., 2017, p.1). Despite the likelihood that all nurses are presented with situations regularly that could incite such research questions, Marion et al. (2017) indicate that research investigating culturally congruent nursing to improve health care is "sparse." These authors also assert that nurse researchers will improve the health and quality of life of different cultures with research programs that move beyond descriptive investigation into designing and testing culturally meaningful interventions. Given the extra challenges associated with mental health interventions in general, encouragement of mental health nurses to identify culturally congruent research questions, as well as supporting research programs that design and test culturally specific interventions, is essential to the improvement of the culturally nondominant population's mental health and quality of life.

## EDUCATIONAL AND CLINICAL IMPLICATIONS

Raman (2015) asserted the need for academic programs to not only include cultural competency in their curriculum but also include diverse educators as well as engage students from nondominant cultures in their learning. There are qualms about the inconsistency in culturally competent care curriculum among academic nursing programs (Byrne, 2016). Additional suggestions for cultural competence include exposure to the cultures, including immersion into the environment and people from a specific culture such as study abroad experiences or simulations, although not readily available or affordable for students (Byrne, 2016). A separate nursing course on cultural competence has been shown to be more effective compared to courses with cultural content or a non-nursing course (Mesler, 2014). Recommendations for nursing programs to include incorporating competency courses and nursing professions to require continuing education workshops have been evoked (Albougami, Pounds, & Alotaibi, 2016).

Providing culturally competent mental health care is a standard for professional nursing care. Nardi and Waite (2012) recommend some ways to do this by including mandatory educational in-services or required continued education credits specifically directed toward enhancing cultural competency skills. Continued development and measurement of policies and practice standards that will integrate culturally competent mental health promotion, disease prevention, and treatment for patients, and within the workplace, examination of best practice initiatives for cultural awareness and improving mental health literacy, implementation of evolving federal and state policies regarding more equitable models of health-care delivery, along with increased activism related to providing mental health, are all ways culturally competent care in mental health can be improved (Nardi & Waite, 2012).

Rosa (2017) asserts that to be of "optimal and sustainable service," nurses must "pause and embrace a transcultural stance" that includes the admittance that nurses need to accept the idea of a lifetime of learning in the "realm of socially responsible transcultural care" (p. 117). Ethnic diversity of healthcare consumers continues to grow. This growth increases the gap in knowledge for nurses caring for a variety of nondominant cultures. Mental health nurses have a professional and ethical obligation to continue to learn about their patients and then incorporate this knowledge into their practice so that culturally competent care is given to an ever-increasingly diverse population. To gain insight and understanding to improve the likelihood of giving appropriate culturally competent care, nurses may read available publications, ask professionals who identify with the nondominant culture, as well as ask questions of the patient and family. At times these resources are not available to nurses who are struggling to provide the best care for their patients and it can leave nurses feeling overwhelmed or frustrated. The same nurses may also be gaining knowledges through their hard work to provide the best care for a diverse population and this knowledge is not being disseminated farther then their own work environment.

## POLICY IMPLICATIONS

Legislation addressing disparities in health-care access for nonminority groups and for people who suffer from mental illness has been introduced at increasing rates over the past 10 years. Insurance coverage for mental health treatment is a significant barrier to receiving necessary and appropriate mental health care. The Mental Health Parity Act of 1996 (MHPA) stipulated that large group health plans could not impose dollar limits on mental health benefits that were less favorable than those imposed on medical/surgical benefits, and then the Mental Health Parity and Addiction Equity Act of 2008 (MHPAEA) protected and added to this federal law by extending the parity requirements to substance use disorders (U.S. Centers for Medicare & Medicaid Services, n.d.). Although the law requires equivalence in the way mental health/substance abuse and medical/surgical benefits are handled, MHPAEA does not require that issuers cover mental health/substance abuse benefits. The law only applies to large group health plans and health insurance issuers that choose to include mental health/substance abuse benefits in their benefit packages. However, the Affordable Care Act builds on MHPAEA and requires coverage of mental health and substance use disorder services as one of the categories in non-grandfathered individual and small group plans (U.S. Centers for Medicare & Medicaid Services, n.d.). Maintaining and continuing to supplement mental health legislation is imperative, as well as supporting disparity legislation. Life expectancy and overall health have improved in recent years for most Americans, but disparities persist, specifically for racial and ethnic minorities, as good health is more difficult to attain for this group because appropriate care is often associated with an individual's economic status, race, and gender (National Conference of State Legislatures, 2014). Policy makers are responding by introducing legislation in several states aimed at eliminating health disparities through a variety of bills that address the social determinants of health for the underserved populations (National Conference of State Legislatures, 2014). Nurses are in a great position to recognize health-care barriers, propose solutions, and be involved in preparing bills, as well as supporting and testifying for bills that increase access of mental health care for minorities.

Racial and ethnic diversity is increasing in the United States. It is predicted that by 2042, racial/ethnic minorities are expected to surpass non-Hispanic Whites as the majority population in the United States, yet minority populations are underserved in the American mental healthcare system (Primm et al., 2010). Primm et al. (2010) note this to be due to limited English proficiency, remote geographic settings, stigma, fragmented services, cost, comorbidity of mental illness and chronic diseases, cultural understanding of health-care services, and incarceration. McGuire and Miranda (2008) noted that some contributions to these disparities also include providers' bias and stereotyping, providers' statistical discrimination, provider and geographic differences, and health insurance differences. Primm et al. (2010) recommend enhanced surveillance, research, evidence-based practice, and public policies that set standards for tracking and reducing disparities. Policy implications to help eliminate these disparities include improving access to care, improving the quality of care, and creating a greater diverse mental health workforce and culturally appropriate provider and patient education (McGuire & Miranda, 2008).

## CONCLUSION

Cultural diversity continues to grow in this country with expanding nondominant population numbers. Awareness of the importance to provide culturally appropriate care has grown since the inception of Dr. Madeleine Leininger's work in developing what we have come to know as transcultural nursing. The importance of providing mental health care alongside physical health care has grown with public awareness as well. Despite the growth in these areas, barriers continue to hinder culturally nondominant persons from seeking the care they need as well as preventing mental health nurses from providing the care they want to give. Mental health nurses have an interest in providing culturally competent mental health care as well as a professional and an ethical obligation to do so. Many useful transcultural frameworks and tools are available to nurses, as well as to researchers, to assist them in learning about and providing culturally competent mental health care. Many researchers and nurses have utilized these tools, and progress has been made toward the inclusion of culturally competent care in mental health environments. This review of literature acknowledges researchers has expanded cultural knowledge available to nurses, although there is no doubt that more inclusion and knowledge regarding cultural mental health beliefs and practices specifically is needed. Mental health nurses, researchers, and educators are encouraged to identify, investigate, and disseminate cultural knowledge learned and to continue to grow transcultural mental health nursing and promote culturally competent mental health care.

## REFERENCES

Albougami, A. S., Pounds, K. G., & Alotaibi, J. S. (2016). Comparison of four cultural competence models in transcultural nursing: A discussion paper. *International Archives of Nursing and HealthCare, 2*(4).

American Psychiatric Association. (2013). *Diagnostic and statistical manual of mental disorders* (5th ed.). Arlington, VA: Author.

Andrews, M. (2017). Some reflections on transcultural nursing's contributions when cultures clash. *Journal of Transcultural Nursing, 28*(6), 625.

Andrews, M. & Boyle, J. (2016). *Transcultural concepts in nursing care* (7th ed.). Philadelphia, PA: Wolters Kluwer.

Beeber, L. (2018). President's message. In *APNA News: The Psychiatric Nursing Voice*. Retrieved from https://www.apna.org/files/public/APNANewsletter-Winter2018.pdf

Byrne, D. (2016). Cultural competency in baccalaureate nursing education: A conceptual analysis. *International Journal for Human Caring, 20*(2), 114–119.

Campinha-Bacote, J. (2011). Coming to know cultural competence: An evolutionary process. *International Journal for Human Caring, 15*(3), 42–48.

Dieujuste, C. (2016). The concept of stigma in mental illness applied to Haitian Americans. *International Nursing Review, 63*(2), 200–207. https://doi.org/10.1111/inr.12267

Doornbos, M. M., Zandee, G. L., & DeGroot, J. (2014). Attending to communication and patterns of interaction: Culturally sensitive mental healthcare for groups of urban, ethnically diverse, impoverished, and underserved women. *Journal of the American Psychiatric Nurses Association, 20*(4), 239–249. https://doi.org/10.1177%2F1078390314543688

Giger, J. (2017). *Transcultural nursing: Assessment and intervention* (7th ed.). St. Louis, MO: Elsevier.

Harding, S. (2016). Self-stigma and veteran culture. *Journal of Transcultural Nursing, 28*(5), 438–444. https://doi.org/10.1177/1043659616676319

Hudson, C. C., Adams, S., & Lauderdale, J. (2015). Cultural expressions of intergenerational trauma and mental health nursing implications for U.S. healthcare delivery following refugee resettlement: An integrative review of the literature. *Journal of Transcultural Nursing, 27*(3), 286–301. https://doi.org/10.1177/1043659615587591

Jeffreys, M. (2016). *Teaching cultural competence in nursing and healthcare: Inquiry, action, and innovation* (3rd ed.). New York, NY: Springer.

Kahn, C. (2017). A brief introduction to mass migration: Then and now. *Psychoanalytic Review, 104*(6), 643–660.

Leininger, M., & McFarland, M. (2006). *Culture care diversity and universality: A worldwide nursing theory* (2nd ed.). Sudbury, MA: Jones and Bartlett.

Long, C. O. (2011). Culture and spiritual consideration in palliative care. *Journal of Pediatric Hematology/Oncology, 33 Suppl2*, S96–S101. https://doi.org/10.1097/mph.0b013e318230daf3

Marion, L., Douglas, M., Lavin, M. A., Barr, N., Gazaway, S., Thomas, E., et al. (2017). Implementing the new ANA standard 8: Culturally congruent practice. *Online Journal of Issues in Nursing, 22*(1), 1.

McGuire, T., & Miranda, J. (2008). New evidence regarding racial and ethnic disparities in mental health: policy implications. *Health Affairs, 27*(2), 393–403.

Mesler, D. M. (2014). A comparative study of cultural competence curricula in baccalaureate nursing programs. *Nurse Educator, 39*(4), 193–198. https://doi.org/10.1097/nne.0000000000000040

Millender, E. (2012). Acculturation stress among Maya in the United States. *Journal of Cultural Diversity, 19*(2), 58–64.

Nardi, D. & Waite, R. (2012). Establishing standards for culturally competent mental healthcare. *CPNP Journal of Psychosocial Nursing and Mental Health Services, 50*(7), 3–5.

National Conference of State Legislatures. (2014). *2014 Health Disparities Legislation.* Retrieved from http://www.ncsl.org/research/health/2014-health-disparities-legislation.aspx

Nguyen, T., Hellebuyck, M., Halpern, M., & Fritze, D. (2017). *The state of mental health in America 2018.* Alexandria, VA: Mental Health America, Inc. Retrieved from http://www.mentalhealthamerica.net/sites/default/files/2018%20The%20State%20of%20MH%20in%20America%20-%20FINAL.pdf

O'Brien, A. (2006). Moving toward culturally sensitive services for Indigenous people: a non-indigenous mental health nursing perspective. *Contemporary Nurse: A Journal for the Australian Nursing Profession, 21*(1), 22–31. https://doi.org/10.5172/conu.2006.21.1.22

Patchell, B. A., Robbins, L. K., Hoke, M. M., & Lowe, J. A. (2012). Circular model of cultural tailoring: An intervention adaption. *The Journal of Theory Construction & Testing, 16*(2), 45–51.

Patchell, B. A., Robbins, L. K., Lowe, J. A., & Hoke, M. M. (2015). The effect of a culturally tailored substance abuse prevention intervention with Plains Indian adolescents. *Journal of Cultural Diversity, 22*(1), 3–8.

Primm, A., Vasquez, M., Mays, R., Sammons-Posey, D., McKnight-Eily, L, Presley-Cantrell, L, et al. (2010). The role of public health in addressing racial and ethnic disparities in mental health and mental illness. *Preventing Chronic Disease, 7*(10), A20. http://www.cdc.gov/pcd/issues/2010

Purnell, L. (2013). *Transcultural healthcare: A culturally competent approach* (4th ed.). Philadelphia, PA: F.A. Davis.

Raman, J. (2015). Improved health and wellness outcomes in ethnically/culturally diverse patients through enhanced cultural competency in nurse educators. *Online Journal of Cultural Competence in Nursing and Healthcare, 5*(1), 104–117. http://dx.doi.org/10.9730/ojccnh.org/v5ila8

Ray, M. (2012). Remembering Madeleine M. Leininger, 1925–2012. *International Journal for Human Caring, 16*(4), 6–8.

Rosa, W. (2017). Immersing in context: A requisite for socially responsible transcultural nursing. *Journal of Transcultural Nursing, 28*(2), 117–118.

Scuglik, D. L., Alarcón, R., Lapeyre, A. C., Williams, M. D., & Logan, K. M. (2007). When the poetry no longer rhymes: Mental health issues among Somali immigrants in the USA. *Transcultural Psychiatry, 44*(4), 581–595. Retrieved from http://search.ebscohost.com/login.aspx?direct=true&db=cin20&AN=2009769914&site=ehost-live

Singleton, K., & Krause, E. M. S. (2009). Understanding cultural and linguistic barriers to health literacy. *Online Journal of Issues in Nursing, 14*(3), 2–2.

Substance Abuse and Mental health Services Administration. (2003). *Developing cultural competence in disaster mental health programs: Guiding principles and recommendations.* DHHS Publication No. SMA 3828. Rockville, MD: Author. Retrieved from https://store.samhsa.gov/shin/content//SMA03–3828/SMA03–3828.pdf

Substance Abuse and Mental health Services Administration. (2015). *Racial/ethnic differences in mental health service use among adults.* HHS Publication No. SMA-15–4906. Rockville, MD: Author. Retrieved from https://www.samhsa.gov/data/sites/default/files/MHServicesUseAmongAdults/MHServicesUseAmongAdults.pdf

Transcultural Nursing Society. (2018). Retrieved from http://www.tcns.org

U.S. Centers for Medicare & Medicaid Services. (n.d.). *The mental health parity and addiction equity act (MHPAEA).* Retrieved from https://www.cms.gov/CCIIO/Programs-and-Initiatives/Other-Insurance-Protections/mhpaea_factsheet.html

Warren, B. (2007). Cultural aspects of bipolar disorder: Interpersonal meaning for clients & psychiatric nurses. *Journal of Psychosocial Nursing & Mental Health Services, 45*(7), 32–53.

Warren, B. J. (2013). How culture is assessed in the *DSM-5. Journal of Psychosocial Nursing 51*(4), 40–45.

Williams, K. A., & Hamilton, K. (2009). Culturally competent assessment and care of self-mutilation in urological nursing. *Urological Nursing, 29*(3), 191–194.

Wilson, D. W. (2010). Culturally competent psychiatric nursing care. *Journal of Psychiatric and Mental Health Nursing, 17*, 715–724.

Wolf, K., Zoucha, R., McFarland, M., Salman, K., Dagne, A., & Hashi, N. (2014). Somali immigrant perceptions of mental health and illness: An ethnonursing study. *Journal of Transcultural Nursing, 27*(4), 349–358. https://doi.org/10.1177/1043659614550487

Yurkovich, E. E., & Lattergrass, I. (2008). Defining health and unhealthiness: Perceptions held by Native American Indians with persistent mental illness. *Mental Health, Religion & Culture, 11*(5), 437–459. https://doi.org/10.1080/13674670701473751

Zoucha, R., & Wolf, K. (2018). Cultural implications. In Halter, M. J. (Ed.), *Varcarolis' foundations of psychiatric-mental health nursing* (8th ed., pp. 77–90). St. Louis, MO: Elsevier.

CHAPTER 8

# Culture and Consent in Clinical Care

## *A Critical Review of Nursing and Nursing Ethics Literature*

Michael J. Deem and Felicia Stokes

**ABSTRACT**

The duty to obtain informed consent carries significant weight within the dominant normative frameworks for healthcare research and clinical care. Informed consent is seen as an important expression of a patient's freedom of choice in healthcare decision-making. However, some clinicians and researchers have raised concerns that the implementation of a normative framework in clinical care that assigns considerable moral weight to patient autonomy and informed consent for all patients, regardless of their cultural identities and values, might be incompatible or in tension with culturally congruent care. The authors of this chapter conducted a review of 83 peer-review nursing and nursing ethics articles that focus on cultural identity and informed consent for treatment within clinical practice settings. The purpose of this review is to identify salient themes in nurses' characterizations of the influence of cultural identity and values on clinicians' and patients' perceptions of informed consent in clinical contexts, as well as of elements of the consent process such as truth-telling and decisional authority. The authors identify and describe multiple themes running


http://dx.doi.org/10.1891/0739-6686.37.223

through this literature, and provide a critical analysis of these characterizations and ways to rethink how cultural considerations modulate communication of clinical information and affect clinicians' interpretation of patient autonomy and informed consent.

## INTRODUCTION

The duty to obtain informed consent carries significant weight within the dominant normative frameworks for medical research and clinical care. From the perspective of many bioethicists, nurses, and clinical researchers, a patient's informed consent to treatment and care is an important expression of freedom of choice in healthcare decision-making (Faden & Beauchamp, 1983; Grace, 2018; Wear, 1998). Working to ensure that patients are accurately informed and free to make their own decisions is an important way in which clinicians promote and protect patient autonomy. Traditionally, four elements are considered necessary to ensure that clinicians obtain informed consent; namely, patient competence for making healthcare decisions, full and accurate disclosure of diagnostic, prognostic, and treatment information to the patient, patient understanding of this information, and a voluntary decision by the patient. These conditions, it is commonly argued, must be met in order to obtain a patient's informed consent, though some bioethicists also underscore the importance of relationships of trust between clinicians and patients for the consent process (O'Neill, 2002).

Some bioethicists, clinicians, and researchers have raised questions regarding the compatibility of informed consent, and the principle of respect for patient autonomy broadly, with recognition and respect for cultural identities and traditions that do not give prominent places to these values (e.g., Candib, 2002; Levine, 1991). This concern often arises when considering the implementation of a normative framework in clinical care that assigns considerable moral weight to patient autonomy and informed consent for all patients, regardless of their cultural identities and values. One might be concerned that this amounts to a sort of normative imperialism, unfairly burdening patients who do not hold a Western conception of individual autonomy or who are accustomed to making important clinical decisions with friends, families, or their broader communities.

This burden might be especially acute when it involves the communication of diagnostic or prognostic information that is potentially distressing. For example, patients who come from cultural backgrounds in which families or prominent community members are the primary decision-makers about serious medical matters, or in which direct communication about such information is considered inappropriate or harmful, might experience an array of negative psychosocial effects. Thus, any discussion of the role of informed consent in clinical care, as well as of elements of informed consent such as truth-telling and decisional responsibility, must include consideration of patients' cultural identities, values, and practices.

The goal of this critical review is twofold (Grant & Booth, 2009). First, the review aims to provide a broad overview of how the nursing and nursing ethics literature characterizes the influence of cultural identity and values on clinicians' and patients' perception of informed consent in clinical contexts, as well as on elements of the consent process such as truth-telling and decisional authority. Second, the review provides both a critical analysis of this characterization and ways to rethink how cultural considerations modulate communication of clinical information and affect clinicians' interpretation of patient autonomy and informed consent.

## METHOD

We conducted a review of the peer-review nursing and nursing ethics literature in April 2018, to identify articles that focus on cultural identity and informed consent for treatment within clinical practice settings. We conducted the literature search utilizing CINAHL and PubMed databases. We restricted the search to peer-reviewed, English-language articles published between 2007 and 2018 (roughly one decade), and further limited the search through the use of keywords selected in consultation with the head of research engagement at a university library.

The following keywords limited the search of the CINAHL database:

> ((MH "Cultural Competence") OR (MH "Culture+") OR (MH "Religion and Religions+") OR (MH "Transcultural Care") OR Cultur* OR Religion*)
> AND
> ((MH "Consent+") OR (MH "Patient Autonomy") OR (MH "Treatment Refusal") OR Consent* OR "Patient Autonomy" OR "Treatment Refusal" OR "Patient autonomy")
> AND
> (Nurs* OR (MH "Nurses+") OR (MH "Nursing Care+") OR (MH "Nursing Role"))

The following keywords limited the search of the PubMed database:

> ("Informed Consent"[Mesh] OR "Personal Autonomy"[Mesh] OR "Treatment Refusal"[Mesh] OR Consent*[ot] OR Consent*[tiab] OR "Patient Autonomy"[ot] OR "Patient Autonomy"[tiab] OR "Treatment Refusal"[ot] OR "Treatment Refusal"[tiab])

AND
("Culture"[Mesh] OR "Religion"[Mesh] OR "Transcultural Nursing"[Mesh] OR Cultur*[ot] OR Cultur*[tiab] OR Religion*[ot] OR Religion *[tiab])
AND
(Nurs*[ot] OR Nurs*[tiab] OR "Nurses"[Mesh] OR "Nursing Care"[Mesh] OR "Nursing"[Mesh])
AND
(bioethics[sb] OR jsubsetn[text])

The searches identified 423 citations, of which we identified 356 as unique. We uploaded these citations, and any accompanying abstracts were uploaded to Covidence for screening.

Through Covidence, we employed a four-stage screening process. The first screening stage consisted of independent review of all 356 article abstracts. For citations that were not accompanied by an abstract, we pulled and reviewed the full text. We independently voted "Yes," "Maybe," or "No" for inclusion of each article in the review. The second screening stage involved discussion and resolution of any discrepancies in first-stage voting. At the end of the second screening stage, we excluded 213 citations, thereby reducing the number of citations for additional screening to 143. We uploaded the full text of these 143 citations to EndNote X7 for the next screening stage.

During the third screening stage, we independently reviewed 143 full-text articles. We agreed on the following inclusion criteria:

- An article must substantively discuss patient informed consent for treatment or a constitutive aspect of patient informed consent for treatment (e.g., clinician truth-telling; patient understanding)
- An article must substantively discuss the relation between patient informed consent for treatment and cultural identity or cultural issues
- An article must be authored or coauthored by a nurse, or contain explicit implications for nursing practice

We agreed to exclude any article that did not clearly meet these three criteria, including articles primarily focused on pediatric care, surrogate-decision-making, and informed consent in research contexts. After reviewing each of the 143 remaining articles, we independently voted "Include" or "Exclude" through Covidence for the review. At the fourth screening stage, we discussed and resolved any discrepancies that resulted from the voting. At the conclusion of the fourth screening stage, 83 articles remained for the review (see Figure 8.1).

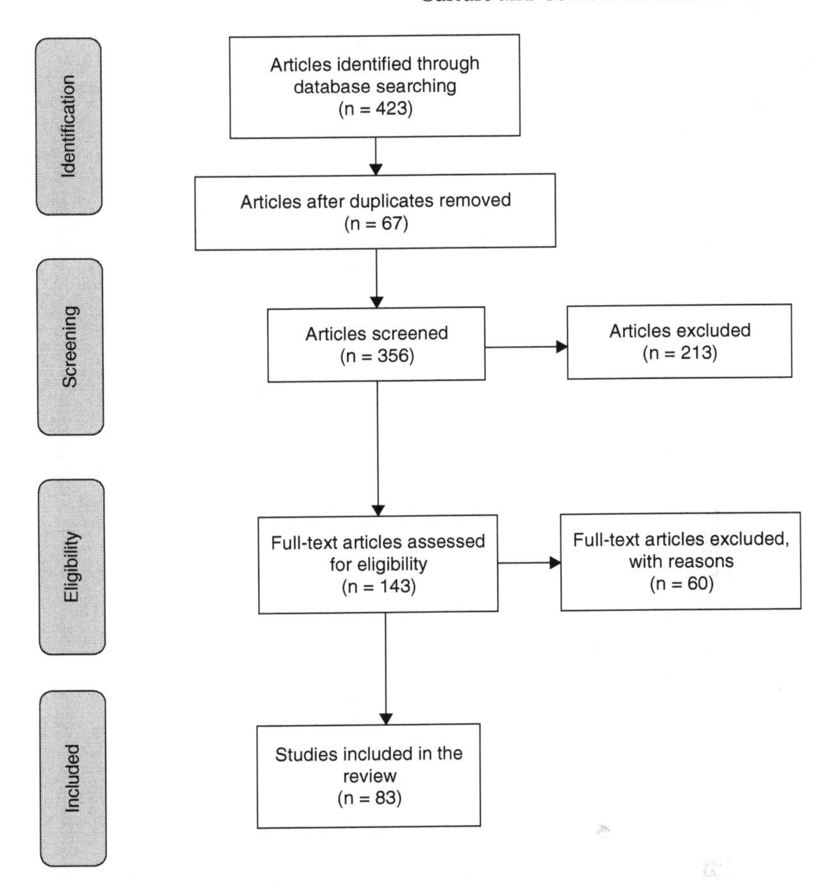


**FIGURE 8.1** PRISMA 2009 flow diagram: Culture and consent in clinical care: A critical review of the nursing and nursing ethics literature. From "Preferred Reporting Items for Systematic Reviews and Meta-Analyses: The PRISMA Statement," by D. Moher, A. Liberati, J. Tetzlaff, D. G. Altman, and The PRISMA group, 2009, *PLoS Med, 6*(6), e1000097. http://dx.doi.org/10.1371/journal.pmed1000097
For more information, visit www.prisma-statement.org.

## RESULTS

We reviewed 83 peer-reviewed articles from nursing and nursing ethics journals. Of these 83 articles, 17 were quantitative studies (see Table 8.1), 26 were qualitative studies (see Table 8.2), and 40 are conceptual, ethics, or case-based discussion. Following Halkoaho et al. (2016), we classified this last group as "theoretical" articles (see Table 8.3).

**TABLE 8.1**
*Selected Quantitative Studies ($n$ = 17)*

| Author/Year | Aim | Method | Location |
|---|---|---|---|
| Bentwich, Dickman, and Oberman (2017) | To explore perspectives of different cultural groups on human dignity and autonomy of dementia patients | Questionnaire study ($n$ = 197) of caretakers | Israel |
| Bülow et al. (2012) | To explore differences in end-of-life decisions and respect for patient autonomy among clinicians who are religious and those who are only affiliated with a religion | Questionnaire ($n$ = 1,268) of clinicians and patients | Sweden, The Netherlands, UK, Czech Republic, Israel, Portugal |
| Carolan, Steele, and Margetts (2010) | To examine attitudes and beliefs of multiethnic sample of women with gestational diabetes | Questionnaire study ($n$ = 143) of patients with gestational diabetes | Australia |
| Chang et al. (2008) | To identify how older Korean people seek information and desire to participate in healthcare decisions | Questionnaire study ($n$ = 165) of men and women aged 65 or older | South Korea |
| Chima (2013) | To determine whether the quality of informed consent obtained by clinicians in South Africa is consistent with international ethical standards and local regulations | Questionnaire study ($n$ = 946) of clinicians | South Africa |
| Clark (2007) | To examine informed consent process from perspectives of intensive care patients | Secondary analysis of quantitative data | N/A |
| Demirsoy, Elcioglu, and Yildiz (2008) | To investigate nurses' and patients' attitudes regarding truth-telling and patient needs and wants regarding information about diagnosis and prognosis | Survey study ($n$ = 465) of nurses and patients | Turkey |

| | | | |
|---|---|---|---|
| Gorden et al. (2010) | To assess the extent of training in culturally and linguistically competent care in US transplantation centers | Survey study ($n$ = 280) of kidney transplant administrators | United States |
| Holt et al. (2009) | To examine the effectiveness of spiritually based education on informed decision-making about prostate cancer screening among African American men | Survey study ($n$ = 49) of African American man with no prostate cancer diagnosis | United States |
| Ingravallo et al. (2017) | To investigate nurses' views and practices in providing information to patients in a global context | Cross-sectional study ($n$ = 295) of Korean and Italian nurses | Italy, Korea |
| Ito, Tanida, and Turale (2010) | To explore perspectives of Japanese patients their families on participation in ethical decision-making during hospitalization | Descriptive survey study ($n$ = 169) of patients and family members | Japan |
| Lillie et al. (2014) | To characterize the perspectives of partners of patients with breast cancer in treatment decisions and describe racial and ethnic differences in decisional outcomes | Cross-sectional survey study ($n$ = 517) of partners of patients with breast cancer | United States |
| Lopez-McKee, McNeill, Bader, and Morales (2008) | To examine the level of cancer fatalism and other behavioral determinants in Mexican American women identified as regular or infrequent mammography screeners | Cross-sectional, descriptive study ($n$ = 68) of Mexican American women | United States |
| Lowther et al. (2014) | To assess the effectiveness of a nurse-led palliative care intervention for HIV positive patients on antiretroviral therapy: recruitment, refusal, randomisation and missing data | Randomized control trial and interview study ($n$ = 120) of HIV positive patients on antiretroviral therapy | Kenya |

(Continued)

**TABLE 8.1**
*Selected Quantitative Studies ($n$ = 17) (Continued)*

| Author/Year | Aim | Method | Location |
| --- | --- | --- | --- |
| Neary, Cahill, Kirwan, Kiely, and Redmond (2008) | To examine the impact a signature on a consent form has on patients' perception of the quality of the informed consent process | Randomized, prospective clinical trial of ($n$ = 37) outpatient clinic patients | Ireland |
| Peretti-Watel et al. (2008) | To assess French district nurses' attitudes toward terminally ill patients' autonomy | Questionnaire study ($n$ = 602) of French district nurses | France |
| Valente (2010) | To investigate cultural influences on HIV patients' preferences for end-of-life care | Survey study ($n$ = 95) of veterans living with HIV disease | United States |

**TABLE 8.2**
*Selected Qualitative Studies (n = 26)*

| Author/Year | Aim | Method | Location |
|---|---|---|---|
| Alpers (2018) | To examine factors that build trust or create distrust between healthcare professionals and ethnic minority patients | Interview study ($n = 10$) of immigrant patients | Norway |
| Bentwich, Dickman, and Oberman (2017) | To explore differences among caretaker attitudes toward patient dignity and autonomy in dementia care | Interview study ($n = 20$) of caretakers | Israel |
| Davies Elwyn, Papadopoulos, Fleming, and Williams (2009) | To explore how clinicians view patient decision-making from an ethical perspective | Interview study ($n = 13$) of clinicians | UK |
| Davoudi, Nayeri, Zokaei, and Fazeli (2017) | To examine processes of and challenges to informed consent in the emergency ward | Field work, participant observation, and interview study of clinicians | Iran |
| Fernández-Sola et al. (2012) | To examine participation and responsibility assigned to nurses in end-of-life decision-making according to the *Rights to and Guarantee of Dignity for the Individual During the Process of Death Act* | Discourse analysis | Spain |
| Fitch, Beaudoin, and Johnson (2013) | To gain increased understanding about dialogue between cancer care clinicians and cancer patients regarding the topic of sexuality | Interview study ($n = 44$) of clinicians | Canada |
| Goodman, Edge, Agazio, and Prue-Owens (2015) | To describe cultural factors that impact military nursing care for Iraqi patients | Focus groups ($n = 15$) of military nurses and licensed nurses | Iraq |

(Continued)

**TABLE 8.2**

*Selected Qualitative Studies ($n = 26$) (Continued)*

| Author/Year | Aim | Method | Location |
|---|---|---|---|
| Granero-Molina, Fernández-Sola, and Aguilera-Manrique (2009) | To present and discuss findings of application of sociolinguistic SPEAKING model to informed consent documents for laparoscopic surgery | Documentary analysis | Spain |
| Harrison, Logar, Le, and Glass, (2016) | To identify global health ethics issues in professional training with resource-limited regions | Focus groups and one interview ($n = 18$) of healthcare professionals | United States |
| Jafree, Zakar, Fischer, and Zakar (2015) | To identify aspects of the hidden curriculum that encourage ethical violations | Interview and focus group study ($n = 42$) | Pakistan |
| Lee, Li, Arai, and Puntillo (2009) | To describe a formal process of translating documents for use by research participants and patients | Translation process utilizing 3-point Flaherty scale | United States |
| Lee, Lee, Kong, Kim, and Kim (2009) | To investigate nurses' perceptions of informed consent and role in improving consent processes in Korea | Interview study ($n = 12$) of nurses | Korea |
| Lin, Huang and Chen (2016) | To discover reasons for family involvement in adult patients' decision-making about surgery | Interview study ($n = 24$) of family members and surgery patients | Taiwan |
| Lowther et al. (2014) | To assess the effectiveness of a nurse-led palliative care intervention for HIV positive patients on antiretroviral therapy: recruitment, refusal, randomisation and missing data | Randomized control trial and interview study ($n = 120$) of HIV positive patients on antiretroviral therapy | Kenya |

| | | | |
|---|---|---|---|
| McLaughlin, Elahi, Ciesielski, and Pomerantz (2016) | To explore attitudes of Muslims living in the United States toward long-term care decision-making | Interview study ($n$ = 167) of members of Muslim mosques | United States |
| Oliveira and Oliveira (2013) | To investigate factors that interfere with follow-up of treatment for hypertensive patients | Interview study ($n$ = 25) of hypertensive patients | Brazil |
| Rio-Valle et al. (2009) | To explore clinicians' perspectives on communication of terminal prognosis to patients | Interview study ($n$ = 42) of clinicians | Spain |
| Sialubanje, Massar, Hamer, and Ruiter (2015) | To identify reasons that women give birth at home and seek the assistance of traditional birth attendants | Focus group and interview study ($n$ = 130) of women of reproductive age | Zambia |
| Sneesby, Satchell, Good, and van der Riet (2011) | To obtain information to support palliative care healthcare workers in end-of-life care for Sudanese patients | Focus group study ($n$ = 15) of members of a Sudanese community in Australia | Australia |
| Sullivan (2017) | To examine informed consent and disclosure practices among Japanese healthcare professionals | Interview study ($n$ = 15) of Japanese healthcare professionals | Japan |
| Sun, Hsia, and Sheu (2008) | To understand patterns and interpretations of women's experiences of amniocentesis in Taiwan | Interview study ($n$ = 20) of women 35 years of age or older | Taiwan |
| Susilo, van Dalen, Chenault, and Scherpbier (2014) | To investigate clinicians' views about the informed consent process and nurse' roles in this process | Questionnaire study ($n$ = 745) of clinicians | Indonesia |
| Susilo et al. (2013) | To investigate clinicians' views about the informed consent process and nurse' roles in this process | Focus group study ($n$ = 27) of hospital managers | Indonesia |

(Continued)

**TABLE 8.2**
*Selected Qualitative Studies ($n$ = 26) (Continued)*

| Author/Year | Aim | Method | Location |
|---|---|---|---|
| Toda, Sakamoto, Tagaya, Takahashi, and Davis (2015) | To explore implications of Japanese psychiatric nurses' decisions to intervene as patient advocates | Interview study ($n$ = 21) of nurses | Japan |
| Watts et al. (2017) | To identify oncology clinicians' challenges in communicating to patients from minority backgrounds | Interview study ($n$ = 38) of oncology clinicians | Australia |
| Zhang, Wong, and Zheng (2017) | To explore the experience of rectal cancer patients who will undergo colostomy surgery | Interview study ($n$ = 18) of patients with diagnosis of primary rectal cancer and expectation of colostomy surgery | China |

**TABLE 8.3**
*Selected Theoretical Studies (n = 40)*

| Author/Year | Aim |
|---|---|
| Baeke, Wils, and Broeckaert (2011) | To explore Jewish perspectives on withholding and withdrawing life-sustaining treatment |
| Barwell (2011) | To examine issues surrounding truth-telling in cancer care |
| Blackman (2009) | To discuss importance of role of nurses in diminishing negative effects of perceived racism felt by patients |
| Braithwaite, Chichester, and Reid (2010) | To examine issues in care for Jehovah's Witness patients and multicultural approaches to care |
| Brown (2014) | To explore impact of religion and culture on truth-telling and futile treatment in end of life care |
| Brownie, Horstmanshof, and Garbutt (2014) | To identify factors that impact residents' transition and adjustment to, and experience of, long-term care |
| Browning (2009) | To address key issues in spiritual assessment in end-of-life care |
| Calloway (2009) | To examine applicability of informed consent requirements from a multicultural perspective |
| Chater and Tsai (2008) | To examine the notion of truth telling and its place in nursing care for patients from minority cultures |
| Chichester (2007) | To provide information on cultural and religious groups to nurses seeking consent for perinatal autopsy |
| Clabots (2012) | To identify strategies to overcome barriers to end-of-life discussions in acute care |
| Clancy (2013) | To consider how cultural awareness and sensitivity relate to genetics in nursing practice |
| Collins et al. (2018) | To synthesize nursing knowledge regarding cultural perspectives of end-of-life care and advance care planning among African Americans |
| Cooper, Chidwick, Cybulski, and Sibbald (2015) | To demonstrate effectiveness of the *Checklist for meeting Ethical and Legal Obligations* in the intensive care unit |
| Coyle (2014) | To provide background for addressing dilemmas in palliative and end-of-life care from a Western ethical perspective |
| Doolen and York (2007) | To describe cultural differences that nurses might encounter in end-of-life care |

(*Continued*)

**TABLE 8.3**

*Selected Theoretical Studies (n = 40) (Continued)*

| Author/Year | Aim |
|---|---|
| Druml et al. (2016) | To provide a critical summary of the ethics of artificial nutrition and hydration therapy |
| Effa-Heap (2009) | To examine legal and consent issues surrounding blood transfusion in Jehovah's Witness patients |
| Evans and Ndirangu (2009) | To provide an overview of provider-initiated HIV testing and counseling policy guidance and examine its implication for nursing in sub-Saharan Africa |
| French and Narayanasamy (2011) | To develop a discourse on the ethics of prayer as a spiritual intervention in clinical care |
| Greenberger (2011) | To describe how ethical issues in healthcare are approached within a Jewish bioethical framework |
| Guven (2010) | To examine critically the "cultural incompatibility" argument about disclosure of information to cancer patients in Turkey |
| Hodge (2015) | To describe and evaluate rationales for administering spiritual assessment in clinical care |
| Johnstone and Kanitsaki (2009) | To explore cross-cultural considerations in end-of-life care planning |
| Kidd, Colbert, and Jatoi (2015) | To describe issues related to mammography screening in young African American women |
| Lech (2008) | To consider how sexual assault nurse examiners can provide culturally competent care to victims of sexual assault |
| Leever (2011) | To explore the moral normative foundations of cultural competence and their relationship to patient autonomy and welfare |
| Ling, Yu, and Guo (2017) | To provide ethical guidance to Chinese nurses regarding truth-telling to patients about terminal illness |
| Marrone (2016) | To examine the concept of informed consent in care for Saudi patients and families in the United States |
| Mor and Oberle (2008) | To explore the moral direction of Jewish law to women regarding decision-making about genetic testing |
| Narruhn & Schellenberg (2013) | To examine how care ethics can be applied to a cross-cultural reproductive dilemma |

(Continued)

**TABLE 8.3**

*Selected Theoretical Studies (n = 40) (Continued)*

| Author/Year | Aim |
|---|---|
| Ortiz and Casey (2017) | To explore a case in which cultural beliefs impact a patient's ability to exercise autonomy |
| Padela Malik, Curlin, and De Vries (2015) | To analyze two accounts of surrogate decision-making with little input sought from patient |
| Pugh (2014) | To discuss the ethical and legal issues surrounding care for dying patients in Australia |
| Rising (2017) | To examine history and assumptions of preference for truth-telling in the United States, and to introduce the concept of cultural humility |
| Sagbakken, Frich, Bjune, and Porter (2013) | To consider ethical implications of directly observed treatment of in a cross-cultural perspective |
| Starr (2015) | To explore legal considerations when a patient refuses treatment on cultural or religious grounds |
| Thompson (2011) | To describe cultural differences regarding truth-telling to patients |
| Wilson et al. (2014) | To examine understandings of autonomy and choice in palliative and end-of-life care |
| Zalon, Constantino, and Andres (2008) | To illustrate ethical and practical conflicts nurses might experience in critical care |

Through our review and analysis of these 83 articles, we extrapolated six dominant themes in studies and discussions of the influence of cultural identity and values on perceptions of informed consent and its constitutive elements:

(1) cross-cultural applicability of dominant conceptions of patient autonomy and informed consent
(2) culture and barriers to informed consent in clinical contexts
(3) influence of culture on clinicians' perspectives on patient autonomy and informed consent
(4) influence of culture on patients' perspectives on patient autonomy and informed consent
(5) culturally appropriate communication
(6) professional codes of ethical conduct

### Theme 1: Cross-Cultural Applicability of Dominant Conceptions of Patient Autonomy and Informed Consent

A recurring theme raised in the peer-review nursing and nursing ethics literature is the degree to which dominant conceptions of patient autonomy and the ethical requirement to obtain informed consent fit within cultural value systems in which individual autonomy and decision-making do not occupy prominent places. Some clinicians abstractly suggest that there is incompatibility between "Western," individualistic notions of individual autonomy and some cultural traditions. One frequently finds expression of such doubts over their compatibility like the following:

> "The Western traditions based on concepts of individual autonomy, informed consent, and truth telling do not fit all cultures and societies." (Coyle, 2014, p. 6).
>
> "Respecting patient choices may be foreign and even antithetical to patients and families from cultural groups who do not share or accept the principles and value assumptions that under pin much of mainstream Western bioethics discourse on end-of-life decision making." (Johnstone & Kanitaski, 2009, p. 407)
>
> "Is the Anglo-American ethic of individual autonomy the right value that should be incorporated into other cultural belief systems in order to elevate their ethical standards?" (Calloway, 2009, p. 69)

Other clinicians and researchers are more specific with regard to where the conflict of values possibly lies. Some locate the potential tension arising from Western medicine's commitment to disclosure of medical information directly to the patient (Clabots, 2012; Clark, 2007; Doolen & York, 2007; Rising, 2017; Watts et al., 2017). Insofar as informed consent is typically conceptualized as involving accurate disclosure of information to the patient, there is potential value conflict in cases in which patients and their families are accustomed to family- or community-oriented disclosure and decision-making. Others suggest that Western perceptions of urgency in care undergird the assumption that a patient wants diagnostic and prognostic information in order to make a decision quickly about care. However, patients who do not identify with this Western notion of time might not perceive a similar urgency in deciding how to respond to such information and resolve a health condition (Clark, 2007).

Researchers suggest that in some cultures individuals are shielded from information about terminal diagnosis or end-of-life care planning. Instead, within these cultures there is a tendency to defer to the patient's family or cultural leaders regarding decisions about both care planning and communication of health information to a patient. For example, researchers found that families of Taiwanese and Chinese cultural backgrounds often seek to make clinical decisions for their loved-ones, or protect them from potential harm of distressing diagnoses, such as terminal cancer, by concealing that information (Lin, Huang, & Chen, 2017; Ling et al., 2017). In the context of end-of-life care, African American patients often express a desire to forego control over clinical decision-making, delegating authority over care to family members, close friends, or community leaders (Collins et al., 2018). Researchers have also observed that some distinct cultures, including Somali and Mexican-American cultures, tend to see important decision-making in clinical contexts to be a family-oriented or communitarian process, as opposed to the more individualistic process that seems tied to the ethical requirement to obtain informed consent from patients themselves (Lopez-McKee et al., 2008; Narruhn & Schellenberg, 2013).

Researchers have also noted tensions arising within some countries undergoing shifts in healthcare values and policies, particularly where the ethics education of clinicians is modelled on Western pedagogical models and normative frameworks. For example, Chang et al. (2008) note that nurses in Korea are now taught basic nursing ethics from a Western viewpoint. This has led to challenges for younger clinicians in implementing a normative framework in care that promotes individual autonomy within a culture that traditionally values the protection of individuals from distressing information (Chang et al., 2008). This challenge is especially acute in countries with multicultural populations, such as Australia, where Western bioethics has progressively dominated ethics education for clinicians (Chater & Tsai, 2008; Padela et al., 2015).

Clinicians, researchers, and ethicists differ, however, with respect to recommended responses to potential tensions between the ethical requirement of informed consent and multicultural values among patient populations. One study found that some clinicians perceive a need to abandon a commitment to informed consent and respect for patient autonomy when caring for patients whose cultural identities and values assign little importance to individualistic decision-making (Harrison et al., 2016). Some instead recommend that despite some tension, clinicians should ultimately respect the dominant ethical framework of the institution in which they practice (Coyle, 2014). The recommendation that clinicians generally, and nurses particularly, ought to be aware of cultural differences among patients and seek ways to accommodate patient preferences remains a dominant view in the literature (Fernández-Sola et al., 2012; Mor & Oberle, 2008).

### Theme 2: Culture and Barriers to Informed Consent in Clinical Contexts

Some researchers and ethicists note that aspects of culture might indirectly contribute to the formation of barriers to informed consent within certain clinical contexts. For example, Fitch et al., (2013) note that critical discussions of sexuality are considered to be taboo in some cultures. Patients who identify with this cultural norm might be reticent to discuss sexual health with a nurse or other healthcare provider, or with a healthcare provider of a different gender (McLaughlin et al., 2016). This can make clinical discussions about conditions and treatments that affect sexual identity and behavior difficult. Some cultures might have taboos relative to discussions about death and risk of harm, creating challenges to discussion of high-risk interventions or end-of-life care planning with patients (Calloway, 2009; Sun, Hsia, & Seu, 2008). These and similar taboos might generate barriers to disclosing health information and explaining risks of treatments to patients, thereby precluding patient informed consent.

Language barriers between patients and clinicians can also generate difficulties in obtaining informed consent (Lee et al., 2009). A study of military nurses providing care to Iraqi patients found that nurses saw language barriers that resulted in suboptimal communication with patients, even when a translator assisted. This is because nurses may not be able to verify that health information is accurately translated, or whether a translator might be biased regarding what the patient needs to know (Goodman et al., 2015). A national survey of US transplantation centers shows that few provide culturally and linguistically competent care training to their nurses, despite often having multicultural or large Hispanic transplant patient populations (Gordan, Caicedo, Ladner, Reddy, & Abecassis, 2010). About a third of the survey responses in this study reported that staff receive some form of cultural competency training. Perception of linguistic difficulties, including complex wording or difficult terminology, might lead nurses or other healthcare professionals to bypass consent procedures when initiating testing or treatment for patients (Granero-Moline et al., 2009; Ortiz & Casey, 2017).

Breakdowns in trust due to cultural identity and tradition can also create obstacles to informed consent. Nurses are the among the most trusted professionals and are thus well suited for patient advocacy in informed consent and healthcare decision-making (Brenan, 2017). Trust is a mutual fundamental characteristic of the nurse–patient relationship and should be respected by all parties (Zalon et al., 2008). However, discrimination and lack of access to high quality health care have resulted in a historical distrust of healthcare professionals by minority populations (Isaacson & Lynch, 2018; Johnstone, Rawson, Hutchinson, & Redley, 2018).

This review revealed a significant subtheme concerning patients of a minority culture or language who fear that decision-making in mainstream health care may leave them disadvantaged or denied proper access to healthcare interventions (Johnstone & Kanitsaki, 2009). Historical circumstances where a lack of consent occurred have contributed to long term patient distrust, hostility and feelings of lack of control (Jafree et al., 2015). This has an adverse effect on informed consent, communication and shared decision-making (Blackman, 2009; Neary et al., 2008). Some minority cultures automatically view the informed consent process with distrust. Others still have confidence, not specific to the provider, but in the institution where care is being delivered (Neary et al., 2008). Extra time must be taken to establish trust in these instances to ensure that informed consent is fully appreciated (Lech, 2008). For example, many Muslim patients value interpersonal relationships, and trust must be developed before decision-making and meaningful communication occur (Marrone, 2016).

A lack of cultural competence in healthcare professionals, real or perceived, may cause wavering trust or distrust from patients (Alpers, 2018). Research suggests that shared cultural identity between the healthcare professional and the patient strengthens the patient–provider relationship (Alpers, 2018; Blackman, 2009). Patients are more likely to trust healthcare professionals who are the same gender, age, race, and culture (Alpers, 2018). Lee et al. (2009) discovered that nurses can be instrumental in cultivating trust between patients and the entire healthcare team and are valuable advocates in the informed consent process. Truth telling and ensuring patients are fully informed according to their preference are obligations of trust that nurses must deliberately meet in order to balance the principles of beneficence and autonomy in practice (Ling et al., 2017; Thompson, 2011).

### Theme 3: Influence of Culture on Clinicians' Perspectives on Informed Consent

Empirical studies show that the cultural identities and values of nurses can significantly influence the way in which they perceive and discharge the duty to obtain informed consent from patients. The peer-review nursing and nursing ethics literature suggests that clinicians bring these identities and values to bear either consciously or tacitly in their assessments of patient competence, what information is appropriate to disclose and withhold, and whom to inform about health information. Lack of awareness of this influence and refusal to take critical distance from culturally entrenched biases might negatively impact patient buy-in and lead to failure in providing holistic and culturally congruent care (Hodge, 2015; Lech, 2008; Ortiz & Casey, 2017).

Researchers have found that nurses in certain countries and geographical regions often carry underlying assumptions about a patient's ability to comprehend health information based on the patient's cultural, racial, or religious background. For example, the discussion sections of two unrelated studies—one of Australian clinicians and another of American intensive-care patients—suggest that clinicians sometimes assume that a patient's comprehension of conditions and risk assessments varies according the cultural or racial group in which the patient is assumed to belong (Carolan et al., 2010; Clark, 2007). The Australian study in particular generalizes this assumption, suggesting that women from "non-Caucasian" backgrounds are at risk of poorer self-management and lower health literacy regarding gestational diabetes than Caucasian patients.

In a study of maternity clinicians in the UK, some participants characterized "Asian" and "Muslim" patients as having limited cognitive capacity to understand information, constrained choice in their decisions to marry, failing to regulate fertility due to cultural values and practices, and taking little responsibility in their child-bearing decisions. In contrast, participants tended to valorize the choices of white, wealthy patients who made the same child-bearing decisions as Asian and Muslim mothers. Participants characterized the former's decisions to be autonomous and responsible, while characterizing the latter's decisions about pregnancy and child-raising as less informed and passively made (Davies et al., 2009). Such assumptions about patients' competence based on their cultural identity or background might affect clinician decisions about when and to what degree health information is communicated to patients. Furthermore, stereotyping patients' responsibility, control, and competence strictly on the basis of cultural classification might lead to differential provision of health information within multicultural patient populations (Davies et al., 2009).

Some researchers and ethicists also discuss tendencies among clinicians from non-Western cultures to withhold information from patients, especially in end-of-life care settings or when information is about a serious condition or terminal diagnosis (Browning, 2009; Doolen & York, 2007). Withholding information in this context, however, is not considered to be deceptive or inappropriate. In some non-Western cultures, beneficent care sometimes outweighs the duty to disclose complete and accurate information to the patient, and withholding information that is potentially distressing for a patient is thought to be a way to promote patient well-being and avoid psychological and emotional harm (Barwell, 2011; Doolen & York, 2007; Harrison et al., 2016).

However, such broad theoretical claims about how non-Western cultures view patient autonomy and informed consent might miss important nuances of individual cultures. For example, an empirical study of Indonesian nurses' perspectives on clinical authority and informed consent shows that the participants regard obtaining informed consent to be a duty attached to the nursing profession, but hierarchical structures in healthcare organizations sometimes prevent them discharging this duty (Susilo et al., 2013). A more detailed picture of clinicians' perspectives on truth-telling and information provision also emerges from a large study of Turkish nurses and patients in a university hospital. This study shows that there is considerable support among nurses for providing accurate information to patients, considering truth-telling to be a moral duty of clinicians. In cases in which distressing information is communicated, the nurses advocated not for withholding information, but for tailoring communication according to individual patients' preferences about disclosure and decision-making (Demirsoy et al., 2008). Interestingly, this perspective appears to conflict with prominent clinical textbooks utilized in the training of clinicians in Turkey. A prominent ethics textbook asserts that clinicians ought not to engage in direct communication to patients about serious conditions (e.g., terminal cancer) because, unlike European patients, Turkish patients are not psychologically or emotionally capable of handling this information (Guven, 2010). These two studies suggest that broad generalizations about truth-telling and information disclosure in non-Western cultures should be more nuanced than is often supposed in nursing and nursing ethics literature.

Researchers have also found that the cultural identities and values of nurses and other healthcare professionals influence their decisions about to whom they communicate health information. Studies of clinicians in Italy, Korea, and Japan report that they frequently deliver complex health information to a patient's family rather than to the patient (Ingravallo et al., 2017; Toda et al., 2015). Cultural values might also influence a nurse's perception of patient autonomy in certain healthcare fields. A study of Israeli-born nursing home staff found that Arab caretakers tended to view nursing home and dementia patients as possessing autonomy and to involve their patients in decision-making about care, whereas their Sabra and Russian peers did so to a much lesser extent. (Bentwich, et al. 2017; Bentwich & Oberman, 2018). This study shows that cultural identities, values of clinicians, and geographic region do not always covary with respect to influence on perception of patient autonomy and informed consent.

A minor subtheme that emerged in this review is the way in which the informed consent process might be impacted by nurses' religious identities or their view of a patient's religious identity. Nurses who endorse a particular religious or spiritual identity might feel compelled to pray over or with their patients as a form of healing. However, initiating prayer without a patient's consent not only disregards a patient's consent to participate in such "treatment," but might impose spiritual views that are not held in common (French & Narayanasamy, 2011). With respect to the religious views of patients, nurses should not assume that spiritual beliefs and religious views are well-integrated in a patient's deliberation about health care, particularly complex decisions about critical or end-of-life care. Exploration of patients religious beliefs might enable nurses to assist patients in connecting religious views with decisions about care (Browning, 2009; Hodge, 2015).

### Theme 4: Influence of Culture on Patients' Perspectives on Informed Consent

Patients' cultural identity and values might influence how they view their own role in clinical decision-making about care. Cultures may differ considerably from one another with respect to the value they place on individual autonomy generally and informed consent in clinical contexts specifically. Researchers frequently contrast American, UK, and Australian promotion of individual decision-making and patient empowerment with non-Western cultures' non-individualistic approaches to these outcomes (Chater & Tsai, 2008; Chichester, 2007; Rising, 2017; Sullivan, 2007). For instance, in a study of patients with gestational diabetes in Australia, Caucasian and Filipino women reported greater valuing of patient autonomy than Indian and Vietnamese women, with educational background having little effect on participants' responses (Carolan et al., 2010).

This review revealed that not all cultures value individual autonomy and decision-making to the same degree as dominant medical communities in the United States, UK, and Australia. Broadly speaking, this review showed that several cultures traditionally value family decision-making in clinical contexts (especially critical care and end-of-life care circumstances) more than individual patient decision-making, or promote respect and deference to healthcare professionals in decisions about care. For example, researchers have found that desires among Korean elderly patients to participate in decisions about their health care was relatively low compared to their desire to include family members in decision-making (Chang et al., 2008), and that discounting the family's input for end-of-life care decisions can be isolating and emotionally distressing for the patient (Doolen & York, 2007). Researchers and clinicians have also found that in Chinese traditional culture the family is considered to be a single unit rather than a group of related individuals, and each member is integrally involved in important decisions for the other members (Chater & Tsai, 2008; Jafree et al., 2015).

In some cultures, the disclosure of potentially distressing health information to the patient is considered to be harmful and inappropriate (see Theme 5). In such scenarios, nurses and other health professionals might experience moral distress over fulfilling families' preferences for information disclosure at the potential cost of violating patient autonomy (Jafree et al., 2015; Lee et al., 2009; Starr, 2015; Watts et al., 2017).

Some nurses and ethicists caution their peers regarding whether to withhold information from patients whose cultural background is one in which decision-making and information disclosure is family-oriented. Barwell (2011), for instance, advocates accurate disclosure of information to patients and autonomy promotion in serious or terminal cases, unless the patient expressly declines to receive that information. Padela et al. (2015) warn that a patient's passive delegation of decision-making to family might appear to be informed by the patient's values, but might in fact be compelled by external familial or social expectations. Similarly, Sialubanje et al. (2015) note that Zambian women's deference to their husbands and other family members in decision-making about childbirth may be a function of cultural disempowerment and social barriers rather than strict cultural identity. A study of ICU patients in the United States found no significant correlation between racial identity and patients' evaluations of the informed consent process (Clark, 2007). In light of these nuances, nurses are advised to refrain from initially deferring to families and to assess and respond to the values and preferences of the individual patient in order to prevent as much as possible the patient's experience of guilt, distress, or shame (Browning, 2009).

This review also showed that the family-oriented and individualistic models of decision-making do not track with "non-Western" and "Western" cultural distinctions. Hispanic, African American, and Native American cultures, for example, also place great importance on the participation of family and even close associates in important healthcare decisions (Clark, 2007; Doolen & York, 2007). A study of Japanese patients' perspectives of medical decision-making shows that some patients in Japanese hospitals sometimes regard important healthcare decision-making to be a process between the patient and the physician, and much less so a process between the family and patient (Ito, Tanida, & Turale, 2010). A systematic review of the literature on patient transition and adjustment to long-term care shows that patients from multiple cultural backgrounds who were transferred to long-term care without consent or participation in decision-making were more likely to experience negative psychosocial effects, including sadness, depression, and anger (Brownie et al., 2014; Wilson, Ingleton, Gott, & Gardiner, 2014).

Some cultures promote strong deference to healthcare professionals with respect to decisions about clinical care. Rather than seek information about their condition or wish to make their own healthcare decisions, some patients might instead view the clinician as the authoritative decision-maker about care. Deference to clinical authority in decisions about care has been associated abstractly with Asian cultures and Iranian, Iraqi, and Somali patient populations (Davoudi et al., 2017; Goodman et al., 2015; Narruhn & Schellenberg, 2013; Sun, Hsia, & Sheu, 2008).

Other studies, however, show that within commonly identified cultures and geographic regions there is considerable variation in the degree to which clinically paternalistic decision-making is endorsed. A study of immigrant patient populations in Norway shows that while some African and Asian immigrant patients were hesitant to participate in healthcare decisions, others expressed preference for the more egalitarian and shared decision-making approach of Norwegian clinicians (Alpers, 2018). Deference to clinician authority in decision-making is also strongly exhibited among patients in southern European countries, Portugal, and Sweden (Brown 2014; Doolen & York, 2007), where northern European clinicians tend to respect patient preferences to a higher degree, particularly with regard to end-of-life care decisions (Bülow et al., 2012). However, Peretti-Watel et al. (2008) found that a significant proportion of French district nurses tend to overlook patient wishes in clinical contexts, such as care for patients with advanced amyotrophic lateral sclerosis.

Thus, deference to clinician authority or culturally endorsed autocratic decision processes do not appear to map neatly onto the conventional distinction between "Western" and "non-Western" understandings of informed consent. Further, deference to clinician authority might not always be an expression of a patient's actual preferences, but instead conformity to cultural and social expectations, or even institutional structures. Accordingly, some researchers warn that patients within cultures that ascribe great respect and authority to healthcare professionals might be subject to a significant power imbalance that is reinforced by organizational practice. This might make patients feel they must acquiesce to healthcare professionals' recommendations (Evans & Ndirangu, 2009; Kidd et al., 2015). Moreover, patients from regions that are resource-impoverished or experience political oppression and violence might be forced into assuming dependent roles on authority figures (Goodman et al., 2015; Harrison et al., 2016; Sagbakken et al., 2013).

Religious and spiritual traditions also impact how the moral weight of informed consent is perceived. Orthodox Jewish patients who follow *Halacha* (Jewish Law) might follow closely the Halachic responsibility for self-care, which extends to seeking all information available in order to make a decision for oneself

(Greenberger, 2011). However, on some Orthodox Jewish interpretations, the duty of self-preservation outweighs patient autonomy, even to the extent that the family or religious leaders ought to attempt to coerce a patient to accept life-sustaining interventions (Baeke et al., 2011; Mor & Oberl 2015). In a study of three religious views, Protestant clinicians more frequently respected patient refusal of life-sustaining treatment, while Jewish professionals were least likely to follow patient refusals and most likely to go against patient refusal (Bülow et al., 2012). However, Reformed Jewish patients might not hold the same view on the moral weight of sustaining life as Orthodox Jewish patients (Baek, Wils & Broeckaert 2011). In contrast to both forms of Jewish practice, a major study of attitudes of Muslims living in the United States showed that half of the participants favored informing the family of the patient about a cancer or terminal diagnosis without the individual's consent (McLaughlin et al., 2016). Accordingly, clinicians should be cautious about making assumptions regarding what a patient's faith tradition means for care, or making broad generalizations about the preferences of patients who identify with a religious tradition.

Spiritual and religious identity and practices can also modulate communication between clinicians and patients. One study found that African American men who attend church regularly reported reading more carefully printed educational materials from healthcare providers that were provided at a spiritually based education session as opposed to a non-spiritually based session (Holt et al., 2009). As noted above (Theme 2), some Muslim patients expect interpersonal relationships and trust with clinicians to be established before important healthcare decisions and significant communication about health information commences (Marrone, 2016). Similarly, on some interpretations of the Confucian directive to preserve one's health, it is believed that the manner in which clinicians communicate health information will affect the quality of a patient's life (Zhang et al., 2017).

### Theme 5: Culturally Appropriate Communication

Attitudes toward truth telling and communication of poor prognosis vary depending on religious and cultural factors in different countries and ethnic communities (Brown, 2014). This review emphasized the importance of healthcare providers critically assessing cultural values and norms of patients and families. Family autonomy and family decision-making is the accepted cultural norm for many patients, families, and communities. For example, clinicians must be cognizant that families and community members, such as priests or rabbis, might play a significant role in decision-making (Baeke et al., 2011).

Some African and Asian patients are accustomed to health information being delivered primarily and directly to the family (Alpers, 2018; Brown, 2014).

Disclosure of healthcare information directly to the family is often done to protect the patient, especially in circumstances of poor prognosis, such as terminal illness (Chater & Tsai, 2008). This is consistent with Vietnamese and traditional Chinese culture, and congruent with the Confucian practice of benevolence and compassion (Calloway, 2009; Chater & Tsai, 2008). Doolen and York (2007) identified that Afghan American elders believed that healthcare decision-making is the responsibility of the head of the family. Conventional findings of autonomy and self-determination for families, rather than patients, are identified in the following:

> "Some cultures see autonomy as directed by the group, not the individual. This has to be respected by the treatment team as long as the collective autonomy does not harm the patient's voluntary will" (Druml et al., 2016, p. 9).
>
> "Unlike in western countries, where patients' self-determination in medical decision-making is respected, it is common in China for the family to be fully engaged in the decision-making process" (Zhang et al., 2017, p. 111).

In some circumstances patients may not receive information about the poor diagnosis first, or even at all. In Russia, families are often notified prior to the patient regarding terminal diagnosis (Calloway, 2009). Yet in some cultures, patients do not receive any communication about a poor prognosis or terminal illness. For example, in Spain and other Mediterranean countries, it is common to conceal a diagnosis from the patient (Rio-Valle et al., 2009).

Although family decision-making is sometimes the cultural norm in non-western communities, research suggests that some patients prefer direct and primary truth telling and disclosure. In a study of Japanese patients and families, almost half of patients believed that healthcare professionals should disclose everything to the patient, even if the family is opposed it (Ito, Tanida, & Turale, 2010). A similar study of Korean elders found that patients desired information concerning health, contrasting the traditional idea that families should receive information on their behalf (Chang, et al., 2008). McLaughlin (2016) also found that the majority of healthcare professionals felt that patients should be directly and primarily informed of a poor diagnosis or imminent death, before family members.

Western healthcare professionals disclose terminal diagnosis to patients out of respect for patient autonomy; yet this principle is not universally shared among Muslims, some of whom emphasize that families and physicians are responsible for healthcare decision-making (McLaughlin et al., 2016). Some of the literature suggests that Caucasian Americans communicate end of life decisions through formal advance directives, yet African Americans are more likely to confide in family members and trusted clergy to communicate preferences at end of life (Collins et al., 2018). However, in both populations, self-determination and decision-making autonomy remain with the patient.

Another aspect of the communication theme emerged in this review, regarding the manner in which healthcare professionals deliver information in a culturally sensitive manner. Some clinicians do not feel comfortable or proficient in effective emoting in cultural contexts, resulting in misunderstandings (Alpers, 2018). For example, in Canada, minority cultures want information to be delivered in culturally sensitive ways (Thompson, 2011). However, because communication and expression across cultures vary, gestures such as eye contact or questioning an authority figure may preclude a patient from truly being informed and result in the perception of an uninterested or incompetent patient by Western healthcare professionals (Alpers, 2018). Communication can be impacted further by rules around verbal and nonverbal communication within a culture, such as tone, volume, inflections, pauses, eye contact, and emotional expressions (Clancy, 2013; Pugh, 2014). For example, Saudi Arabian women who communicate with a male healthcare professional often speak directly and try to avoid eye contact, yet erudite Saudis generally respect eye contact as a sign of honesty and integrity (Marrone, 2016). Some Iranian women find that communication, especially delicate information, can be delivered too directly and can crush the spirit (Thompson, 2011).

Based on these findings, healthcare professionals must not make assumptions about a patient's cultural preference. A proper assessment is necessary to obtain the patient's preference for truth telling and information disclosure. Nurses communicate beliefs consciously and unconsciously to their patients and therefore must be cognizant of verbal and nonverbal communication and behavior to understand the delicate nature of conveying healthcare information (Lech, 2008). If preferences in relation to truth telling are not known, nurses might be unable to properly care for patients in a culturally appropriate and sensitive manner (Ling et al., 2017). Expectations and preferences for truth telling, disclosure and communication vary drastically and must occur in light of recognized differences in beliefs and values that patients hold (Clark, 2007; Sneesby et al., 2011).

### Theme 6: Professional Codes of Ethical Conduct

Globally, nurses recognize the professional ethical obligations to advocate for patient's rights during the informed consent process. The ethical duty to advocate for patients applies in multiple facets of informed consent, including the respect for patient autonomy, protection of human rights, safeguarding patients from inappropriate paternalistic situations, respecting confidentiality and self-determination, duty for primary commitment to the patient and high quality nursing care, respect for kindness in self and others, and respect for the cultural diversity in patient care (Ingravallo et al., 2017; Jafree et al., 2015; Marrone, 2016; Pugh, 2014; Susilo et al., 2013; Susilo et al., 2014; Toda et al., 2015; Wilson et al., 2014).

Nurses frequently confront these ethical obligations, especially in cultures where families have a significant role in healthcare decision-making. The nurse's role in advocacy in decision-making is valuable in the protection of dignity and human rights. For example, the Japanese code of ethics for nurses does not expressly exclude the obligation to advocate for individual patient decision-making; yet, decision-making in the Japanese culture is often a family decision rather than solely a patient decision (Toda et al., 2015). Nurses are essential in educating families about confidentiality and respect of patient autonomy (Toda et al., 2015). Cultural norms do not justify a breach in confidentiality. Therefore, Japanese nurses often face this ethical dilemma in practice. The American code of ethics for nurses identifies the nurse's responsibilities in medical interpretation through cultural humility (Ortiz & Casey, 2017). Western culture is reflected in the American ethical code for nurses, which outlines the nurse's primary commitment to the patient through delivery of care with compassion and respect for dignity (Marrone, 2016). Additionally, nurses have a significant role in establishing that patients participate in the planning and implementation of their care (Mor & Oberle, 2008). The Korean and Italian codes of ethics for nurses emphasize the nurse's role in ensuring that patients have necessary and sufficient information so that they are supported in decision-making (Ingravallo et al., 2017). In addition, the Nursing Midwifery Council Code of Conduct, which governs nursing practice in the United Kingdom, states that nurses must uphold a patient's right to be fully informed and participate in decision-making (Clancy, 2013; Wilson et al., 2014). The ethical code of conduct governing Australian nurses requires respect and kindness for the diversity of people, in addition to culturally sensitive and appropriate advocacy for patient self-determination and autonomy (Pugh, 2014). Failure to comply challenges the ability to provide ethically sound care (Pugh, 2014).

Although nurses may be aware of professional ethical obligations, the actual or perceived inability to follow through can result in neglect of cultural competence or avoidance of patient advocacy during informed consent. For instance, nurses in India were reluctant to advocate on behalf of patients subjected to inappropriate paternalism during the informed consent process, and feared being blamed or unsupported by their hospital (Susilo et al., 2013).

Notably, a study of Pakistani nurses revealed that although nurses were aware of the ethical obligations of informed consent and patient advocacy, a near absence of consent existed in nonsurgical procedures (Jafree et al., 2015). The lack of consent was originally hypothesized to be due to the cultural norm of family decision-making in Asian countries, but this study revealed that the rationale for failure to obtain consent was actually due to time constraints, patient health illiteracy, and the assumption that patient admission to a teaching hospital was a de facto consent for treatment (Jafree et al., 2015). The absence of obtaining proper consent significantly impacted the nurses' emotional and psychological well-being, resulting in a reduced commitment to high quality patient care (Jafree et al., 2015).

While some articles in the review acknowledged the ethical code applicable to the nurses in their respective countries, several articles highlighted the significance of the International Council of Nurses Code of Ethics and its broad application to nurses globally (Hodge, 2015; Ingravallo et al, 2017; Marrone, 2016; Susilo et al., 2013; Wilson et al., 2014). Nurses recognize both the global ethical obligations of providing sufficient information for adequate decision-making in a culturally sensitive manner and the significance of respecting patients cultural and religious beliefs (Hodge, 2015; Susilo et al., 2013; Wilson et al., 2014).

## CRITICAL DISCUSSION

This review provides the first published analysis of how nurses and nurse researchers perceive the impact of aspects of culture on the process of obtaining patient informed consent. The review clearly shows that the cultural identities and values of both clinicians and patients, as well as assumptions and generalizations about a patient's cultural background, impact a number of elements in this process. These elements include whether and to whom patient health information is disclosed, whether patients wish to receive full and accurate diagnostic and prognostic information, whether clinicians differentially disclose information or seek patient consent due to classifying or stereotyping patients on the basis of cultural or religious identity, and whether barriers to consent due to cultural or linguistic differences are recognized and removed.

This review reveals wide consensus among clinicians and researchers that nursing care for multicultural patient populations demands that nurses cultivate competence and knowledge regarding patients' cultural and spiritual identities (Browning, 2009; Calloway, 2009; Doolen & York, 2007; Valente, 2010). Sensitivity to and awareness of different cultural perspectives on health, illness and death, on appropriate means for disseminating information, and on procedures and contexts for making important personal decisions will assist nurses in tailoring their care to individual patients' needs, preferences, and expectations (Brownie et al., 2014; Calloway, 2009; Clabots, 2012; Clancy, 2013; Martin, 2016; Oliveira & Oliveira, 2013).

However, the literature contains far less consensus regarding how cultural competence and sensitivity would bear on clinicians' understanding of informed consent, including deliberation over whether to disclose information directly to the patient or to expect patients to make their own decisions about care. As we note above (Theme 1), some of the articles we reviewed claim that dominant conceptions of respect for patient autonomy and informed consent are incompatible with respecting the cultural values and practices of some patients. However, this claim is ambiguous.

On the one hand, the claim might mean that there will be occasions in clinical practice when nurses and other clinicians either will not be able to secure informed consent from a patient while also respecting that patient's cultural beliefs and values, or will not be required to obtain informed consent when caring for a patient whose cultural identity and traditions do not regard individual decision-making or direct disclosure of health information to be appropriate. However, several articles point out that respect for these cultural preferences need not preclude respecting a patient's autonomous decision-making and consent. One way to avoid possible practical conflict between a patient's cultural values and a nurses' sense of the importance of informed consent is for the nurse to conduct initial discussions with the patient regarding what information the patient wishes to have disclosed and whether the patient, the patient's family, or the family unit will be making healthcare decisions (Chater & Tsai, 2008; Goodman et al., 2015). As we noted above (Themes 4 and 6), such putative conflicts among clinicians' duties might occur more frequently in scenarios involving a terminal diagnosis, advanced care planning, and end-of-life care. But even in these scenarios, nurses and clinicians should not assume that cultural barriers are present in the care of multicultural patient populations, but instead should initiate discussion of patients' preferences for communication, information disclosure, and decision-making (Collins et al., 2018; Cooper et al., 2015; Lech, 2008). Through individualized consultation with patients, a nurse is respecting the autonomy and decisional authority of the patient, even when a patient confers that decisional authority to a family member or other close associate (Childress, 1993; Clabots, 2012; Guven, 2010; Leever, 2011). Empowering patients to express their cultural and spiritual beliefs and values, and subsequently respecting those beliefs and values, is an important way in which a nurse respects the exercise of a patient's autonomy to determine how consent processes will proceed. While it is important for nurses to be knowledgeable to some degree of different cultural and religious beliefs and values (Browning, 2009; Clabots, 2012), it is also important that nurses not assume that patients endorse every belief and value of the culture with which they identify (Chang et al., 2018; Effa-Heap, 2009; Guven, 2010). Indeed, as we note above (Theme 4) there can be considerable variation among individuals from similar cultural and spiritual backgrounds in endorsement of cultural beliefs and values. Thus, nurses ought to couple culturally competent care with respect for individual patients' beliefs, values, and preferences.

On the other hand, the claim of incompatibility might be pointing to a conceptual tension between respect for patient autonomy and cultural preferences for non-disclosure or family- or community-oriented decision-making. For example, Calloway (2009) contrasts family-centered decision-making with individualistic notions of patient autonomy and informed consent. Padela et al. (2015) likewise trace the ethical principle of respect for patient autonomy and the requirement to obtain informed consent to individualistic conceptions of persons. One might accordingly infer that informed consent and the principle of respect for patient autonomy are conceptually tied to an overly individualistic picture of autonomy. This inference, however, would be incorrect. The conception of the individual as an atomistic, self-sufficient decision-maker is logically independent of a conception of individual autonomy and the duty to obtain a patient's informed consent. That is, one could endorse either conception and reject the other (Deem, 2016). Indeed, some of the articles we reviewed suggest that a broader view of individual autonomy—that is, a view of autonomy that does not simply take the individual to be a self-sufficient decision-maker—is compatible with respect for cultural preferences for nondisclosure or family-centered decision-making (Calloway, 2009; Chater & Tsai, 2008). One resource from which nursing ethics might to draw to fill in this broader notion of autonomy is the feminist philosophical literature on relational autonomy (Mackenzie & Stoljar, 2000).

According to some relational conceptions of autonomy, autonomous decision-making is the product of social and cultural scaffolding. Our social relations and cultural backgrounds play determinant roles in the formation of our desires, preferences, and decisions. On a relational view of the principle of respect for patient autonomy, what matters is whether patients regard healthcare decisions as their own and not whether they complete the process of forming a decision in isolation from social and cultural influences. Even if healthcare decisions are made by family or community members without full disclosure of information to a patient, a patient's autonomy can still be respected and promoted whenever clinicians ensure that the patient endorses such decisions or processes for decision-making, and regards the outcome of the process as truly her/his own. When we view autonomy relationally, as opposed to individualistically, then we might find that the conceptual tensions that some articles identity between informed consent and some cultural values are only apparent.

## CONCLUSION

The nursing and nursing ethics literatures reveals the potential difficulties that arise for many patients, families, and healthcare professionals when recognizing patient cultures and values during the informed consent process. Cultures, religions, and spiritual traditions may vary regarding the value placed on individual autonomy and the involvement of families and communities in healthcare decision-making. Healthcare professionals who are accustomed and trained to respect individual patient autonomy are challenged when healthcare decision-making, truth telling, and information disclosure are modulated by a patient's cultural identity and values. These challenges can contribute to barriers or reluctance to obtain informed consent, dissolution of trust in the patient–provider relationship, and moral conflict from healthcare professionals who seek to safeguard patients' cultural identity.

This review emphasizes the role of nurses and the significance of identifying, respecting, and acknowledging the culture, needs and values of every patient. Nurses have a global ethical obligation to advocate for patients in healthcare decision-making and informed consent. They must also tailor communication of health information in a culturally appropriate and sensitive manner. In doing so, nurses will promote patient autonomy and empowerment in healthcare decision-making.

## ACKNOWLEDGMENT

We are grateful to David A. Nolfi for valuable assistance in conducting the literature search for this review.

## REFERENCES

Alpers, L.-M. (2018). Distrust and patients in intercultural healthcare: A qualitative interview study. *Nursing Ethics, 25*(3), 313–323.

Baeke, G., Wils, J. -P., & Broeckaert, B. (2011). Orthodox Jewish perspectives on withholding and withdrawing life-sustaining treatment. *Nursing Ethics, 18*(6), 835–846.

Barwell, J. (2011). Should the truth always be told in colorectal cancer care? *Gastrointestinal Nursing, 9*(3): 28–31.

Bentwich, M. E., Dickman, N., & Oberman, A. (2017). Dignity and autonomy in the care for patients with dementia: Differences among formal caretakers of varied cultural backgrounds and their meaning. *Archives of Gerontology and Geriatrics, 70*, 19–27.

Bentwich, M. E., & Oberman, A. (2018). Autonomy and dignity of patients with dementia: Perceptions of multicultural caretakers. *Nursing Ethics, 25*(1), 37–53.

Blackman, R. (2009). Knowledge for practice: Challenges in culturally safe nursing practice. *Contemporary Nurse, 32*(1–2), 211–214.

Braithwaite, P., Chichester, M., & Reid, A. (2010). When the pregnant Jehovah's Witness patient refuses blood: Implications for nurses. *Nursing for Women's Health*, *14*(6), 463–470.

Brenan, M. (2017, December 26). *Nurses keep healthy lead as most honest, ethical profession*. Gallup. Retrieved from https://news.gallup.com/poll/224639/nurses-keep-healthy-lead-honest-ethical-profession.aspx

Brown, E. A. (2014). Ethnic and cultural challenges at the end of life: Setting the scene. *Journal of Renal Care, 40*(Suppl. 1), 2–5.

Brownie, S., Horstmanshof, L., & Garbutt, R. (2014). Factors that impact residents' transition and psychological adjustment to long-term aged care: A systematic literature review. *International Journal of Nursing Studies, 51*(2014), 1654–1666.

Browning, A. M. (2009). Incorporating spiritual beliefs into end-of-life care. *Journal of Christian Nursing, 26*(1), 10–17.

Bülow, H. -H., Sprung, C. L., Baras, M., Carmel, S., Svantesson, M., Benbenishty, J. et al. (2012). Are religion and religiosity important to end-of-life decisions and patient autonomy in the ICU?: The Ethicatt study. *Intensive Care Medicine, 38*:1126–1133.

Calloway, S. J. (2009). The effect of culture on beliefs related to autonomy and informed consent. *Journal of Cultural Diversity, 16*(2), 68–70.

Candib, L. M. (2002). Truth telling and advance planning at the end of life: Problems with autonomy in a multicultural world. *Families, Systems, & Health, 20*(3), 213–228.

Carolan, M., Steele, C., & Margetts, H. (2010). Attitudes toward gestational diabetes among a multiethnic cohort in Australia. *Journal of Clinical Nursing, 19*, 2446–2453.

Chang, S. J., Lee, K. J., Kim, I. S., & Lee, W. H. (2008). Older Korean people's desire to participate in healthcare decision making. *Nursing Ethics, 15*(1), 73–86.

Chater, K., & Tsai, C. -T. (2008). Palliative care in multicultural society: A challenge for western ethics. *Australian Journal of Advanced Nursing, 26*(2), 95–100.

Chichester, M. (2007). Requesting perinatal autopsy: Multicultural considerations. *MCN: The American Journal of Maternal Child Nursing, 32*(2), 81–86.

Childress, J. F. (1993). The place of autonomy in bioethics. *Hasting Center Report, 20*(1), 12–17.

Chima, S. C. (2013). Evaluating the quality of informed consent and contemporary clinical practices by medical doctors in South Africa: An empirical study. *BMC Medical Ethics, 14*(Suppl 1), S3.

Clabots, S. (2012). Strategies to help initiate and maintain the end-of-life discussion with patients and family members. *MEDSURG Nursing Journal, 21*(4), 199–204.

Clancy, T., & Morgan, R. (2013). Tailoring genetic/genomic services and information to the individual. *Nursing Standard, 28*(10), 37–43.

Clark, P. A. (2007). Intensive care patients' evaluations of the informed consent process. *Dimensions of Critical Care Nursing, 26*(5), 207–226.

Collins, J. W., Zoucha, R., Lockhart, J. S., & Mixer, S. J. (2018). Cultural aspects of end-of-life care planning for African Americans: An integrative review of the literature. *Journal of Transcultural Nursing*. https://doi.org/10.1177/1043659617753042

Cooper, A. B., Chidwick, P., Cybulski, P., & Sibbald, R. (2015). *Checklist to meet Ethical and Legal Obligations in the consent pathway for critically ill patients (ChELO): A quality improvement project and case studies. Canadian Journal of Critical Care Nursing, 26*(3), 16–24.

Coyle, N. (2014). Palliative care, hospice care, and bioethics. *Journal of Hospice and Palliative Nursing, 16*(1), 6–12.

Davies, M., Elwyn, G., Papadopoulos, I., Fleming, L., & Williams, G. (2009). Can promoting patient decision making be exclusionary? Moral expectations and cultural difference in the narratives of UK maternity clinicians. *Communication and Medicine, 6*(1), 39–48.

Davoudi, N., Nayeri, N. D., Zokaei, M. S., & Fazeli, N. (2017). Challenges of obtaining informed consent in emergency ward: A qualitative study in one Iranian hospital. *The Open Nursing Journal, 11*, 263–276.

Deem, M. J. (2016). Microbes and medical decisions. *American Journal of Bioethics, 16*(2), 55–56.

Demirsoy, N., Elcioglu, O., & Yildiz, Z. (2008). Telling the truth: Turkish patients' and nurses' views. *Nursing Science Quarterly, 21*(1), 75–79.

Doolen, J., & York, N. L. (2007). Cultural differences with end-of-life care in the critical care unit. *Dimensions of Critical Care Nursing, 26*(5), 194–198.

Druml, C., Ballmer, P. E., Druml, W., Oehmichen, F., Shenkin, A., Singer, P., et al. (2016). ESPEN guideline on ethical aspects of artificial nutrition and hydration. *Clinical Nutrition, 35*, 545–556.

Effa-Heap, G. (2009). Blood transfusion: Implications of treating a Jehovah's Witness patient. *British Journal of Nursing, 18*(3), 174–177.

Evans, C., & Ndirangu E. (2009). The nursing implications of routine provider-initiated HIV testing and counselling in sub-Saharan Africa: A critical review of new policy guidance from WHP/UNAIDS. *International Journal of Nursing Studies, 46*, 723–731.

Faden, R., & Beauchamp, T. (1986). *A history and theory of informed consent*. Oxford, UK: Oxford University Press.

Fernández-Sola, C., Granero-Molina J., Manrique, G. A., Castro-Sánchez, A. M., Hernández-Padilla J. M., et al. (2012). New regulation of the right to a dignified dying in Spain: Repercussions for nursing. *Nursing Ethics, 19*(5), 619–628.

Fitch, M. I., Beaudoin, G. & Johnson, B. (2013). Challenges having conversations about sexuality in ambulatory settings: Part II – Healthcare provider perspectives. *Canadian Oncology Nursing Journal, 23*(3), 182–196.

French, C., & Narayanasamy, A. (2011). To pray or not to pray: A question of ethics. *British Journal of Nursing, 20*(18), 1198–1204.

Goodman, P., Edge, B., Agazio, J., & Prue-Owens, K. (2015). Cultural awareness: Nursing care of Iraqi patients. *Journal of Transcultural Nursing, 26*(4), 395–401.

Gordan, E. J., Caicedo, J. C., Ladner, D. P., Reddy, E. & Abecassis M. M. (2010). Transplant center provision of education and culturally and linguistically competent care: A national study. *American Journal of Transplantation 10*, 2701–2707.

Grace, P. J. (2018). *Nursing ethics and professional responsibility in advanced practice* (3rd ed.). Burlington, MA: Jones and Bartlett.

Granero-Molina, J., Fernández-Sola, C., & Aguilera-Manrique, G. (2009). Applying a sociolinguistic model to the analysis of informed consent documents. *Nursing Ethics, 16*(6), 797–812.

Grant, M. J., & Booth, A. (2009). A typology of reviews: An analysis of 14 review types and associated methodologies. *Health Information and Libraries Journal, 26*, 91–108.

Greenberger, C. (2011). The hierarchy of values in Jewish bioethics. *Nursing Ethics, 18*(4), 537–547.

Guven, T. (2010). Truth-telling in cancer: Examining the cultural incompatibility argument in Turkey. *Nursing Ethics, 17*(2), 159–166.

Halkoaho A, Pietilä A. -M., Ebbesen M., Karki S., Kangasniemi M. (2016). Cultural aspects related to informed consent in health research: A systematic review. *Nursing Ethics, 23*(6), 698–712.

Harrison, J. D., Logar, T., Le, P., & Glass, M. (2016). What are the ethical issues facing global-health trainees working overseas? A multi-professional qualitative study. *Healthcare, 4*(3), 43.

Hodge, D. R. (2015). Administering a two-stage spiritual assessment in healthcare settings: A necessary component of ethical and effective care. *Journal of Nursing Management 23*: 27–38.

Holt, C. L., Wynn, T. A., Litaker, M. S., Southward, P., Jeames, S. E., & Schulz, E. K. (2009). A comparison of a spiritually based and non-spiritually based educational intervention for informed decision making for prostate cancer screening among church-attending African-American men. *Urological Nursing, 29*(4), 249–258.

Isaacson, M. J., & Lynch, A. R. (2018). Culturally relevant palliative and end-of-life care for U.S. indigenous populations: An integrative review. *Journal of Transcultural Nursing, 29*(2), 180–191.

Ingravallo, F., Kim, K. H., Han, Y. H., Volta, A., Chiari, P., Taddia, P., et al. (2017). Difficulties and practices regarding information provision among Korean and Italian nurses. *International Nursing Review, 64*, 528–535.

Ito, M., Tanida, N., & Turale, S. (2010). Perceptions of Japanese patients and their family about medical treatment decisions. *Nursing and Health Sciences, 12*, 314–321.

Jafree, S. R., Zakar, R., Fischer, F., & Zakar, M. Z. (2015). Ethical violations in the clinical setting: The hidden curriculum learning experience of Pakistani nurses. *BMC Medical Ethics, 16*,16.

Johnstone, M.-J., & Kanitsaki, O. (2009). Ethics and advance care planning in a culturally diverse society. *Journal of Transcultural Nursing, 20*(4), 405–416.

Johnstone, M. J., Rawson, H., Hutchinson, A. M., & Redley, B. (2018). Fostering trusting relationships with older immigrants hospitalised for end-of-life care. *Nursing Ethics, 25*(6), 760–772.

Kidd, A. D., Colbert, A. M., & Jatoi, I. (2015). Mammography: Review of the controversy, health disparities, and impact on young African American women. *Clinical Journal of Oncology Nursing, 19*(3), E52–E58.

Lech, R (2008). Getting inside their skin – improving SANE's cultural competence. *On the Edge, The Official Newsletters of the International Association of Forensic Nurses, 14*(3).

Lee, C. -C., Li, D., Arai, S., & Puntillo, K. (2009). Ensuring cross-cultural equivalence in translation of research consents and clinical documents: A systematic process for translating English to Chinese. *Journal of Transcultural Nursing, 20*(1), 77–82.

Lee, S., Lee, W. -H., Kong, B. H., Kim, I. -S. & Kim, S. (2009). Nurses' perceptions of informed consent and their related roles in Korea: An exploratory study. *International Journal of Nursing Studies, 46*, 1580–1584.

Leever, M. G. (2011). Cultural competence: Reflections on patient autonomy and patient good. *Nursing Ethics, 18*(4), 560–570.

Levin, R. J. (1991). Informed consent: Some challenges to the universal validity of the Western model. *Journal of Law, Medicine, and Ethics, 19*(3–4), 207–213.

Lillie, S. E., Janz, N. K., Friese, C. R., Graff, J. J., Schwartz, K., Hamilton, A. S., et al. (2014). Racial and ethnic variation in partner perspectives about the breast cancer treatment decision-making experience. *Oncology Nursing Forum, 41*(1), 13–20.

Lin, M. -L., Huang, C. -T., & Chen, C. -H. (2016). Reasons for family involvement in elective surgical decision-making in Taiwan: A qualitative study. *Journal of Clinical Nursing, 26*, 1969–1977.

Ling, D. -L., Yu, H. -J. & Guo, H. -L. (2017). Truth-telling, decision-making, and ethics among cancer patients in nursing practice in China. *Nursing Ethics*. doi.org/10.1177/0969733017739783

Lopez-McKee, G. -L., McNeill, J. A., Bader, J., & Morales, P. (2008). Comparison of factors affecting repeat mammography screening of low-income Mexican American women. *Oncology Nursing Forum, 35*(6), 941–947.

Lowther, K., Higginson, I. J., Simms, V., Gikaara, N., Ahmed, A., Ali, Z., et al. (2014). A randomized controlled trial to assess the effectiveness of a nurse-led palliative care intervention for HIV positive patients on antiretroviral therapy: Recruitment, refusal, randomization and missing data. *BMC Research Notes ,7*, 600.

MacKenzie, C., & Stoljar, N. (ed.) (2000). *Relational autonomy: Feminist perspectives on autonomy, agency, and social self*. Oxford, UK: Oxford University Press.

Marrone, S. R. (2016). Informed consent examined within the context of culturally congruent care: An interprofessional perspective. *Journal of Transcultural Nursing, 27*(4), 342–348.

Martin, E. M., & Barkley, T. W. (2016). Improving cultural competence in end-of-life pain management. *Nursing, 46*(1), 32–41.

McLaughlin, M. H., Elahi, A., Ciesielski, J., & Pomerantz, S. (2016). Attitudes of Muslims living in the United States toward long-term care decisions and diagnosis disclosure for elderly family matters. *Journal of the American Geriatrics Society, 64*(10), 2132–2137.

Mor, P., & Oberle, K. (2008). Ethical issues related to BRCA gene testing in Orthodox Jewish Women. *Nursing Ethics, 15*(4), 512–522.

Narruhn, R., & Schellenberg, I. R. (2013). Caring ethics and a Somali reproductive dilemma. *Nursing Ethics, 20*(4), 366–381.

Neary, P., Cahill, R. A., Kirwan, W. O., Kiely, E., & Redmond, H. P. (2008). What a signature adds to the consent process. *Surgical Endoscopy, 22*, 2698–2704.

O'Neill, O. (2002). *Autonomy and trust in bioethics*. Cambridge, UK: Cambridge University Press.

Oliveira, E. C. T., & Oliveira, J. D. S. (2013). Hypertension: Factors that interfere in the follow-up to the therapeutic regimen. *Journal of Nursing UFPE on line, 7*(11), 6488–6497.

Ortiz, J., & Casey, D. (2017). Dead wrong! The ethics of culturally competent care. *MEDSURG Nursing Journal, 26*(4), 279–282.

Padela, A. I., Malik, A. Y., Curlin, F., & De Vries, R. (2015). [Re]Considering respect for persons in a globalizing world. *Bioethics, 15*(2), 98–106.

Peretti-Watel, P., Bendiane, M. -K., Galinier, A., Favre, R., Ribiere, C., Lapian, J. -M., et al. (2008). District nurses' attitudes toward patient consent: The case of mechanical ventilation on amyotrophic lateral sclerosis patients: Results from a French national survey. *Journal of Clinical Care, 23*, 332–228.

Pugh, D. M. (2014). Ethics at the end of life: An Australian perspective. *Clinical Nurse Specialist: The Journal for Advanced Nursing Practice, 28*(4), 201–204.

Rio-Valle, J. S., Caro, M. P. G., Juarez, R. M., Peña, D. P., Vinuesa, A. M., Pappous, A., Quintana, F. C. (2009). Bad news for the patient and family? The worst part of being a health care professional. *Journal of Palliative Care, 25*(3). 191–196.

Rising, M. L. (2017). Truth telling as an element of culturally competent care at end of life. *Journal of Transcultural Nursing, 28*(1), 48–55.

Sagbakken, M., Frich, J. C., Bjune, G. A., & Porter, J. D. H. (2013). Ethical aspects of directly observed treatment for tuberculosis: A cross-cultural comparison. *BMC Medical Ethics, 14*, 25.

Sialubanje, C., Massar, K., Hamer, D. H., & Ruiter, R. A. C. (2015). Reasons for home delivery and use of traditional birth attendants in rural Zambia: A qualitative study. *BMC Pregnancy and Childbirth, 15*, 216.

Sneesby, L, Satchell, R., Good, P. & van der Riet, P. (2011). Death and dying in Australia: Perceptions of a Sudanese community. *Journal of Advanced Nursing, 67*(12), 2696.

Starr, K. T. (2015). The curious case of the cultural or religious 'no' to standard medical care. *Nursing, 45*(11), 13.

Sullivan, L. S. (2017). Dynamic axes of informed consent in Japan. *Social Science and Medicine 174*, 159–168.

Sun, J. -C., Hsia, P.-H., & Sheu, S. -J. (2008). Women of advanced maternal age undergoing amniocentesis: A period of uncertainty. *Journal of Clinical Nursing, 17*, 2829–2837.

Susilo, A. P., van Dalen, J., Chenault, M. N., & Scherpbier A. (2014). Informed consent and nurses' roles: A survey of Indonesian practitioners. *Nursing Ethics, 21*(6), 684–694.

Susilo, A. P., van Dalen, J., Scherpbier, A., Tanto, S., Yuhanti, P., & Ekawati, N. (2013). Nurses' roles in informed consent in a hierarchical and communal context. *Nursing Ethics, 20*(4), 413–425.

Thompson, J. (2011). Truth-telling. . .even when the news is bad. *World Council of Enterostomal Therapists Journal, 31*(4), 18–21.

Toda, Y., Sakamoto, M., Tagaya, A., Takahashi, M., & Davis, A. J. (2015). Patient advocacy: Japanese psychiatric nurses recognizing necessity for intervention. *Nursing Ethics, 22*(7), 765–777.

Valente, S. (2010). HIV, culture and end-of-life issues. *JOCEPS: The Journal of Chi Eta Phi, 54*(1), 15–22.

Watts, K. J., Meiser, B., Zilliacus, E., Kaur, R., Taouk, M., Girgis, A., et al. (2017). Communicating with patients from minority backgrounds: Individual challenges experienced by oncology health professionals. *European Journal of Oncology Nursing, 26*, 83–90.

Wear, S. (1998). *Informed consent: Patient autonomy and clinician beneficence within healthcare* (2nd ed.). Washington, DC: Georgetown University Press.

Wilson, F., Ingleton, C., Gott, M., & Gardiner, C. (2014). Autonomy and choice in palliative care: Time for a new model? *Journal of Advanced Nursing, 70*(5), 1020–1029.

Zalon, M. L., Constantino, R. E., & Andrews, K. L. (2008). The right to pain treatment: A reminder for nurses. *Dimensions of Critical Care Nursing, 27*(3), 93–101.

Zhang, J., Wong, F. K. Y., & Zheng, M. (2017). The preoperative reaction and decision-making process regarding colostomy surgery among Chinese rectal cancer patients. *European Journal of Oncology Nursing, 28*, 107–113.

CHAPTER 9

# Cultural Factors Influencing Suicidal Ideation and Behaviors in Puerto Ricans

## *An Integrative Review*

Griselle Batista Estrada, Rick Zoucha, and Yovanska Duarté-Vélez

**ABSTRACT**

Deaths by suicide are the 10th leading cause of death for Latinxs in the United States. Given the heterogeneity of the Latinx population, additional focus on Latinx mental health is needed at the subgroup level. Puerto Ricans comprise the second largest Latinx subgroup in the nation. Their American citizenship, ethnohistory, and unique migration patterns to and from the U.S. mainland point to the need for further understanding of the impact of culture on Puerto Rican mental health. Guided by Leininger's Culture Care Theory, an integrative review examined cultural factors influencing suicidal ideation and behaviors in Puerto Ricans in the United States and in Puerto Rico; a total of 24 articles from the past 10 years were reviewed. There is a dearth of current research literature addressing suicide and suicide prevention in Puerto Ricans, particularly those living in the continental United States. Further focus on the cultural and social factors that impact suicide risk is warranted. Advancing the evidence regarding the culture care needs of Puerto Ricans and other Latinx subgroups can guide future research


http://dx.doi.org/10.1891/0739-6686.37.261

efforts and the development of culturally congruent nursing strategies aimed at mental health promotion and suicide prevention in the Latinx population.

## INTRODUCTION

Suicide was reported to be the 10th leading cause of death for *Latinxs*[1] in the United States in 2016 (Centers for Disease Control and Prevention [CDC], National Center for Injury Prevention and Control, 2017a); it was ranked 11th from 2012 to 2015 (CDC, 2017b, 2017c, 2017d, 2017e; Heron, 2017). This raises concern not only regarding the number of individuals who die by suicide but also regarding the number of Latinxs who experience suicidal ideation (SI) or a suicide attempt (SA). Although suicide has been identified as "an important public health problem in the United States and a tragedy for all involved" (Piscopo, Lipari, Cooney, & Glasheen, 2016, p. 2), there is a dearth of research studies focusing on suicide and suicide prevention within the Latinx population and its many subgroups, including Puerto Ricans. Given that the Latinx population is projected to grow and comprise 27.5% of the total U.S. population by 2060 (Vespa, Armstrong, & Medina, 2018), assessment and management of suicide risk within Latinx subgroups is a critical issue for nursing practice not just in the psychiatric–mental health setting but in every healthcare setting.

Even though Latinxs may be considered by some to be a homogeneous population, they represent many different cultures, countries, and sociopolitical backgrounds (Gonzales, Germán, & Fabrett, 2012). Just as individuals who originate from different English-speaking countries can differ in their accents, ethnohistory, and affinity for specific foods and dishes, so too can Latinxs. The National Latino and Asian American Study (NLAAS), a first-of-its-kind national survey providing needed information about the mental health of Latinxs and Asians in the United States (Alegría et al., 2004), considered sociocultural differences when investigating the prevalence of mental health issues among specific Latinx subgroups. Not only were variations identified within the sociodemographic characteristics of Mexicans, Puerto Ricans, Cubans, and Other Latinxs, but variations were also identified in the rates of psychiatric conditions within these four subgroups (Alegría, Mulvaney-Day, Woo, & Viruell-Fuentes, 2012). In fact, NLAAS revealed reports of higher prevalence of psychiatric disorders from what Alegrí et al. (2012) identified as "certain vulnerable subgroups" (p. 299), one of which was Puerto Ricans.

Given the heterogeneity of the Latinx population in the United States, it is essential for nurses to foment continued discovery of the sociocultural elements

---

1 *Latinx* is used as a gender-inclusive term throughout this chapter. Latinx was also included as a substitute for the terms Hispanic and Latino that were used in most studies.

that can influence the mental health of Latinx individuals, families, and communities. In its first comprehensive report addressing the global impact of suicide, the World Health Organization (WHO, 2014) identified a complex interplay of factors that can impact suicide risk. Recommendations for national prevention efforts included consideration for strategies that address the specific needs in each country, since "suicide depends on a number of factors, and its expression is influenced by social and cultural contexts" (WHO, 2014, p. 58). Building the evidence related to cultural factors that influence suicide risk, particularly in underserved racial and ethnic minority groups such as the Latinx population and its subgroups, can serve to inform culturally congruent nursing care aimed at preventing suicide.

## BACKGROUND

The 5-year population estimate for 2012 to 2016 from the U.S. Census Bureau (2016b) conveyed that out of the total Latinx population (55.2 million), Mexicans (35.1 million) constituted the largest Latinx subgroup in the United States, followed by Puerto Ricans (5.3 million) and Cubans (2.1 million). Puerto Rico's island population was estimated to be 3.5 million during the same 5-year range (U. S. Census Bureau, 2016a), indicating that the number of Puerto Ricans living in the U.S. mainland is larger than the island's population.

### Brief Ethnohistory of Puerto Ricans

The island of Puerto Rico became a U.S. colony in 1898; in 1952, it gained the political status of U.S. commonwealth (Garcia-Preto, 2005). Although Puerto Ricans are American citizens by birth and can freely migrate within the United States, their roots lie deep within their Spanish, African, and native Taíno heritage. This cultural inheritance, along with the influence of Roman Catholicism, has helped to shape their spirituality and religious beliefs (Garcia-Preto, 2005). Puerto Ricans encourage the pursuit of education (Purnell, 2013), promote respect for those who are older (Purnell, 2013), and cherish interpersonal relationships (Garcia-Preto, 2005; Purnell, 2013). Family unity plays a central role in the Puerto Rican culture and care of the family is prioritized (Purnell, 2013). Family members and extended family are sought for assistance and support (Garcia-Preto, 2005). Zayas, Lester, Cabassa, and Fortuna (2005) expanded on the central role that family plays in the Latinx culture and how *familism*, a cultural value, "emphasizes maintenance of family cohesion, obligation and intense attachment to relatives, and primacy of the family in the individual's self-identity and social world" (p. 278). Garcia-Preto (2005) suggested that socioeconomic factors and acculturation may influence gender roles, presenting possible challenges within the Puerto Rican family. Machismo can still impact these roles

(Purnell, 2013); however, Zayas (2011) cautioned against negative connotations of this concept, adding that in Latinxs it can also represent a regard for honor and protection of the family.

Primarily using 2012 population data from the U.S. Census Bureau, Cohn, Patten, and Lopez (2014) compared Puerto Ricans on the island to those on the U.S. mainland and reported several differences that included the following: (a) a higher percentage (24%) of adult Puerto Ricans on the island aged 25 years and over obtained a bachelor's degree compared to those on the mainland (17%), (b) a lower percentage of Puerto Ricans on the island (15%) *speak English very well* versus those on the mainland (45%), and (c) a higher percentage of Puerto Ricans on the island (45% of all ages) identified as *living in poverty* when compared to those on the mainland (27%). The number of Puerto Ricans who migrated from the island to the mainland in recent years has been the largest "since the Great Migration after World War II" (p. 4); Florida was a common destination (Cohn et al., 2014). Most recently, though, Puerto Rico received a direct hit from Hurricane María, one of the most costly and devastating storms to impact the United States (Pasch, Penny, & Berg, 2018). The full impact of this natural disaster on the mental health of Puerto Ricans on the island and those who migrated to the mainland after the hurricane is yet to be determined.

### Mental Health Concerns

Findings from research studies targeting the U.S. Latinx population point to differences among subgroups that generate concern about the higher rates of mental health issues found in Puerto Ricans: (a) statistically significant differences in the past year prevalence of alcohol abuse and alcohol dependence across four male Latinx subgroups, with Mexican Americans and Puerto Ricans having higher rates than two other Latinx subgroups (Caetano, Ramisetty-Mikler, & Rodríguez, 2008); (b) statistically significant differences when comparing the unadjusted 12-month rates of *any anxiety disorder* and *any disorder* (psychiatric) among Puerto Ricans (15.8%; 24.3%, respectively), Cubans (11.3%;16.6%), Mexicans (9.2%;15.6%), and Other Latinxs (7.8%; 15.2%; Alegría et al., 2007); and (c) statistically significantly higher estimated rates of reported lifetime SAs among Puerto Ricans (9.1%) compared to Mexican Americans (3.1%; Oquendo, Lizardi, Greenwald, Weissman, & Mann, 2004). In addition, Lucas, Freeman, and Adams (2016) reported that Puerto Ricans were more likely to report *serious psychological distress* in the past month compared to three other Latinx subgroups. Furthermore, there is some evidence that raises caution regarding the generalization of the Latinx immigrant paradox to all subgroups and for all psychiatric conditions (Alegría et al., 2008; Alegría et al., 2012). Thus, additional focus on the sociocultural elements that impact the mental health and well-being of Puerto Ricans is warranted.

National mortality data for 2016 signal the need for further examination of factors that impact suicide risk in the Latinx population and its subgroups. In terms of the overall U.S. Latinx population, suicide was ranked as the third leading cause of death for those between the ages of 10 and 34 years (Heron, 2018). The age-adjusted death rate for suicide (per 100,000 standard population) for U.S. Latinxs was 6.7 compared to 6.3 for non-Latinx Blacks; however, the estimated age-adjusted suicide death rate among U.S. Latinx males was 10.9 compared to 2.6 for their female counterparts (Xu, Murhpy, Kochanek, Bastian, & Arias, 2018). For Puerto Rico, an estimated age-adjusted death rate for suicide of 5.1 was reported for 2016 (Xu et al., 2018). Preliminary government data from Puerto Rico also conveys differences by sex; for 2016, over 80% of suicide deaths occurred in males (Gobierno de Puerto Rico, Departamento de Salud, 2018).

Surveillance data pertaining to SI and suicidal behavior (SB) also point to concerns among U.S. Latinx high school students. In 2017, findings revealed that (a) a statistically significantly higher percentage of Latinx male students (9.9%) made a plan for a SA in the past year compared to non-Latinx Black males (6.5%; CDC, n.d.-c); (b) a statistically significantly higher percentage of Latinx female students (10.5%) made a SA in the past year compared to Latinx males (5.8%; CDC, n.d.-b); and (c) an estimated 22.2% of Latinx females considered a SA during the past year compared to 17.2% of all students nationwide (Kann et al., 2018). Additionally, an estimated 10.5% of Latinx female students reported a past year SA compared to 7.3% of non-Latinx White and 12.5% non-Latinx Black females (Kahn et al., 2018). However, previous survey findings have reported statistically significantly higher rates of past year SAs for Latinx female adolescents in comparison to both non-Latinx White and non-Latinx Black females (Kann et al., 2014; Kann et al., 2016); consequently, researchers have identified them as an at-risk group for SAs (Zayas, 2011; Zayas et al., 2005). For Puerto Rico, the prevalence of past year SAs reported by high schoolers (13.7%) was statistically significantly higher in 2017 than the estimated nationwide prevalence for students in the United States (7.4%; CDC, n.d.-a). In sum, these findings call for research studies aimed at understanding the risk and protective factors for Latinx adolescents by subethnic groups and by gender.

## PROBLEM

Latinx suicide is an understudied topic in research (Silva & Van Orden, 2018); moreover, there is paucity in the literature relative to Latinx subgroups such as Puerto Ricans. Although caution is advised when examining self-reports of SI and SA (WHO, 2014) and comparing the mortality rates of certain minority groups due to inconsistencies in the designation of race/ethnicity on death certificates (Xu et al., 2018), the need for research efforts to specifically target Latinx subgroups must be addressed. Puerto Ricans have unique historical, economic, and cultural ties to the United States that differentiate them from other Latinx groups. Since understanding the influence of culture on health supports nursing research and the provision of effective nursing care (Marion et al., 2016), expanding current knowledge pertaining to the influence of culture on the mental health of Puerto Ricans is necessary.

### Purpose

Given the dearth of current research addressing the relationship between culture and suicide in Puerto Ricans, the purpose of this integrative review (IR) is to synthesize research findings that address cultural factors that influence SI and SB in Puerto Ricans across the life span. The review of the current literature is guided by the following research question: What cultural factors influence SI and SB in Puerto Ricans? American citizenship grants Puerto Ricans the opportunity to travel without restrictions between the island and the U.S. mainland leading to a unique pattern of *circular migration* (Guarnaccia, Martinez, & Acosta, 2005; Purnell, 2013). Thus, this IR will target the literature addressing both Puerto Ricans on the island and the mainland.

## LITERATURE REVIEW METHOD

A literature review was conducted following Whittemore and Knafl (2005) and their specific recommendations for guiding and strengthening the IR process. These strategies include identifying the targeted problem, population, and purpose of the IR; detailing a specific process for searching the literature; implementing a method for evaluating the quality of the reports selected for review; determining techniques for data analysis; and reporting findings.

The databases used to carry out the literature search were CINAHL, PsycINFO, PubMed, Scopus, and Sociological Abstracts. A health sciences research librarian assisted with identifying the appropriate headings, operators, and functions that would allow a broad search strategy of the keyword *suicide* in each database. The search was combined with the term *Puerto Rican* and its different variations, including *Puerto Rico, Puertorrique,** and *Boricua*. The time frame was limited to the past 10 years to offer current trends and perspectives on the research focus of the IR that may not be present in older items in the literature. With the exception of Scopus, findings from each database were limited to publications from January 2007 to January 2018. Findings from Scopus were limited from 2007 to 2017 since 2018 was not available at the time the search was conducted.

Articles were selected for the IR if they addressed SI and SB (e.g., study variable) and were published in a peer-reviewed journal (e.g., books and dissertations were not included). Articles could be written in English or Spanish since the first and third authors are fully bilingual. Since the focus of the review is specifically on the Puerto Rican culture, articles were included if the study was carried out in Puerto Rico, greater than 50% of the study sample was identified as Puerto Rican, or the study made comparisons in relation to SI and SB between Puerto Ricans and other subgroups. Articles were excluded from selection if they (a) focused on assisted suicide, (b) targeted pharmacological interventions, (c) focused on participants with psychotic features, (d) provided information on SI and SB to describe the sample without any clear implications specifically for Puerto Ricans, or (e) did not address cultural elements related to SI and SB. Studies were also excluded if the majority of participants had cognitive impairment or a psychotic disorder.

The first author was responsible for carrying out the literature search and conducting the review; questions about the inclusion/exclusion of articles were addressed by the second and third authors. A database search performed on February 3, 2018, resulted in a total of 298 articles found. The third author provided 22 articles, including one accepted for publication in January 2018. An additional 12 records were identified by reviewing the reference list of all selected articles and relevant items found in excluded articles or references used. After applying the time limit, the total amount of records was reduced to 181 articles. Duplicates were removed and an initial screen of titles, abstracts, and sample descriptions was conducted. Articles that did not meet the selection criteria were excluded ($n$ = 33); another two could not be confirmed as peer-reviewed. The full text of all remaining articles was read. Six articles were excluded from the review due to lack of confidence in the statistical analyses; errors on the presentation of data on tables or lack of clarity on methods undertaken to analyze the data were the primary reasons. An additional 34 articles were not eligible based on the inclusion criteria; however, one of these was used as a reference within the discussion section of the IR. Therefore, the final number of articles included in the IR was 24. A flow diagram of the article selection process is found in Figure 9.1.

The Quality Assessment Tool for Studies of Diverse Design (QATSDD; Sirriyeh, Lawton, Gardner, & Armitage, 2012) was used to evaluate the quality of selected records. Designed for use with health research studies implementing different methodologies, the QATSDD delineates 16 criteria (e.g., use of theoretical framework, reliability and validity of instruments, description of recruitment

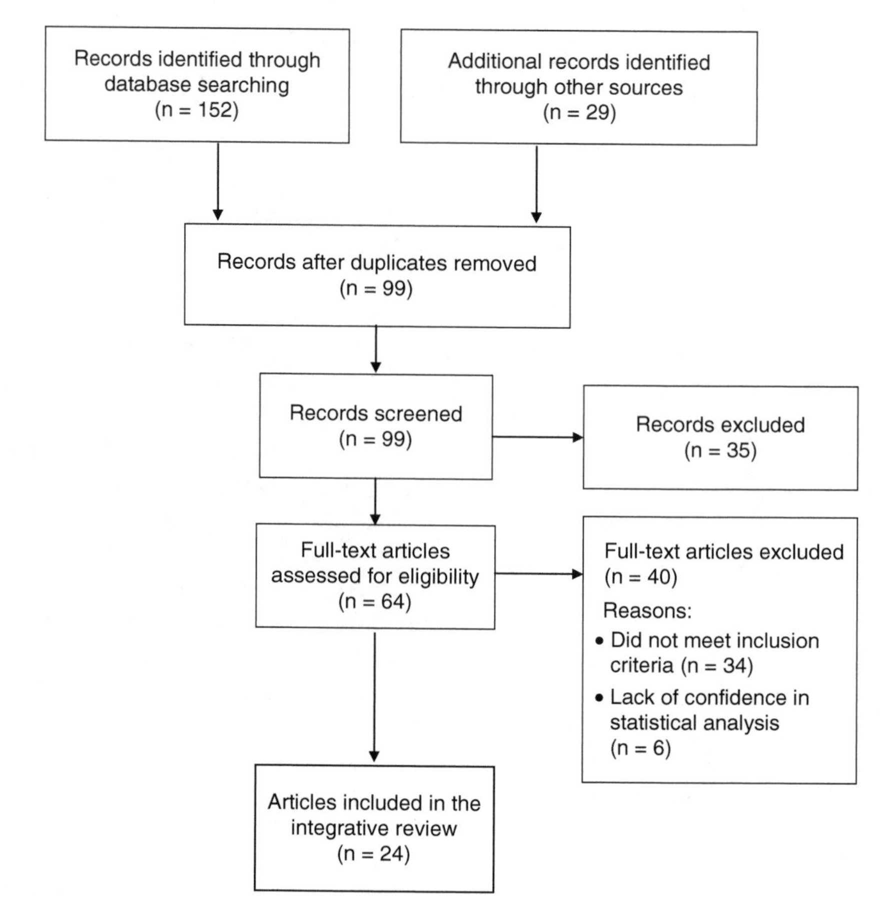


**FIGURE 9.1** Flow diagram of article selection for the integrative review.
Adapted from PRISMA 2009 flow diagram. "Preferred Reporting Items for Systematic Reviews and Meta-analyses: The PRISMA Statement," by D. Moher, A. Liberati, J. Tetzlaff, D. G. Altman, and The PRISMA Group, 2009, *PLoS Medicine, 6*(7), e1000097. https://doi.org/10.1371/journal.pmed.1000097

process) that can be assigned scores on a 4-point scale (0 to 3). All 16 items can be used to assess mixed methods studies, 14 items can be used to assess quantitative research, and 14 items can be used for qualitative research. A quality score expressed as a percentage of the total possible score allows for comparison between studies; articles receiving a lower quality score were given less weight in the IR analysis.

The complexity of cultural influence can present a challenge in understanding its role. Leininger's Culture Care Theory (CCT; McFarland, 2018) was used in this IR to provide a holistic approach to the identification and extraction of

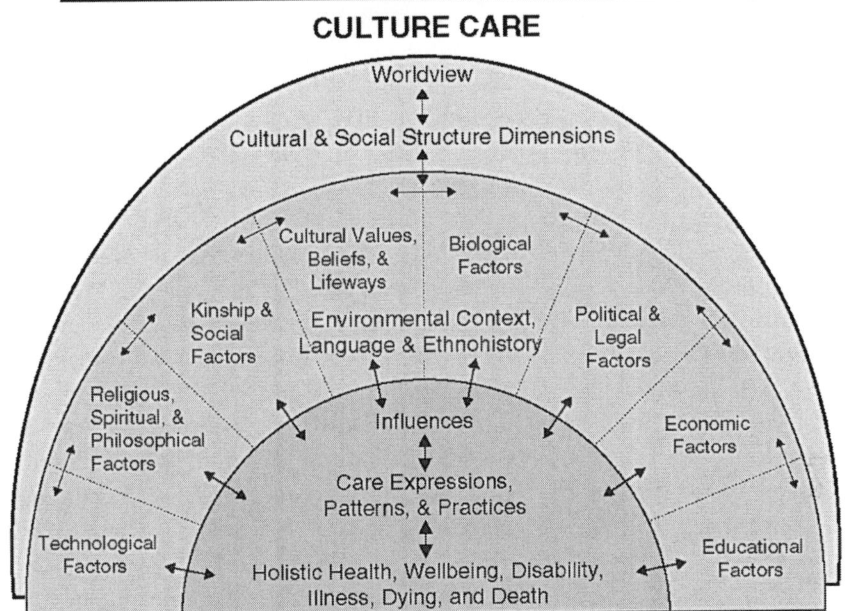


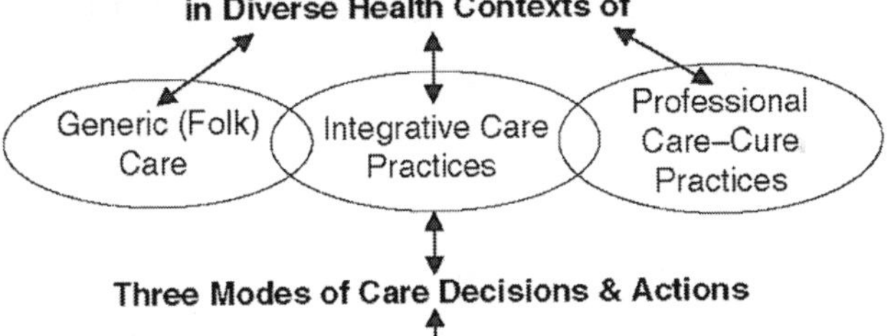


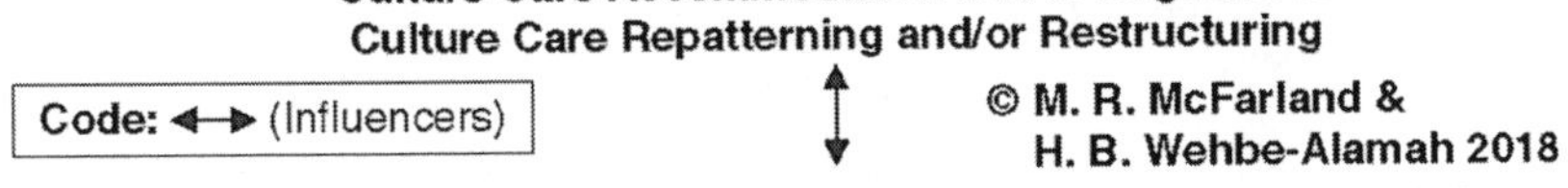


**FIGURE 9.2** Leininger's Sunrise Enabler to Discover Culture Care.
From McFarland, M., & Wehbe-Alamah, H. (2018). *Transcultural Nursing Concepts, Theories, Research, & Practice* (4th ed.). New York, NY: McGraw-Hill Education. Used with permission.

cultural factors found in the literature. The CCT can serve as a guide for nursing research efforts since it can help identify cultural aspects of care, from an emic and etic perspective, that may influence health (Leininger, 2002; McFarland, 2018). The Sunrise Enabler to Discover Culture Care (see Figure 9.2) provides a visual representation of the CCT and facilitates cultural discovery relative to a domain of inquiry (Wehbe-Alamah, 2018); it displays *cultural and social structure dimensions* that represent "the dynamic, holistic, and interrelated patterns of structured features of a culture" (Leininger, 2002, p. 83). These features, in a sense, represent cultural elements that can influence beliefs, practices, and meanings related to different aspects of care for different groups (McFarland, 2018). Some of the different factors identified by Leininger include economics; education; kinship and social factors; cultural values, beliefs, and lifeways; and religion (McFarland, 2018; McFarland & Wehbe-Alamah, 2015). Biological factors were added to the Sunrise Enabler at a later time (Wehbe-Alamah, 2018). Data were extracted from pertinent findings and inferences that carried cultural implications for Puerto Ricans; major categories were identified and organized by the cultural elements represented in the Sunrise Enabler (Wehbe-Alamah, 2018).

Definitions for suicide-related terms are provided to offer clarity for the review. Except when referencing variable names specified by research articles, the terms suicide, SB, and SI are defined in this IR as follows:

- Suicide: "Death caused by self-directed injurious behavior with any intent to die as a result of the behavior" (Crosby, Ortega, & Melanson, 2011, p. 23).
- Suicidal behaviors: "Behaviors related to suicide, including preparatory acts, as well as suicide attempts and deaths" (U. S. Department of Health and Human Services [HHS], Office of the Surgeon General, National Action Alliance for Suicide Prevention, 2012, p. 142).
- Suicidal ideation: "Thoughts of engaging in suicide-related behavior" (HHS, 2012, p. 143).

## RESULTS

A review of the literature resulted in the identification of four major cultural factors: biological factors; cultural values, beliefs, and lifeways; kinship and social factors; and educational factors (see Table 9.1). Most studies reviewed were conducted in Puerto Rico ($n$ = 16); only seven articles were written in Spanish. Participants were predominantly female in many studies and the majority of articles focused on the adolescent population ($n$ = 13). The items included in the IR were primarily psychology research and/or published in psychology journals;

**TABLE 9.1**

*Summary of Records Related to Suicidal Ideation and Behaviors in Puerto Ricans*

| Author/ Year | Purpose | Design/Sample/Location | Pertinent Findings Related to SI/SB | Cultural Factors[a] | Quality Score (%) |
|---|---|---|---|---|---|
| Baca-García et al. (2011) | Examine prevalence rates of SI and SA among Latinx subgroups in the United States during 1991–1992 and 2001–2002. | Secondary analysis of data from two epidemiologic surveys with representative sample of U.S. adults ≥ 18 years of age (first survey $n = 42,862$ [Puerto Ricans $n = 312$]; second survey $n = 43,093$ [Puerto Ricans $n = 962$]). Additional Latinx categories: Mexican, Cuban, and Other Latinx<br>Location: United States | Puerto Ricans had the highest estimated crude rates of both lifetime SA and lifetime SI (without attempts) among Latinx subgroups in both surveys. | Biological factors | 47.6 |
| Bandiera et al. (2013) | Examine the relationship between asthma and SI/SB in Puerto Rican youth and explore possible factors that influence this relationship. | Secondary analysis (data from longitudinal epidemiologic study); Puerto Rican adolescents aged 11–18 years ($n = 1,550$)<br>Location: New York City and Puerto Rico | The variable SI/SB was identified as a *global construct* composed of four variables: SI, thoughts of death, plan for suicide, and SA. After logistic regression analyses and controlling for other variables, an association was reported between SI/SB and the following: a history of asthma, lifetime history of cigarette use, history of life stressors, and MDD. | Biological factors | 40.5 |

(*Continued*)

**TABLE 9.1**

*Summary of Records Related to Suicidal Ideation and Behaviors in Puerto Ricans (Continued)*

| Author/ Year | Purpose | Design/Sample/Location | Pertinent Findings Related to SI/SB | Cultural Factors[a] | Quality Score (%) |
|---|---|---|---|---|---|
| Diefenbach et al. (2009) | Compare prevalence rates and effect of anxious depression (MDD depression (MDD with symptoms of generalized anxiety disorder [GAD]) in older Puerto Ricans and African Americans. | Descriptive; Puerto Ricans (*n* = 218) and African Americans (*n* = 206) aged 60 years and over<br>Location: Connecticut | Puerto Ricans reported greater rates of anxious depression (18.3%) and MDD without symptoms of GAD (11.9%) compared to the African American group (7.2%; 7.8%, respectively). They also reported greater SI. | Cultural values, beliefs, and lifeways | 47.6 |
| Duarté-Vélez and Bernal (2007) | Describe relevant findings in studies pertaining to SI and SB in Latinx adolescents. | A review of the literature from 1990 to 2006, focusing primarily on the Latinx adolescent population. Most studies were conducted in the United States; a few looked at Latinx subgroups | Gender and variables related to family functioning were reported to be factors for consideration in understanding Latinx adolescent SB; prevalence and risk factors varied by subgroups. Authors identified the use of different definitions for SI/SB, an absence of a theoretical framework in most studies, and a dearth of studies comparing Latinx subgroups. | Kinship and social factors | 59.5 |

(*Continued*)

| | | | | | |
|---|---|---|---|---|---|
| Duarté-Vélez et al. (2017) | Guided by a socio-cognitive vulnerability model, examine factors hypothesized to influence SI in Latinx adolescents in Puerto Rico. | Path analyses (survey data); Latinx adolescent students in Puerto Rico aged 11–19 years ($n$ = 233); majority were born in Puerto Rico ($n$ = 195)<br>Location: Puerto Rico | Severe level of SI reported by 9% of students. Standardized parameter estimates in the total model were statistically significant at $p < .10$ (age, parental status [together or not], school were controlled). Proposed factors related to SI included (a) direct effects of *depressive symptoms*, *externalizing behaviors*, and *negative life events* for both males and females; (b) a direct effect of hopelessness only for males; and (c) indirect effects of *family dysfunction* and perceived *social support* via symptoms of depression. | Biological factors<br>Kinship and social factors | 69.0 |

(*Continued*)

**TABLE 9.1**

*Summary of Records Related to Suicidal Ideation and Behaviors in Puerto Ricans (Continued)*

| Author/ Year | Purpose | Design/Sample/Location | Pertinent Findings Related to SI/SB | Cultural Factors[a] | Quality Score (%) |
|---|---|---|---|---|---|
| Duarté-Vélez et al. (2012) | Explore the effect of depression, coping skills, and cognitive factors on SI in Puerto Rican adolescents. | Descriptive (survey); adolescent students in Puerto Rico aged 13–18 years (*n* = 179)<br>Location: Puerto Rico | SI was reported by 16.4% of the total sample; a lifetime SA was reported by 12.4%.<br>Significant differences reported for teens belonging to the SI group compared to those in the non-SI group included the following: higher mean scores for depressive symptoms and cognitive dysfunction as well as lower mean scores for the *seeking family support* measure. | Biological factors<br>Kinship and social factors | 57.1 |
| Duarté-Vélez et al. (2015) | Assess feasibility and further development of an innovative socio-CBT for SB protocol targeting Puerto Rican adolescents. | Case study (quantitative and qualitative data) from a study developing a psychotherapeutic protocol; 15-year-old Puerto Rican female with SI, history of two SAs, diagnosed with recurrent MDD (among other diagnoses)<br>Location: Puerto Rico | Reduced scores reported for depression and hopelessness measures at posttreatment.<br>Slight increase reported in posttreatment score for SI measure but SI denied; SI score decreased at 12-month follow-up. Changes to the protocol included the addition of a caregiver session and a module to address family communication. | Biological factors<br>Kinship and social factors | 50.0 |

(Continued)

| | | | | | |
|---|---|---|---|---|---|
| Duarté-Vélez et al. (2016) | Develop and test a socio-CBT for SB protocol targeting Puerto Rican adolescents after hospitalization for SI or SA. | Pilot test (qualitative and quantitative data); Puerto Rican adolescents aged 13–17 ($n$ = 11). All were diagnosed with psychiatric disorders; all were taking medication<br>Location: Puerto Rico | At pretreatment, teens who did not meet the clinical cutoff point on the SI measure ($n$ = 6) remained below the cutoff score at posttreatment; teens with scores higher than the cutoff point ($n$ = 2) had lower scores at posttreatment (reported as a reliable change). Refinements to the protocol included additional sessions to address family communication. | Biological factors<br>Cultural values, beliefs, and lifeways<br>Kinship and social factors | 72.9 |
| Duke and Mateo (2008) | Gain understanding of the barriers and disparities related to the behavioral health needs of Puerto Rican adolescents. | Qualitative study; Puerto Rican adolescents between the ages of 13 and 18 years ($n$ = 40) categorized into two groups: counseling ($n$ = 20) and not in counseling but met aggression and depression criteria ($n$ = 20). Five experienced behavioral health providers were also interviewed.<br>Location: Connecticut | Three main categories were identified: common behavioral health issues, treatment challenges, and barriers to care (e.g., language barrier, socioeconomic status). For participants, SI/SB represented a sense of despair, a need for attention, or a cry for help. One participant expressed a sense of ambivalence related to suicide intent. | Kinship and social factors | 47.6 |

*(Continued)*

**TABLE 9.1**

*Summary of Records Related to Suicidal Ideation and Behaviors in Puerto Ricans (Continued)*

| Author/ Year | Purpose | Design/Sample/Location | Pertinent Findings Related to SI/SB | Cultural Factors[a] | Quality Score (%) |
|---|---|---|---|---|---|
| Fortuna et al. (2007) | Examine prevalence rates of SI and SA among Latinx subgroups in the United States and risk factors associated with SI and SB in these groups. | Descriptive study (national survey); representative sample of U.S. Latinx adults ($n$ = 2,554). Latinx categories: Puerto Rican, Mexican, Cuban, and Other Latinx<br>Location: United States | The estimated prevalence rate of *lifetime history of SI* for Puerto Ricans was 14.2%; for *lifetime history of SA,* it was 6.9%. Findings point to the need for further research among different Latinx subgroups to address the relationship between SB and sociocultural factors (e.g., English-speaking ability, birthplace), as well as family-related variables. | Biological factors | 52.4 |
| Holloway et al. (2015) | Explore the sexual identity and effects of concealment patterns of sexual relationships on the mental health of males who have sex with men and women. | Qualitative study; Latinx adult males who acknowledged a same-sex sexual relationship while in a primary sexual relationship with a woman ($n$ = 20; 70% Puerto Rican, 30% Dominican).<br>Location: United States | Themes related to the stress associated with (a) living up to social expectations surrounding masculinity, (b) efforts to keep sexual relationships with men a secret from female partners and others, and (c) possible impact on mental health if disclosure occurred (e.g., anxiety, suicide). | Cultural values, beliefs, and lifeways Kinship and social factors | 54.8 |

(*Continued*)

| | | | | | |
|---|---|---|---|---|---|
| Jiménez-Chafey. (2008) | Describe prevalence and risk factors for SI and SB in college students. | A review of the literature of the past 10 years, focusing primarily on college students in the United States and Puerto Rico | There is very limited research addressing suicide prevalence and risk factors among college students in Puerto Rico; additional knowledge is needed to address prevention in this group. | Educational factors | 38.1 |
| Jiménez-Chafey et al. (2009) | Examine factors related to CBT response and challenges faced. | Case study (qualitative and quantitative data) from an RCT on psychotherapy; 15- year-old Puerto Rican female with SI, diagnosed with MDD (among other diagnoses). Location: Puerto Rico | After completion of standard treatment, participant still met MDD criteria, requiring additional sessions; parental marital conflict was identified as a major stressor. At conclusion of treatment, MDD criteria were not met and score on SI measure decreased. | Biological factors Kinship and social factors | 37.5 |
| Jiménez-Chafey et al. (2011) | Describe family interactions and their impact on adolescent treatment response to a CBT protocol. | Two case studies (qualitative and quantitative data) from an RCT on psychotherapy; two 14-year-old Puerto Rican females with SI and diagnosed with MDD (among other diagnoses) Location: Puerto Rico | After completion of standard treatment, both females required additional sessions. Issues addressed included depression symptoms and mother–daughter conflict. At posttreatment, one female did not present symptoms of depression or SI; the other reported decreased depression and SI but MDD criteria were met again at 12-month follow-up. | Biological factors Kinship and social factors | 54.2 |

(*Continued*)

**TABLE 9.1**

*Summary of Records Related to Suicidal Ideation and Behaviors in Puerto Ricans (Continued)*

| Author/ Year | Purpose | Design/Sample/Location | Pertinent Findings Related to SI/SB | Cultural Factors[a] | Quality Score (%) |
|---|---|---|---|---|---|
| Jones et al. (2008) | Explore the relationship between psychiatric disorders, psychosocial factors, and SB in adolescents in Puerto Rico. | Secondary analysis; representative probability samples of adolescents aged 12–17 years. One sample is from the community (*n* = 1,896), the other is a clinical sample (*n* = 736)<br>Location: Puerto Rico | The variable SB was composed of two variables: past year SI and lifetime history of SA. SB was reported by 10.3% of teens in the total community sample; SB was reported by 37.9% of teens in the clinical sample. Logistic regression analyses revealed statistically significant associations for both samples between SB and several factors, including any psychiatric disorders and psychiatric comorbidity. | Biological factors | 47.6 |

(*Continued*)

| | | | | | |
|---|---|---|---|---|---|
| Jovet-Toledo et al. (2014) | Describe the rates of suicide in patients with HIV in Puerto Rico. | Descriptive; participants ≥ 16 years of age recruited from a specialty clinic for screening/treatment of HIV and sexually transmitted infections ($n$ = 1,185)<br>Location: Puerto Rico | The study focused on SA, not suicide. In the overall sample, 20.4% of participants reported a history of at least one SA. No association was found between HIV status and lifetime SA. In both the general sample and the subgroup of patients who self-reported HIV-positive status, an association was reported between lifetime SA and the following: gender (female), job status (unemployment), and those reporting lifetime history of drug use. | Biological factors | 38.1 |
| Moscoso Alvarez et al. (2016) | Explore rates of mental health issues among adolescents in Puerto Rico and their relationship with school and family factors. | Secondary analysis of survey data; students from 7th to 12th grade ($n$ = 10,235)<br>Location: Puerto Rico | The estimated prevalence of past year SI was 8.3%; for depression in the past year, it was 13.4%. Several family-related factors were reported to be associated with SI. | Kinship and social factors | 42.9 |

(Continued)

**TABLE 9.1**

*Summary of Records Related to Suicidal Ideation and Behaviors in Puerto Ricans (Continued)*

| Author/ Year | Purpose | Design/Sample/Location | Pertinent Findings Related to SI/SB | Cultural Factors[a] | Quality Score (%) |
|---|---|---|---|---|---|
| Pedroso (2013) | Examine trends in mortality rates and the main causes of death by sex in Puerto Rico from a gender perspective. | Descriptive research using population, mortality, and life expectancy data for Puerto Rico from 2005 to 2010 | The report focuses on 2008 mortality rates by age and gender; a greater suicide mortality rate (per 100, 000 population) was identified for males (13.2) compared to females (2.3). Trends relative to a higher rate of death for young adult males, due to external causes (e.g., homicide, suicide), are suggested to contribute to premature loss of life. | Cultural values, beliefs, and lifeways | 50.0 |
| Reyes-Rodríguez et al. (2010) | Estimate the prevalence of eating disorder symptoms and depressive symptoms in college freshmen in Puerto Rico. | Cross-sectional survey; college freshmen aged 15–38 years from several campuses in a university system ($n$ = 2,163) Location: Puerto Rico | Of those who screened positive for symptoms of eating disorders (ED Screen +), 5.9% were identified as *high suicidal risk*. Females in the ED Screen (+) group were found to have statistically significantly higher mean scores on the depressive symptoms measure than those in the ED Screen (–) group ($p$ < .001). A similar pattern was reported for males ($p < .001$). | Biological factors | 61.9 |

(Continued)

| | | | | | |
|---|---|---|---|---|---|
| Reyes-Rodríguez et al. (2013) | Examine the prevalence of depression and SI in college freshmen in Puerto Rico. | Secondary analysis of questionnaire data; representative sample of college freshmen from several campuses in a university system ($n$ = 2,163)<br>Location: Puerto Rico | An estimated 9% of students reported moderate-to-severe depressive symptoms. Of students with severe depressive symptoms, 73.3% ($n$ = 11) *would like to attempt suicide* and 76.9% ($n$ = 10) *would do it if given the opportunity*. Multiple regression analyses revealed that SI, a romantic breakup, illness, and moving away for college were statistically significant predictors of depressive symptoms in females; only SI, illness, and relocation were significant predictors in males. | Biological factors<br>Educational factors | 69.0 |
| Rosselló et al (2011) | Explore the effect of a CBT intervention (including a suicide risk protocol); identify predictors for SI and how SI affects treatment response. | Quasi-experimental (one group pre/post); adolescents aged 13–17.5 years, diagnosed with MDD ($n$ = 121); majority Puerto Rican ($n$ = 114)<br>Location: Puerto Rico | A high level of SI (above the clinical cutoff) was reported for 20.7% of teens. Findings indicated that CBT treatment statistically significantly reduced SI severity scores from pretreatment to posttreatment: $t$ (114) n = 7.96, $p < .001$. In terms of a reduction in SI scores, a reliable change was reported for 34.8% of teens and a significant clinical change for 89.6%. | Biological factors | 52.4 |

(*Continued*)

**TABLE 9.1**

*Summary of Records Related to Suicidal Ideation and Behaviors in Puerto Ricans (Continued)*

| Author/Year | Purpose | Design/Sample/Location | Pertinent Findings Related to SI/SB | Cultural Factors[a] | Quality Score (%) |
|---|---|---|---|---|---|
| Rosselló et al (2008) | Explore differences in adolescents reporting SI; explore the relationship between SI and several factors classified as *cognitive*, *family*, and *diagnostic* variables. | Descriptive; youth aged 12–17 years and met criteria for MDD ($n$ = 121) Location: Puerto Rico | A significantly higher mean score for the SI measure was reported for females (17.14) compared to males (10.59). Significant differences were reported on several variables when comparing youth in two different categories of SI (severe; none/moderate) | Biological factors Kinship and social factors | 50.0 |
| Vélez-Pérez et al. (2017) | Examine the rates of SI and SA in students at a college campus in Puerto Rico. | Descriptive (questionnaire); college students aged 17–25 years ($n$ = 507) Location: Puerto Rico | Of the 50 students (9.9%) who reported lifetime SA, 90% were female, 30% were first-year students, and 42% were in the College of Sciences. Of the 43 students (8.5%) who reported past year SI: 74.4% were female, 37.2% were first-year students, and 67.4% were in the College of Sciences. A statistically significant association was found between SA and gender ($p$ = .004) but not between SI and gender ($p$ = .79). | Cultural values, beliefs, and lifeways Educational factors | 42.9 |

(Continued)

| | | | | | |
|---|---|---|---|---|---|
| Vera et al. (2011) | Explore the prevalence of SI and risk factors for SI in general practice patients receiving care in Puerto Rico. | Descriptive; adult patients ≥18 years of age with chronic medical conditions (*n* = 2,068)<br>Location: Puerto Rico | SI in the past 2 weeks was reported by 15.4% of all patients in the sample. These patients were categorized into an SI group that consisted of four categories: *passive ideation, active ideation without a plan, active ideation with a plan, suicide attempt*.<br>The following factors were found to be associated with greater odds of SI: moderately severe and severe levels of depression (compared to none to moderate), being ≤ 64 years of age (compared to ≥ 65 years), and having some college or less years of education (compared to ≥ 4 years of college). | Biological factors<br>Educational factors | 52.4 |

*Note*. CBT = cognitive behavioral therapy; MDD = major depressive disorder; RCT = randomized clinical trial; SA = suicide attempt; SB = suicidal behaviors; SI = suicidal ideation.

[a]Data were categorized into cultural factors according to areas of cultural influence represented in the Sunrise Enabler to Discover Culture Care from Leininger's Culture Care Theory. From Wehbe-Alamah, H. B. (2018). The Ethnonursing Research Method: Major features and enablers. In M. R. McFarland & H. B. Wehbe-Alamah (Eds.). *Leininger's transcultural nursing: Concepts, theories, research & practice* (4th ed., pp. 57–84). New York, NY: McGraw-Hill Education.

none were identified as nursing research. The mention of a theoretical framework was missing from 13 of the selected articles. In relation to suicide, most articles targeted SI; however, many did not specify the question or time frame used to measure the variable.

Only two studies compared adult Puerto Ricans to other Latinx subgroups. Baca-García et al. (2011) carried out a secondary analysis of data from two surveys of representative samples of U.S. adults (National Epidemiological Survey on Alcohol and Related Conditions [NESARC], National Longitudinal Alcohol Epidemiologic Survey [NLAES]), focusing on participants who met the criteria for the depression section of the surveys. They found that among the Latinx subgroups, Puerto Ricans had statistically significantly higher rates of the following: (a) lifetime SI in the NLAES (7.9%, 95% CI [3.8, 12.0]) compared to Cubans (1.7%, 95% CI [0.0, 3.7]); lifetime SI in the NESARC (8.0%, 95% CI [5.3, 10.7]) compared to Mexicans (2.8%, 95% CI [2.2, 3.4]); and (c) lifetime SA in the NESARC (4.4%, 95% CI [3.0, 5.8]) compared to Cubans (1.1%, 95% CI [0.5, 1.7]), Mexicans (1.7%, 95% CI [1.1, 2.3]), and Whites (2.4%, 95% CI [2.2, 2.6]). However, a report from the NLAAS indicated that although a greater proportion of Puerto Ricans reported a lifetime history of SI and SA, no statistically significant differences were found among the Latinx subgroups (Fortuna, Perez, Canino, Sribney, & Alegria, 2007).

Another study based in the United States compared Puerto Rican and African American older adults and found higher rates of major depressive disorder with and without symptoms of generalized anxiety disorder among the Puerto Rican group; Puerto Ricans also reported more SI severity (Diefenbach, Disch, Robison, Baez, & Coman, 2009). A majority of Puerto Rican participants (97.2%) were interviewed in Spanish. Although age and socioeconomic status were included as factors that could influence prevalence rates in this sample, the authors also noted that conducting the majority of interviews in Spanish for Puerto Rican participants could have been an influential factor; cultural variations may impact how symptoms of depression and anxiety are identified, expressed, and reported by racial/ethnic groups (Diefenbach et al., 2009)

## Gender

Since gender can be related to several of the social structure factors in the Sunrise Model (Leininger, 2002), differences between males and females in relation to SI and SB are reported in this section. In several articles, females were found to report SI in greater proportions than males: in adolescents in Puerto Rico (Jones, Ramirez, Davies, Canino, & Goodwin, 2008; Moscoso Álvarez, Rodríguez-Figueroa, Reyes-Pulliza, Colón, 2016; Rosselló, Duarté-Vélez, Bernal, & Zuluaga 2008); in college students in Puerto Rico (Vélez-Pérez,

Maldonado-Santiago, & Rivera-Lugo, 2017); and in adults with chronic medical conditions living in Puerto Rico (Vera et al., 2011). Recommendations were made by several researchers relative to the need for suicide prevention measures that not only target cultural factors but also address specific gender needs (Reyes-Rodríguez, Rivera-Medina, Camara-Fuentes, Suarez-Torres, & Bernal, 2013; Rosselló et al., 2008; Vélez-Pérez et al., 2017).

Gender differences were also identified by Pedroso (2013), who found a greater suicide mortality rate for males in Puerto Rico for 2008. Using a gender perspective, concerns about high rates of deaths by external causes (e.g., homicides, suicides) in young adult males in Puerto Rico were discussed. The author posited that cultural values related to masculinity and male gender expectations may play a role in risk-taking behaviors by young men; the need for the development of health policies that promote gender equity and equality to reduce disparities were proposed (Pedroso, 2013).

Citing the need for Latinx suicide by specific subgroups, Duarté-Vélez, Jones, and Spirito (2017) studied data from a sample of Latinx teens in Puerto Rico to compare influential factors by sex. Guided by a socio-cognitive vulnerability framework, they conducted path analyses and proposed a model of factors influencing SI. The authors suggested that *externalizing behaviors* and *depressive symptoms* had a larger direct effect on SI for females; *depressive symptoms* and *hopelessness* were found to have a larger direct effect on SI for males. Duarté-Vélez et al. (2017) posited that perceived failure to meet gender role expectations of strength and leadership by adolescent males in Puerto Rico may have a negative impact on their thought patterns.

## Biological Factors

Biological factors represent elements that address how illness (e.g., hereditary) can impact care (McFarland, 2018); thus, several studies that addressed SI and SB in relation to physical and psychiatric disorders are included under this category.

A group of studies suggested a relationship between depressive symptoms and SI for different populations in Puerto Rico. While some recruited adolescent samples (Duarté-Vélez et al., 2017; Duarté-Vélez, Lorenzo-Luaces, & Rosselló, 2012; Rosselló, Duarté-Vélez, Gema-Zuluaga, & Bernal, 2011; Rosselló et al., 2008), a few targeted adults (Reyes-Rodríguez et al., 2013; Vera et al., 2011). Focusing on adults with chronic illness in Puerto Rico, Vera et al. (2011) conducted a multiple logistic regression analysis and found that among other significant factors, moderately severe ($OR$ = 11.46, 95% CI [8.36, 15.71] and severe levels of depression ($OR$ = 18.76, 95% CI [12.53, 28.09]) were statistically significantly associated ($p < .001$) with SI, compared to lower levels of severity.

Reyes-Rodríguez et al. (2013) recruited a representative sample of college students in Puerto Rico and utilized a unique approach to study the relationship between SI and SB in this group. They conducted multiple regression analyses and included SI in some models as a predictor for depressive symptoms. The best fitted model for females included illness, SI, moving away for college, and a romantic breakup; together, these factors explained 31% of the variance in depressive symptoms. Illness, SI, and relocation for college were significant predictors for males and explained 47.6% of the variance (Reyes-Rodríguez et al., 2013).

Findings from a number of other studies suggested the need for further investigation of the relationship between (a) SI/SB and asthma in adolescents (Bandiera, Ramirez, Arheart, Canino, & Goodwin, 2013); (b) SI and eating disorders in college students in Puerto Rico (Reyes-Rodríguez et al., 2010); (c) psychiatric disorders and SB in adolescents in Puerto Rico (Jones et al., 2008); and (d) history of SA and drug use in adults in Puerto Rico (Jovet-Toledo et al., 2014). Baca-García et al. (2011) referred to *ataque de nervios* as a culture-bound syndrome that may impact vulnerability to SAs in adult Puerto Rican women. In addition, several case studies addressed the treatment of female adolescents in Puerto Rico who were diagnosed with depression, reported SI, and had a family history of mental health issues (Duarté-Vélez, Torres Dávila, & Laboy Hernández, 2015; Jiménez Chafey, Bernal, & Rosselló, 2009; Jiménez Chafey, Duarté Vélez, & Bernal, 2011).

As noted, the majority of these articles were conducted with samples in Puerto Rico; several assessed the relationship between depression and SI. Further research focus on Puerto Ricans who live on the U.S. mainland is needed; additional evidence will aid in evaluating the impact of specific biological factors on SI and SB in Puerto Ricans.

## Cultural Values, Beliefs, and Lifeways

Cultural values and beliefs can influence health and how care is expressed (McFarland & Wehbe-Alamah, 2015). Familism (Duarté-Vélez et al., 2017; Jiménez Chafey et al., 2011), gender role expectations (Duarté-Vélez et al., 2015), and the influence of the family system in adolescent development (Duarté-Vélez et al., 2012; Duarté-Vélez et al., 2015; Jiménez Chafey et al., 2009) were discussed as influential factors that must be considered for further understanding of SI and SB in Puerto Rican adolescents. Since these cultural values are closely related to Leininger's kinship and social factors, they are further discussed in the following section.

A few studies made mention of the possible role that expectations surrounding masculine behavior may have on the mental health of Puerto Rican males (Duarté-Vélez et al., 2017; Holloway, Padilla, Willner, & Guilamo-Ramos, 2015; Pedroso, 2013). Perceived social norms surrounding masculinity were described in a qualitative study with a small sample of adult men who acknowledged a same-sex sexual relationship while in a primary sexual relationship with a woman (Holloway et al., 2015). The group was primarily Puerto Rican. Men described the secrecy surrounding their relationships with other men and the stress and fears related to potential discovery. Authors hypothesized that the pressure of failing to meet expectations tied to traditional masculine behaviors endorsed by the Latinx culture could possibly lead to mental health issues in this population (Holloway, Padilla, Willner, & Guilamo-Ramos, 2015).

Addressing multiple factors that may influence SI and SB, Duarté-Vélez, Torres-Dávila, Spirito, Polanco, and Bernal (2016) proposed a socio-cognitive behavioral treatment protocol for Puerto Rican adolescents with SB; it targeted an identified need for theory-driven, culturally tailored interventions for specific Latinx groups. The modality integrated an ecological perspective of SB and allowed for elements related to adolescent development, cultural values and personal beliefs, the family system, and gender. Pilot testing led to the inclusion of sessions that covered adolescent trauma and family communication; teaching communication skills to teens and caregivers was essential. Although benefits regarding suicide risk were reported, the small sample size ($n$ = 11) was a limitation.

Given the potential influence of culture on SI and SB in Puerto Ricans, the research literature addressing cultural values and beliefs is limited for both adolescents and adults on the island and the mainland. While a few articles addressed gender expectations, specific attention to cultural meaning and beliefs regarding suicide and those at risk of suicide was missing.

### Kinship and Social Factors

Leininger (1978) originally referred to kinship and social systems to acknowledge the influence of "relationships by blood, marriage, and other social means" (p. 61). Several studies addressed kinship and social factors pertaining to the central role of family in the Latinx culture, mostly in adolescents at risk for SI and SB. Jiménez Chafey et al. (2011) stressed that "assessing family functioning and values is essential when designing treatment plans with adolescents, particularly for Latino/a adolescents" (p. 65). However, Duarté-Vélez and Bernal (2007) posited that risk factors may vary among Latinx subgroups and cautioned against generalizations for all Latinx adolescents. Other areas that were addressed in relation to family functioning included gender role expectations and how they may influence parent–child interactions and parenting approach (Duarté-Vélez et al., 2015; Rosselló et al., 2008), family conflict (Duarté-Vélez et al., 2015;

Duarté-Vélez et al., 2016; Jiménez Chafey et al., 2009; Jiménez Chafey et al., 2011), and the family's ability to serve as a source of support (Duarté-Vélez et al., 2012).

Given the role of family in the Puerto Rican culture, a variety of measures were recommended to support interventions with teens and their families. They included (a) the family's need for effective communication skills to facilitate interactions and reduce conflict (Duarté-Vélez et al., 2015; Duke & Mateo, 2008; Jiménez Chafey et al., 2011); (b) recognizing the specific needs of single mothers (Duarté-Vélez et al., 2015; Jiménez Chafey et al., 2011); (c) providing individual therapy sessions for parents/caregivers to offer support (Duarté-Vélez et al., 2015; Jiménez Chafey et al., 2011); (d) offering psychoeducation for parents (Duarté-Vélez et al., 2017; Jiménez Chafey et al., 2011); (e) differentiating between assertiveness and disrespect in communication styles (Jiménez Chafey et al., 2011); and (f) offering therapy sessions that include the family (Duarté-Vélez et al., 2015; Duke & Mateo, 2008). Addressing language barriers that may exist for families seeking mental health services on the mainland is a key issue (Duke & Mateo, 2008). Duke and Mateo (2008) suggested the possibility of challenges related to cultural identity for adolescents living stateside and that circular migration patterns of Puerto Rican families may contribute to adolescents feeling "a sense of being neither wholly American nor Puerto Rican" (p. 73).

In summary, consideration and assessment of family-related factors was reflected in several studies addressing the treatment needs of Puerto Rican adolescents. However, most of these were either case studies or studies with a small sample size; the majority were conducted in Puerto Rico.

### Educational Factors

Education, along with other factors included within the cultural and social structure dimensions of the CCT, can also influence health (McFarland & Wehbe-Alamah, 2015). Thus, a few articles that specifically addressed education-related issues in relation to SI and SB are discussed in this section.

In a sample of adults with chronic illness in Puerto Rico, having less years of education was found to be associated with greater odds of SI compared to having a college education of four years or more (Vera et al., 2011). In a survey of undergraduate students in Puerto Rico (*n* = 507), 9.9% of participants reported a history of a lifetime SA; authors inferred that stressors related to finances, transition from high school, relationships, and academic expectations may increase vulnerability among college students in Puerto Rico (Vélez-Pérez et al., 2017). Although a dearth of research specifically targets Puerto Rican college students (Jiménez Chafey, 2008), the few articles found offered recommendations for suicide prevention on college campuses in Puerto Rico that included consideration for gender differences relative to SB (Vélez-Pérez et al., 2017), implementation of innovative methods for screening (Reyes-Rodríguez et al., 2013), and offering support for stress management and college-related transitions (Reyes-Rodríguez et al., 2013).

Although this section includes a small number of articles, these studies point to the need for future research focus on the mental health needs of college students and emerging adults, suicide prevention in schools and college campuses, mental health literacy, and the relationship between educational levels and mental health outcomes.

## DISCUSSION

Since "culture can be viewed as the blueprint for guiding human actions and decisions" (McFarland & Wehbe-Alamah, 2015, p. 10), consideration of the cultural context surrounding mental health and mental illness is a critical element for the provision of culturally congruent mental health care. The CCT (McFarland, 2018) was used to guide an IR of the literature pertaining to SI and SB in Puerto Ricans in the U.S. mainland and in Puerto Rico. The limited amount of research found suggests four cultural factors that may influence SI and SB in this population: biological factors; cultural values, beliefs, and lifeways; kinship and social factors; and educational factors.

Depressive symptoms in relation to SI and SB were studied in several of the records found. Although depression and other mental health issues have been identified as possible risk factors for suicide, it is imperative to note that suicide risk can be influenced by the interaction of many factors that may increase vulnerability to SI and SB, including personal characteristics, sociocultural elements, and environmental context (WHO, 2014). The complexity of these issues further emphasizes the need for additional research with Puerto Rican samples that targets not only depression and mental health issues but different areas of the cultural and social structure dimensions identified in the CCT. For example, the possibility of cultural expressions of distress by teens merits further attention (Goldston et al., 2008). Zayas and Gulbas (2012) proposed that SAs could be "a variant of *ataques de nervios*, or perhaps a developmental variation of this particular idiom" (p. 729). Guarnaccia et al. (2010) postulated that although ataques de nervios may be experienced by individuals from different Latinx subgroups, this idiom of distress is more likely to be reported by Puerto Ricans and can possibly indicate a vulnerability to mental health issues.

Addressing family needs when providing care to Puerto Rican adolescents should be an important consideration, given the cultural value of familism.

Focus on the family can also help identify patterns of interactions and conflict that impact the emotional health of the adolescent (Gulbas & Zayas, 2015). Although many of the articles reviewed addressed family-related factors, most were conducted in Puerto Rico and focused on an adolescent population. Since "culturally sensitive mental healthcare providers assess for and incorporate kinship and social factors in their plans of care" (Vossos & Wehbe-Alamah, 2018, p. 205), a critical need exists for further understanding of the needs of Puerto Rican families living on the U.S. mainland. This can include effective ways to address language barriers, assessing the possible impact of acculturation, and engaging the family in suicide prevention efforts (Goldston et al., 2008).

Another area of consideration in a review of the body of evidence is an evaluation of the methodologies used in research studies (Polit & Beck, 2017). Challenges for the generalization of findings and the drawing of conclusions from the sample of articles reviewed include varying definitions and time reference for the suicide-related variables under study, varying characteristics of the samples and sites used, the absence of a theoretical framework for many studies, and failure to indicate how the sample size was selected. Several studies did not provide sample questions of the suicide measured used; a few others failed to provide the time frame that was being addressed in relation to SI or SB.

The exclusion of six articles due to lack of confidence in the statistical analyses was previously mentioned. Presenting and publishing research are processes involved in disseminating the evidence needed for evidence-based practice. From the submission of a proposal to the analysis and interpretation of results, there are demands placed on time, knowledge, and resources. Space constraints can present challenges in reporting all details involved in the research process. Thus, further discussion is warranted within research, academic, and editorial circles on best practices for the accurate documentation and sharing of relevant data in the literature.

The limited number of items found in a broad search of studies relating to the topic of SI and SB in Puerto Ricans speaks to the overall gap in the current literature. Although some of the cultural factors from the Sunrise Model (Wehbe-Alamah, 2018) were extracted from the literature reviewed, the following factors need to be further addressed: technology (e.g., Internet-based resources, apps), religion and spirituality, political and legal factors, and economic factors. These factors can all serve as potential areas of future research. In addition, Leininger (1991) posited the following: "Cultural care knowledge derived from the people . . . could provide the truest knowledge base for culturally congruent care so that people would benefit from and be satisfied with nursing care practices held to be healthy ways of serving them" (p. 36). From this theoretical perspective, research efforts can target the inclusion of Puerto Rican participants who can provide cultural insight on the following areas: how suicide is spoken about in the culture, the meaning given to suicide, how suicide risk and prevention are addressed in families and communities, gender perspective, mental health promotion, and the role of the nurse in suicide prevention. Given the dearth of research, these areas need to be addressed for Puerto Ricans on the island and on the mainland, particularly those within the range of ages where suicide has been identified as a leading cause of death.

### Implications for Nursing

Suicide prevention not only targets the saving of individual lives but can also serve to prevent the weight of the aftermath faced by families and friends of those who die by suicide. Given the presence of nurses who provide care and education within a wide variety of settings, there is a tremendous opportunity for the nursing profession to raise awareness about suicide prevention, particularly within the Latinx population and other vulnerable groups. Nursing implications of this IR encompass three major areas. First, culturally competent interventions directed toward suicide prevention are imperative. The 2012 National Strategy for Suicide Prevention (HHS, 2012) stressed the importance of addressing cultural context in the development of suicide prevention strategies. Focus must be given not only to adolescents but also to other at-risk groups within the Puerto Rican population. Interventions should address the needs of the family, given its significance within the Puerto Rican culture. Preventive strategies are needed to incorporate not only immediate family members but also the extended family and community.

A second area for nursing implications is research. If nursing is to play a larger role in suicide prevention, it must address the need for research targeting the U.S. Latinx population and its subgroups because "an immense gap exists between mental health risks faced by Latinos and our knowledge of how research can be translated to improved mental health services for this underserved population" (Alegría et al., 2012, p. 298). Goldston et al. (2008) recommended focusing on not just risk factors within specific cultures but also protective factors inherent to the culture. The discovery of cultural knowledge from qualitative studies can aid in further understanding what beliefs and practices exist relative to suicide prevention, what care needs exist for at-risk individuals and their families, and what resources are accessed to address mental health issues and concerns.

A third area for nursing implications is nursing education. Results from the IR point to the continued need for consideration of the cultural context in both mental health promotion and suicide prevention. This entails that education for nurses and students training to be nurses should foster competency in providing culturally congruent care to at-risk individuals, those in need of emergency interventions after an SA, and families facing the death of a loved one.

### Limitations

The wide-ranging samples and settings in this IR limit generalizability; nonetheless, a broad perspective of cultural factors suggested in the current literature is offered. The first author conducted the literature search, evaluated the articles, and made the final selection of items for review. Although concerns and questions were discussed with the other authors, a second reviewer can help to reduce bias in the process of record selection and assessment of quality (Whittemore, 2005). An additional limitation is that the electronic database search may not have produced all articles that are relevant to the topic (Whittemore & Knafl, 2005); however, other sources were also used to find items (e.g., manual search of reference lists, journals written in Spanish). Furthermore, even though there is literature exploring the relationship between psychotic features and SI and SB in Puerto Rican samples (López-Robledo, Cumba-Avilés, & Bernal, 2009; Loue & Sajatovic, 2008), these type of studies were beyond the scope of this IR. A final limitation is the specific focus of this IR on current, peer-reviewed articles from the past 10 years; hence, additional factors within the cultural context (e.g., acculturation, socioeconomic status) may have been addressed in other types of publications or studies from previous years.

## CONCLUSION

There is a marked dearth of research focusing on SI and SB in Puerto Ricans living on the U. S. mainland and the island. Although the existing literature supports the need to consider the cultural context in addressing SI and SB in Puerto Ricans, a better understanding of the role that different cultural factors play is necessary. We argue that a step in this direction is to build the evidence that sheds light on the cultural influences that impact suicide risk within specific Latinx subgroups, including Puerto Ricans.

The rates of SI reported in a few studies addressing adolescents in Puerto Rico are concerning. The broad range of sample characteristics and locations of the studies included in the IR present a challenge in identifying specific at-risk groups within the Puerto Rican community. There is a critical need for research to target prevalence and risk factors for emerging adults in Puerto Rico, as well as the adolescent, emerging adult, and adult populations on the mainland. Epidemiologic studies that reflect current trends and correlates of SI and SB in

Latinx subgroups in the United States can further assist in understanding risk and protective factors that impact Puerto Rican mental health and well-being. Existing gender differences in suicide mortality rates, SA, and SI among Puerto Ricans also warrants research focus.

A noticeable gap exists in the area of primary prevention efforts that address mental health promotion, psychoeducation, and culturally sensitive messages that raise awareness. This is a prime opportunity for nurses to identify and foster innovative strategies that contribute to national suicide prevention efforts, particularly those targeting the growing Latinx population. Advancing the science in the area of cultural knowledge can greatly aid in tailoring nursing assessments of suicide risk, developing community programs to enhance mental health literacy, and supporting culturally congruent nursing care aimed at reducing suicide risk for Puerto Ricans and other Latinx subgroups.

## ACKNOWLEDGMENT

We extend our deepest gratitude to Mr. David A. Nolfi, Head, Research Engagement, Health Sciences/STEM Initiatives, Gumberg Library, Duquense University, for his guidance and assistance in conducting the literature search; and Dr. James B. Schreiber, Professor, School of Nursing, Duquesne University, for his expertise and timely feedback related to the reporting of statistical analysis in the literature.

## DISCLOSURE

Contributions from Dr. Duarté-Vélez were supported by the NIMH (K23 MH097772).

## REFERENCES

Alegría, M., Canino, G., Strout, P. E., Woo, M., Duan, N., Villa, D., et al. (2008). Prevalence of mental illness in immigrant and non-immigrant U.S. Latino groups. *American Journal of Psychiatry, 165*(3), 359–369. https://doi.org/10.1176/appi.ajp.2007.07040704

Alegría, M., Mulvaney-Day, N., Woo, M., & Viruell-Fuentes, E. A. (2012). Psychology of Latino adults: Challenges and an agenda for action. In E. C. Chang & C. A. Downey (Eds.). *Handbook of race and development in mental health* (pp. 279–306). New York, NY: Springer Publishing.

Alegría, M., Shrout, P. E., Woo, M., Guarnaccia, P., Sribney, W., Vila, D., et al. (2007). Understanding differences in past year psychiatric disorders for Latinos living in the US. *Social Science & Medicine, 65*(2), 214–230. https://doi.org/10.1016/j.socscimed.2007.03.026

Alegría, M., Takeuchi, D., Canino, G., Duan, N., Shrout, P., Meng, X. L., et al. (2004). Considering context, place and culture: The National Latino and Asian American Study. *International Journal of Methods in Psychiatric Research, 13*(4), 208–220. https://doi.org/10.1002/mpr.178

Baca-García, E., Perez-Rodríguez, M. M., Keyes, K. M., Oquendo, M. A., Hasin, D. S., Grant, B. F., et al. (2011). Suicidal ideation and suicide attempts among Hispanic subgroups in the United States: 1991–1992 and 2001–2002. *Journal of Psychiatric Research, 45*(4), 512–518. https://doi.org/10.1016/j.jpsychires.2010.09.004

Bandiera, F. C., Ramirez, R., Arheart, K. L., Canino, G., & Goodwin, R. D. (2013). Asthma and suicidal ideation and behavior among Puerto Rican adolescents. *The Journal of Nervous and Mental Disease, 201*(7), 587–591. https://doi.org/10.1097/nmd.0b013e3182982ba4

Caetano, R., Ramisetty-Mikler, S., & Rodríguez, L. A. (2008). The Hispanic Americans Baseline Alcohol Survey (HABLAS): Rates and predictors of alcohol abuse and dependence across Hispanic national groups. *Journal of Studies on Alcohol and Drugs, 69*(3), 441–448. https://doi.org/10.15288/jsad.2008.69.441

Centers for Disease Control and Prevention. (n.d.-a). *1991–2017 High School Youth Risk Behavior Survey data: Puerto Rico 2017 and United States 2017 results: Unintentional injuries and violence, both males and females, all races/ethnicities, all grades, all sexual orientations.* [Youth Online data analysis tool]. Retrieved from http://nccd.cdc.gov/youthonline

Centers for Disease Control and Prevention. (n.d.-b). *1991–2017 High School Youth Risk Behavior Survey data: United States 2017 results: Unintentional injuries and violence, Hispanic or Latino, all grades, all sexual orientations.* [Youth Online data analysis tool]. Retrieved from http://nccd.cdc.gov/youthonline

Centers for Disease Control and Prevention. (n.d.-c). *1991–2017 High School Youth Risk Behavior Survey data: United States 2017 results: Unintentional injuries and violence, male, all grades, all sexual orientations.* [Youth Online data analysis tool]. Retrieved from http://nccd.cdc.gov/youthonline

Centers for Disease Control and Prevention, National Center for Injury Prevention and Control. (2017a). *Web-based Injury Statistics Query and Reporting System (WISQARS), Fatal injury data: Leading causes of death reports, 1981–2016: 10 leading causes of death, United States: 2016, all races, Hispanic, both sexes.* [Online database]. Retrieved from https://webappa.cdc.gov/sasweb/ncipc/leadcause.html

Centers for Disease Control and Prevention, National Center for Injury Prevention and Control. (2017b). *Web-based Injury Statistics Query and Reporting System (WISQARS), Fatal injury data: Leading causes of death reports, 1981–2016: 12 leading causes of death, United States: 2012, all races, Hispanic, both sexes.* [Online database]. Retrieved from https://webappa.cdc.gov/sasweb/ncipc/leadcause.html

Centers for Disease Control and Prevention, National Center for Injury Prevention and Control. (2017c). *Web-based Injury Statistics Query and Reporting System (WISQARS), Fatal injury data: Leading causes of death reports, 1981–2016: 12 leading causes of death, United States: 2013, all races, Hispanic, both sexes.* [Online database]. Retrieved from https://webappa.cdc.gov/sasweb/ncipc/leadcause.html

Centers for Disease Control and Prevention, National Center for Injury Prevention and Control. (2017d). *Web-based Injury Statistics Query and Reporting System (WISQARS), Fatal injury data: Leading causes of death reports, 1981–2016: 12 leading causes of death, United States: 2014, all races, Hispanic, both sexes.* [Online database]. Retrieved from https://webappa.cdc.gov/sasweb/ncipc/leadcause.html

Centers for Disease Control and Prevention, National Center for Injury Prevention and Control. (2017e). *Web-based Injury Statistics Query and Reporting System (WISQARS), Fatal injury data: Leading causes of death reports, 1981–2016: 12 leading causes of death, United States: 2015, all races, Hispanic, both sexes*. [Online database]. Retrieved from https://webappa.cdc.gov/sas-web/ncipc/leadcause.html

Cohn, D., Patten, E., & Lopez, M. H. (2014). *Puerto Rican population declines on island, grows on U.S. mainland*. Washington, D. C.: Pew Research Center. Retrieved from http://www.pewhispanic.org/2014/08/11/puerto-rican-population-declines-on-island-grows-on-u-s-mainland

Crosby, A. E., Ortega, L., & Melanson, C. (2011). *Self-directed violence surveillance: Uniform definitions and recommended data elements, version 1.0*. Atlanta, GA: Centers for Disease Control and Prevention, National Center for Injury Prevention and Control. Retrieved from https://www.cdc.gov/violenceprevention/pdf/Self-Directed-Violence-a.pdf

Diefenbach, G. J., Disch, W. B., Robison, J. T., Baez, E., & Coman, E. (2009). Anxious depression among Puerto Rican and African-American older adults. *Aging & Mental Health, 13*(1), 118–126. https://doi.org/10.1080/13607860802591062

Duarté-Vélez, Y., & Bernal, G. (2007). Suicide behavior among Latino and Latina adolescents: Conceptual and methodological issues. *Death Studies, 31*(5), 435–455. https://doi.org/10.1080/07481180701244579

Duarté-Vélez, Y., Jones, R. N., & Spirito, A. (2017). Understanding suicidal ideation in Latino/a adolescents living in Puerto Rico. *Archives of Suicide Research, 22*(4), 569–583. https://doi.org/10.1080/13811118.2017.1378142

Duarté-Vélez, Y., Lorenzo-Luaces, L., & Rosselló, J. (2012). Ideación suicida: Síntomas depresivos, pensamientos disfuncionales, autoconcepto, y estrategias de manejo en adolescentes puertorriqueños/as. [Suicidal ideation: Depressive symptoms, dysfunctional thoughts, self-concept, and management strategies in Puerto Rican adolescents]. *Revista Puertorriqueña de Psicología, 23*(Suppl.), 1–17.

Duarté-Vélez, Y., Torres Dávila, P., & Laboy Hernández, S. (2015). Retos en la intervención con adolescentes puertorriqueños/as que manifiestan comportamiento suicida. [Challenges in the intervention of Puerto Rican adolescents that show suicidal behavior]. *Revista Puertorriqueña de Psicología, 26*(1), 90–106.

Duarté-Vélez, Y., Torres-Dávila, P., Spirito, A., Polanco, N., & Bernal, G. (2016). Development of a treatment protocol for Puerto Rican adolescents with suicidal behaviors. *Psychotherapy, 53*(1), 45–56. https://doi.org/10.1037/pst0000044

Duke, M. R., & Mateo, W. (2008). Disparities in access to behavioral health services for Puerto Rican-descended adolescents. *Human Organization, 67*(1), 68–76. https://doi.org/10.17730/humo.67.1.d73v2x0x48217rx4

Fortuna, L. R., Perez, D. J., Canino, G., Sribney, W., & Alegria, M. (2007). Prevalence and correlates of lifetime suicidal ideation and attempts among Latino subgroups in the United States. *The Journal of Clinical Psychiatry, 68*(4), 572–581. https://doi.org/10.4088/jcp.v68n0413

Garcia-Preto, N. (2005). Puerto Rican families. In M. McGoldrick, Giordano, J., & Garcia-Preto, N. (Eds.), *Ethnicity and family therapy* (3rd ed., pp. 242–255). New York, NY: The Guilford Press.

Gobierno de Puerto Rico, Departamento de Salud. (2018). *Estadísticas preliminares de casos de suicidio: Puerto Rico, febrero 2018*. Retrieved from http://www.salud.gov.pr/Estadisticas-Registros-y-Publicaciones/Estadisticas%20Suicidio/Febrero%202018.pdf

Goldston, D. B., Molock, S. D., Whitbeck, L. B., Murakami, J. L., Zayas, L. H., & Hall, G. C. N. (2008). Cultural considerations in adolescent suicide prevention and psychosocial treatment. *American Psychologist, 63*(1), 14–31. https://doi.org/10.1037/0003-066x.63.1.14

Gonzales, N. A., Germán, M., & Fabrett, F. C. (2012). US Latino youth. In E. C. Chang & C. A. Downey (Eds.), *Handbook of race and development in mental health* (pp. 259–278). New York, NY: Springer.

Guarnaccia, P. J., Lewis-Fernández, R., Pincay, I. M., Shrout, P., Guo, J., Torres, M., et al. (2010). Ataque de nervios as a marker of social and psychiatric vulnerability: Results from the NLAAS. *International Journal of Social Psychiatry, 56*(3), 298–309. https://doi.org/10.1177/0020764008101636

Guarnaccia, P. J., Martinez, I., & Acosta, H. (2005). Mental health in the Hispanic immigrant community: An overview. In M. J. González & G. González-Ramos (Eds.), *Mental healthcare for new Hispanic immigrants: Innovative approaches in contemporary clinical practice* (pp. 21–46). Binghamton, NY: The Haworth Press, Inc.

Gulbas, L. E., & Zayas, L. H. (2015). Examining the interplay among family, culture, and Latina teen suicidal behavior. *Qualitative Health Research, 25*(5), 689–699. https://doi.org/10.1177/1049732314553598

Heron, M. (2017). *Deaths: Leading causes for 2015*. (National Vital Statistics Reports, Vol. 66, No. 5). Hyattsville, MD: National Center for Health Statistics. Retrieved from https://www.cdc.gov/nchs/data/nvsr/nvsr66/nvsr66_05.pdf

Heron, M. (2018). *Deaths: Leading causes for 2016*. (National Vital Statistics Reports, Vol. 67, No. 6). Hyattsville, MD: National Center for Health Statistics Retrieved from https://www.cdc.gov/nchs/data/nvsr/nvsr67/nvsr67_06.pdf

Holloway, I. W., Padilla, M. B., Willner, L., & Guilamo-Ramos, V. (2015). Effects of minority stress processes on the mental health of Latino men who have sex with men and women: A qualitative study. *Archives of Sexual Behavior, 44*(7), 2087–2097. https://doi.org/10.1007/s10508-014-0424-x

Jiménez Chafey, M. I. (2008). Conducta e ideación suicida en estudiantes universitarios. *Revista Griot, 1*(4), 5–17. Retrieved from http://136.145.11.86/index.php/griot/article/view/1900

Jiménez Chafey, M. I., Bernal, G., & Rosselló, J. (2009). Clinical case study: CBT for depression in a Puerto Rican adolescent: Challenges and variability in treatment response. *Depression and Anxiety, 26*(1), 98–103. https://doi.org/10.1002/da.20457

Jiménez Chafey, M. I., Duarté Vélez, Y. M., & Bernal, G. (2011). Mother-daughter interactions among depressed Puerto Rican adolescents: Two case studies in CBT. *Revista Puertorriqueña de Psicología, 22*, 46–71.

Jones, J., Ramirez, R. R., Davies, M., Canino, G., & Goodwin, R. D. (2008). Suicidal behaviors among adolescents in Puerto Rico: Rates and correlates in clinical and community samples. *Journal of Clinical Child and Adolescent Psychology, 37*(2), 448–455. https://doi.org/10.1080/15374410801955789

Jovet-Toledo, G. G., Clatts, M. C., Rodriguez-Diaz, C. E., Goldsamt, L., & Vargas-Molina, R. L. (2014). Risk factors for suicide attempts in a clinic-based sample of people living with HIV in Puerto Rico. *AIDS Care, 26*(8), 1032–1035. https://doi.org/10.1080/09540121.2014.894618

Kann, L., Kinchen, S., Shanklin, S. L., Flint, K. H., Kawkins, J., Harris, W. A., et al. (2014). Youth Risk Behavior Surveillance--United States, 2013. *Morbidity and Mortality Weekly Report: Surveillance Summaries, 63*(4), 1–168. Retrieved from https://www.cdc.gov/mmwr/pdf/ss/ss6304.pdf

Kann, L., McManus, T., Harris, W. A., Shanklin, S. L., Flint, K. H., Hawkins, J., et al. (2016). Youth Risk Behavior Surveillance-United States, 2015. *Morbidity and Mortality Weekly Report: Surveillance Summaries, 65*(6), 1–174. https://doi.org/10.15585/mmwr.ss6506a1

Kann, L., McManus, T., Harris, W. A., Shanklin, S. L., Flint, K. H., Queen, B., et al. (2018). Youth Risk Behavior Surveillance-United States, 2017. *Morbidity and Mortality Weekly Report: Surveillance Summaries, 67*(SS–8), 1–114. https://doi.org/10.15585/mmwr.ss6708a1

Leininger, M. (1978). Towards conceptualization of transcultural healthcare systems: Concepts and a model. In M. Leininger (Ed.), *Transcultural nursing: Concepts, theories, and practices* (pp. 53–74). New York, NY: John Wiley & Sons.

Leininger, M. (1991). The Theory of Culture Care Diversity and Universality. In M. M. Leininger (Ed.), *Culture Care Diversity and Universality: A theory of nursing* (pp. 5–68). New York, NY: National League for Nursing Press.

Leininger, M. (2002). Part I: The Theory of Culture Care and the ethnonursing research method. In M. Leininger & M. R. McFarland (Eds.), *Transcultural nursing: Concepts, theories, research & practice* (3rd ed., pp. 71–98). New York, NY: McGraw-Hill Medical Publishing Division.

López-Robledo, Y. M., Cumba-Avilés, E., & Bernal, G. (2009). Experiencias atípicas psicóticas y cuasi-psicóticas en adolescentes puertorriqueños/as deprimidos/as: Prevalencia y factores asociados. [Psychotic and quasi-psychotic atypical experiences in Puerto Rican depressed adolescents: Prevalence and related factors]. *Revista Interamericana de Psicología, 43*(2), 350–361.

Loue, S., & Sajatovic, M. (2008). Auditory and visual hallucinations in a sample of severely mentally ill Puerto Rican women: An examination of the cultural context. *Mental Health, Religion & Culture, 11*(6), 597–608. https://doi.org/10.1080/13674670701795971

Lucas, J. W., Freeman, G., & Adams, P. F. (2016). *Health of Hispanic adults: United States, 2010–2014*. (NCHS Data Brief 251). Hyattsville, MD: National Center for Health Statistics. Retrieved from http://www.cdc.gov/nchs/data/databriefs/db251.pdf

Marion, L., Douglas, M., Lavin, M. A., Barr, N., Gazaway, S., Thomas, E., et al. (2016). Implementing the new ANA standard 8: Culturally congruent practice. *Online Journal of Issues in Nursing, 22*(1). doi:10.3912/OJIN.Vol22No01PPT20

McFarland, M. R. (2018). The Theory of Culture Care Diversity and Universality. In M. R. McFarland & H. B. Wehbe-Alamah (Eds.). *Leininger's transcultural nursing: Concepts, theories, research & practice* (4th ed., pp. 39–56). New York, NY: McGraw-Hill Education.

McFarland, M. R., & Wehbe-Alamah, H. B. (2015). The Theory of Culture Care Diversity and Universality. In M. R. McFarland & H. B. Wehbe-Alamah (Eds.). *Leininger's Culture Care Diversity and Universality: A worldwide nursing theory* (3rd ed., pp. 1–34). Burlington, MA: Jones & Bartlett Learning.

Moher, D., Liberati, A., Tetzlaff, J., Altman, D. G., & The PRISMA Group. (2009). Preferred reporting items for systematic reviews and meta-analyses: The PRISMA statement. *PLoS Medicine, 6*(7), e1000097. https://doi.org/10.1371/journal.pmed.1000097

Moscoso Álvarez, M. R., Rodríguez-Figueroa, L., Reyes-Pulliza, J. C., & Colón, H. M. (2016). Adolescentes de Puerto Rico: Una mirada a su salud mental y su asociación con el entorno familiar y escolar. [Puerto Rican youth: A look at their mental health and its association with family and school environment]. *Revista Puertorriqueña de Psicología, 27*(2), 320–332.

Oquendo, M. A., Lizardi, D., Greenwald, S., Weissman, M. M., & Mann, J. J. (2004). Rates of lifetime suicide attempt and rates of lifetime major depression in different ethnic groups in the United States. *Acta Psychiatrica Scandinavica, 110*(6), 446–451. https://doi.org/10.1111/j.1600-0447.2004.00404.x

Pasch, R. J., Penny, A. B., & Berg, R. (2018). *National Hurricane Center Tropical Cyclone Report: Hurricane Maria (AL152017)*. Retrieved from https://www.nhc.noaa.gov/data/tcr/AL152017_Maria.pdf

Pedroso, T. (2013). Gender disparities in mortality: Challenges for health equity in Puerto Rico. [Disparidades de género en mortalidad: Retos para la equidad en salud en Puerto Rico]. *Acta Colombiana de Psicología, 16*(2), 103–114. doi:10.41718/ACP.2013.16.2.10

Piscopo, K., Lipari, R. N., Cooney, J., & Glasheen, C. (2016). *Suicidal thoughts and behavior among adults: Results from the 2015 National Survey on Drug Use and Health*. (NSDUH Data Review). Retrieved from https://www.samhsa.gov/data/sites/default/files/NSDUH-DR-FFR3-2015/NSDUH-DR-FFR3-2015.pdf

Polit, D. F., & Beck, C. T. (2017). *Nursing research: Generating and assessing evidence for nursing practice* (10th ed.). Philadelphia, PA: Wolters Kluwer.

Purnell, L. D. (2013). People of Puerto Rican heritage. In L. D. Purnell (Ed.), *Transcultural health care: A culturally competent approach* (4th ed., pp. 407–425). Philadelphia, PA: F. A. Davis Company.

Reyes-Rodríguez, M. L., Franko, D. L., Matos-Lamourt, A., Bulik, C. M., Von Holle, A., Cámara-Fuentes, L. R., et al. (2010). Eating disorder symptomatology: Prevalence among Latino college freshmen students. *Journal of Clinical Psychology, 66*(6), 666–679. https://doi.org/10.1002/jclp.20684

Reyes-Rodríguez, M. L., Rivera-Medina, C. L., Camara-Fuentes, L., Suarez-Torres, A., & Bernal, G. (2013). Depression symptoms and stressful life events among college students in Puerto Rico. *Journal of Affective Disorders, 145*(3), 324–330. https://doi.org/10.1016/j.jad.2012.08.010

Rosselló, J., Duarté-Vélez, Y., Bernal, G., & Zuluaga, M. G. (2011). Ideación suicida y respuesta a la terapia cognitiva conductual en adolescentes puertorriqueños/as con depresión mayor. [Suicide ideation and response to cognitive behavioral therapy in Puerto Rican adolescents with major depression]. *Interamerican Journal of Psychology, 45*(3), 321–329.

Rosselló, J., Duarté-Vélez, Y., Gema-Zuluaga, M., & Bernal, G. (2008). Características de adolescentes con depresión e ideación suicida en una muestra clínica. [Characteristics of adolescents with depression and suicidal ideation in our clinic]. *Ciencias de la Conducta, 23*(1), 55–86.

Silva, C., & Van Orden, K. A. (2018). Suicide among Hispanics in the United States. *Current Opinion in Psychology, 22*, 44–49. https://doi.org/10.1016/j.copsyc.2017.07.013

Sirriyeh, R., Lawton, R., Gardner, P., & Armitage, G. (2012). Reviewing studies with diverse designs: The development and evaluation of a new tool. *Journal of Evaluation in Clinical Practice, 18*(4), 746–52. https://doi.org/10.1111/j.1365-2753.2011.01662.x

U. S. Census Bureau. (2016a). *Age and sex, 2012–2016 American Community Survey 5-year estimates, Puerto Rico*. Retrieved from https://factfinder.census.gov/bkmk/table/1.0/en/ACS/16_5YR/S0101/0400000US72

U. S. Census Bureau. (2016b). *Hispanic or Latino origin by specific origin, universe: Total population, 2012-2016 American Community Survey 5-year estimates, United States*. Retrieved from https://factfinder.census.gov/bkmk/table/1.0/en/ACS/16_5YR/B03001

U.S. Department of Health and Human Services (HHS), Office of the Surgeon General, National Action Alliance for Suicide Prevention. (2012). *2012 National strategy for suicide prevention: Goals and objectives for action*. Washington, DC: U.S. Department of Health and Human Services. Retrieved from https://www.surgeongeneral.gov/library/reports/national-strategy-suicide-prevention/full-report.pdf

Vélez-Pérez, D., Maldonado-Santiago, N., & Rivera-Lugo, C. I. (2017). Espectro del suicidio en jóvenes universitarios en Puerto Rico. [Spectrum of suicide in young university students in Puerto Rico]. *Revista Puertorriqueña de Psicología, 28*(1), 34–44.

Vera, M., Reyes-Rabanillo, M. L., Huertas, S., Juarbe, D., Pérez-Pedrogo, C., Huertas, A., et al. (2011). Suicide ideation, plans, and attempts among general practice patients with chronic health conditions in Puerto Rico. *International Journal of General Medicine, 4*, 197–205. https://doi.org/10.2147/ijgm.s17156

Vespa, J., Armstrong, D. M., & Medina, L. (2018). *Demographic turning points for the United States: Population projections for 2020 to 2060*. (Current Population Reports, P25–1144). Washington, DC: U. S. Census Bureau. Retrieved from https://www.census.gov/content/dam/Census/library/publications/2018/demo/P25_1144.pdf

Vossos, H. B., & Wehbe-Alamah, H. B. (2018). Using a culturally congruent approach in mental healthcare. In M. R. McFarland & H. B. Wehbe-Alamah (Eds.), *Leininger's transcultural nursing: Concepts, theories, research & practice* (4th ed., pp. 199–213). New York, NY: McGraw-Hill Education.

Wehbe-Alamah, H. B. (2018). The Ethnonursing Research Method: Major features and enablers. In M. R. McFarland & H. B. Wehbe-Alamah (Eds.), *Leininger's transcultural nursing: Concepts, theories, research & practice* (4th ed., pp. 57–84). New York, NY: McGraw-Hill Education.

Whittemore, R. (2005). Combining evidence in nursing research: Methods and implications. *Nursing Research, 54*(1), 56–62. https://doi.org/10.1097/00006199-200501000-00008

Whittemore, R., & Knafl, K. (2005). The integrative review: Updated methodology. *Journal of Advanced Nursing, 52*(5), 546–553. https://doi.org/10.1111/j.1365-2648.2005.03621.x

World Health Organization. (2014). *Preventing suicide: A global imperative*. Retrieved from http://apps.who.int/iris/bitstream/10665/131056/1/9789241564779_eng.pdf?ua=1&ua=1

Xu, J., Murhpy, S. L., Kochanek, K. D., Bastian, B., & Arias, E. (2018). *Deaths: Final data for 2016*. (National Vital Statistics Reports, Vol. 67, No. 5). Hyattsville, MD: National Center for Health Statistics. Retrieved from https://www.cdc.gov/nchs/data/nvsr/nvsr67/nvsr67_05.pdf

Zayas, L. H. (2011). *Latinas attempting suicide: When cultures, families, and daughters collide*. New York, NY: Oxford University Press.

Zayas, L. H., & Gulbas, L. (2012). Are suicide attempts by young Latinas a cultural idiom of distress? *Transcultural Psychiatry, 49*(5), 718–734. https://doi.org/10.1177/1363461512463262

Zayas, L. H., Lester, R. J., Cabassa, L. J., & Fortuna, L. R. (2005). Why do so many Latina teens attempt suicide? A conceptual model for research. *American Journal of Orthopsychiatry, 75*(2), 275–287. https://doi.org/10.1037/0002-9432.75.2.275

CHAPTER 10

# The Lens of Culture and Forensic Nursing Practice

Ashley Smith and L. Kathleen Sekula

## ABSTRACT

Forensic nursing is a relatively new area of nursing practice and one about which little is written regarding the impact of culture on the various areas of forensic nursing practice. Forensic nursing is an evolving nursing specialty that focuses on healthcare when legal issues are involved. When referring to culture related to the practice of forensic nursing one must take into consideration a broad approach to the various cultures that must be taken into consideration. For example, the culture of correction holds many variables in addition to the individual personal cultures that prisoners bring to corrections including the question of *caring versus custody*. The culture within corrections is often addressed through Foucault's theory of power. An additional area for attention is the LGBTQ communities. As has been our history when one refers to gender bias or gender discrimination, we viewed gender as a binary demographic—female and male. Gender identity and culture share a strong connection as they affect daily life in all aspects of a person's life. In this article we address two areas of forensic nursing practice in light of the cultural issues that should be addressed in order to provide the highest standard of care for all victims and perpetrators of violence.


http://dx.doi.org/10.1891/0739-6686.37.301

## INTRODUCTION

Forensic nursing is a relatively new area of nursing practice and one about which little is written regarding the impact of culture on the various areas of forensic nursing practice. Forensic nursing is an evolving nursing specialty that focuses on healthcare when legal issues are involved. The scope and standards of practice for the forensic nurse were established by the American Nurses Association in 2009 and revised in 2017 (American Nurses Association, 2009, 2017). When referring to culture related to the practice of forensic nursing one must take into consideration a broad approach to the various cultures that must be taken into consideration. For example, the culture of correction holds many variables in addition to the individual personal cultures that prisoners bring to corrections including the question of *caring versus custody* (Holmes, 2005). The culture within corrections is often addressed through Foucault's theory of power. Foucault proposes that power is not just a negative, coercive or repressive concept forcing us to do things against our wishes, but can also be a necessary, productive and positive force in society (Gaventa, 2003).

> We must cease once and for all to describe the effects of power in negative terms: it "excludes," it "represses," it "censors," it "abstracts," it "masks," it "conceals." In fact power produces; it produces reality; it produces domains of objects and rituals of truth. The individual and the knowledge that may be gained of him belong to this production. (Foucault, 1991, p. 194)

However, how do we address the individual's cultural needs within a culture of caring versus custody? Forensic nurses in corrections must balance these cultures carefully in order to provide the most culturally sensitive care possible. While individual ethnic cultures play a pivotal role in any area of nursing practice, there are other specific cultural implications, such as the culture of the environment, when interacting with various populations in practice such as corrections, sexual assault, LGBTQ, interpersonal violence, and others.

## METHODS

This article addresses the research literature regarding the impact of culture on both forensic nurses and forensic patients in two populations: corrections, and sexual assault in the LGBTQ population. In preparation for writing the manuscript the authors conducted literature searches using PubMed, Ovid, Cinahl that included the keywords/phrases *culture and forensic nursing, culture and corrections, sexual assault and cultural care,* and *stigmatization and cultural care.* Several hundred articles were found before further narrowing the search to include articles from only the past 10 years and adding *nursing* as a keyword.

Ultimately 62 articles were chosen as possibly being useful in helping to explicate the relationship between culture and the selected forensic environments.

## BACKGROUND

Transcultural nursing is defined as a formal area of study and practice focused on comparative human-care (caring) differences and similarities of the beliefs, values, and patterned lifeways of cultures to provide culturally congruent, meaningful, and beneficial health care to people (Leininger, 2002). While there are excellent models related to transcultural care (Campinha-Bacote, 2002; Giger & Davidhizar, 2002; Leininger, 2002; Purnell, 2002) this author has not identified a model that speaks specifically to cultural issues in the forensic environments. Purnell's model does stress several assumptions of which the nineteenth includes "Professions, organizations, and associations have their own cultures which can be analyzed using a grand theory" such as the Purnell Model for Cultural Competence (Purnell, 2002, p. 194). The model includes *workforce issues* as one of the 12 domains and addresses concepts related to autonomy, acculturation, assimilation, gender roles, ethnic communication styles, individualism, and health care practices from the country of origin. For these reasons, the Purnell model will guide the discussion within the area of forensic nursing practice.

We will explore the cultural *self* in relationship to the cultural *other* and *community*. The question of whether the application of transcultural nursing theory can help us to understand violence within and across cultures. It is imperative that we view the connection between transcultural and forensics in the care of individuals, families, and communities from a global perspective. Issues of violence must be understood in the context of culture for victims and offenders (Zoucha, 2006). Clinicians must work from the context of culture in promoting mental and physical health for those affected by forensic health care issues.

And so, we ask: What is Culture? We believe that it is a common collectivity of beliefs, values and shared understandings and patterns of behavior of a specific group of people and their environments (Leininger, 2002). Culture includes values, beliefs, traditions, family, religion, art, music, language, and other variables. As forensic nurses we must come to know who we are culturally. Where do we come from? What values do we hold dear? How does my culture affect my health and well-being? And how do my cultural values affect how I interact with people who are culturally different? What values are prevalent in my life?

## EXPLORING CULTURE WITHIN CORRECTIONS

Holmes (2005) challenged those who work within the corrections systems to think about how we care for that unique population. He asks whether clinicians within the correction system can distinguish between our roles related to *custody* or *caring*, and more importantly whether we understand how to determine what our role is within this conundrum of custody versus caring. This article will discuss the cultural implications regarding forensic psychiatric and medical care within the distinct practice areas in the correction system. These individuals are *captives* within the authority of those in power (Jacob, Holmes, & Buus, 2008). Their actions are subject to constant observation by professionals working in such settings. Forensic nurses who work in corrections are often torn between the duality of custody and care (Holmes & Federman, 2003).

In an article by Jacob et al. (2008) the issue of humanity in forensic psychiatry was explored. Humanism is an approach that derives from existentialism and is rooted in modernism. In other words, humanism seeks to understand life in personally relevant terms, and the locus of control is situated with the individual. They conducted a critical reflection on how humanism has influenced nursing theories in relationship to forensic nursing. Most importantly, they explored the disconnect between the art of humanism and its incapability to acknowledge the power relationships between individuals and the day-to-day realities of corrections' culture. Sadly, their final tenet was that it is clear that the humanistic philosophy and its models of care are in discordance with the specialty of forensic nursing. And so, how do we create an environment within corrections that is humane for both the nurse and the incarcerated? While that answer is not clear, we will try to address issues related to culture that can help us move forward.

To begin, we must know what our individual biases are? Do we understand the *other* worldview; looking outward, understanding diversity, understanding the sameness, cultural relativism, and ethnocentrism? Most clinicians know that cultural competence is defined as a set of behaviors, attitudes, and policies within a system or professional group that allows those persons to work effectively in cross cultural situations (Leininger & McFarland, 2002). The challenge here is the balance between *custody* and *caring*. How does a forensic nurse balance humanistic care within this environment where care is intertwined with social control? We might begin by carefully reflecting on the two main cultural issues at hand. The overarching and present culture is that of the correction system itself. What role do forensic nurses play in any particular correction setting? Are they tasked with both caring for the incarcerated as well as treating (controlling) them? And the second cultural issue is the culture of each individual within that correction system. How do we address both for the betterment of life for all involved?

In a qualitative study by Holmes, Perron, and Michaud (2007b) a comparison was made between the role of forensic nurses in corrections in Canada when compared with forensic nurses in corrections in France. Four main categories emerged from the data: Logics, Socio-professional identity of nursing staff, Descriptions of prisoners, and Interpersonal relationships among staff. The researchers chose to concentrate on the category of logic because they felt that it clearly highlighted the main differences between the Canadian and French systems. In their words "This merging of health care and correctional concerns, as experienced by the Canadian staff, differs enormously from that which we were able to observe in the French correction environment" (Holmes, Perron, & Michaud, 2007, p. 128). In essence, forensic nurses in France experience a complete separation of their health care role from the role of the penitentiary staff. Records are kept separate: in France, access to medical/nursing files is restricted to health care personnel and criminal files are seen only by staff working in the penitentiary system. Nurses regard them as patients and guards regard them as prisoners. Nursing staff insist on addressing the prisoners with respect by calling them Mr., Ms., and so forth, and as much as possible limit their contact with the corrections officers to that which is necessary. The researchers concluded that in Canada there is a basic problem regarding professional nursing ethics versus penal regulations because of being based on paradoxical ideologies. How do we reconcile this paradox? It appears that France has done exactly that.

When considering the second cultural issue—each individual's culture (both the incarcerated, the corrections officers, as well as the nurse) plays a role in the *theatre* that is corrections. Unless we are aware of our own culture and how it influences how we see others and how we act, then we cannot understand how the culture of *the other* impacts how they interface with us. Do we understand the importance (even the graveness) of what it means to the Muslim inmate to adhere to their dietary restrictions? Can we say that because they are incarcerated they give up their rights to religious teaching? That answer may be nebulous at this point but it is certainly one that we need to consider. What about other cultures? We must acknowledge that in order to provide the best care and ultimately to support the incarcerated in their quest to reenter the world as valuable citizens, then we must acknowledge their humanity—their culture. Are there those who do not deserve this consideration? And who would make this determination? As we consider difficult issues that are presented when we explore the corrections systems then we must think of man's humanity to man. While not an excuse we must consider the culture from which the incarcerated come to the correction system—many have suffered abuse at the hands of those entrusted to raise them, contributing to their abhorrent behavior as they interact with others.

It is only by attending to all cultures involved in every setting in which we work that we can begin to make sense of humanity. Who will make the breakthrough in corrections in order to realize that the conundrum of custody versus caring can be solved by addressing cultural needs? Understanding the other worldview is paramount to good practice: looking outward, understanding diversity, understanding sameness, cultural relativism, and ethnocentrism (Zoucha, 2006).

## SEXUAL ASSAULT IN THE LGDTQ (LGBTQ) COMMUNITY

As has been our history when one refers to gender bias or gender discrimination, we viewed gender as a binary demographic—female and male. Gender identity and culture share a strong connection as they affect daily life in all aspects of a person's life (Black, 2014). Over the past several years we have come to recognize that gender identity includes many other experiences of how we perceive ourselves related to gender and sexuality. However, culture is a major influence in determining what behaviors are acceptable for men and women, as well as constructing *rules* related to what sexual behaviors are deemed as appropriate between men and women. Black (2014) has given us a sound foundation to explore the impact of culture of this community.

The lesbian, gay, bisexual, transsexual, queer (LGBTQ community is at higher risk of victimization as compared with the rest of the general population, and at even higher risk of sexual assault (Stotzer, 2009). While most data is gathered through self-report, it is clear that gender variant individuals are victims of sexualized violence, not only in adulthood but in their youth as well. While most assaults are committed by people known to them, stranger assault and hate crimes also remain prevalent, specifically towards those in the LGBTQ communities.

LGBTQ is an acronym used to refer to gender minorities and includes lesbian, gay, bisexual, transgender and queer. Due to the increase risk of violence this culture faces, it is crucial that forensic nurses understand the culture(s) of gender minorities and strive to improve practices to be inclusive of all. Specifically, it's important for nurses to recognize the spectrum of gender and the difference between that and sexuality. Transgender refers to individuals who do not identify with the sex they were assigned at birth, while cisgender is defined as having a gender identity which parallels the sex you were assigned at birth (World Professional Association for Transgender Health, 2018). Practitioners must incorporate the gender spectrum into practice versus the two-sided binary that lingers in many settings. Transgender individuals may identify at any point on the spectrum and not just at the masculine or feminine ends of the scale. Gender nonconforming is a term used to describe those who don't necessarily identify with male or female but whose identity differs from what the cultural norms tell us it should be. Assessment of violence is a priority in the health care settings by all clinicians who practice in those settings. Identification of cultural values related to violence is integral to a quality assessment (Amar, Stockbridge, & Bess, 2008).

Sexuality is not necessarily associated with one's gender identity. Sexuality is not how we identify with the sex we were assigned at birth, but is a representation of what we are attracted to, physically or sexually, in an intimate manner. Sexuality may be fluid, as maybe one's gender, however the one does not dictate the other. One must also attend to the fact that while we discuss the culture of identification, even between the LGBTQ communities there are cultural differences which are now being defined.

Due to the prevalence of sexual violence among this culture, forensic nurses should review their practices to ensure the settings we work in are not only safe for all individuals, and offer a welcoming environment to disclose and receive treatment. While the self-report of sexual assault is low in the general population, those numbers are even lower in the LGBTQ communities. They not only experience bias within the general community, they also are suspect of the kind of care they might receive if reporting having been sexually assaulted. Will they be further victimized?

Campina-Bacote stresses the importance of understanding the process of cultural competence involving cultural awareness, skill, knowledge, and encounters (Campinha-Bacote, 2003). Examples of where we can address these processes: cultural awareness (understanding gender differences), skill (how to incorporate the implications of those cultural differences), knowledge (understanding the interactions of cultural backgrounds), and encounters (analyzing the communication within a cultural environment). Workplaces should begin with education and look at standards that can be implemented to ensure all staff receives training on the culture of gender, including safety and inclusiveness. The use of advocates should be encouraged in order to provide support for the victim throughout the exam and after as the victim traverses the legal system, while also ensuring that advocates are trained in cultural sensitivity. For instance, what are on the forms and documents in your setting? Are there checkboxes for male and female with no alternative or do you have a line for gender to be more inclusive? In some programs, gender-neutral trauma grams have been adopted, while still keeping detailed anatomical diagrams for documenting genital exams. If we were to explore all health care settings at this time (October of 2018), how many of these settings will have addressed the *current* view of gender and sexuality? How many health care clinicians are knowledgeable in this area?

It is important to ensure that patients are respected and their correct pronouns are used. Regardless of what is on their identification, staff should ask patients how they identify and what pronoun they would like used to decrease dysphoria and affirm their gender role (Donald & Ehrenfeld, 2015). Having a spot on electronic medical records or the patient's chart for the name they go by is also important. Many individuals who identify as transgender may not go by the name listed on their identification. Does this impact the ways we view culture within community? How could it not?

Other areas to consider are how your sexual assault clinic or program is perceived in the community. This is an opportunity to look at what images portray your service. Are they mostly heterosexual or all females? If so, this may not appear to be a welcoming space to others not portrayed. It may be useful to indicate in brochures and patient information that your program sees all genders, as opposed to saying male and female.

Lastly, it is imperative that examiners keep in mind what the goal of service is when assessing gender minorities after sexual assault. What health information is crucial to the visit? Ensure any questions being asked of the patient are medically necessary and not overly curious for nonmedical or forensic reasons. For example, it may not be relevant to ask if someone has had gender affirming surgery if they sexual assault was oral and genitals were not involved. Respect and open communication is key. Examiners should also be sensitive when conducting a health or forensic history with gender minorities. Sometimes using terms that are associated with one gender may cause discomfort. For example when asking about menstruation in transgender males (who are assigned female at birth), it may be more sensitive to ask the patient if they still bleed every month in contrast to asking if they get a period every month. This concept is similar when talking about genital anatomy. Although we may need to identify the correct anatomical location of the assault at one point in the history, of assault during the exam one may be refer to that genital area simply as the patient's bottom when the examination starts. This may cause less dysphoria than repeatedly saying vagina to a patient who is dysphoric about this body part.

The important message to take away when considering the evolving culture(s) of the LGBTQ communities is that we must become knowledgeable about each of the LGBTQ cultures as well as to self-reflect on our own understanding or biases regarding gender differences and sexual preferences. If we find that we cannot, then we must provide that patient with a culturally sensitive clinician and remove ourselves from that encounter.

## DISCUSSION

Forensic nursing provides important new expertise for the patient who is a victim of violence. However, that expertise must be grounded in cultural sensitivity in all settings. Whether it be in corrections, care of sexual assault patients, death investigation, advanced practice forensic nursing practice in the clinical settings, risk management, coroner, mitigation specialist, forensic nurse consultant, or any other area of forensic practice. Both the culture of a person's background (race, nationality, religion, etc.) must be understood as well as their gender and environment. We should *ask* the person about their cultural preferences, not guess what they are. And then we can self-reflect on our own culture and our cultural biases. Only by doing this can we then provide optimal care to all patients and provide a safe and welcoming space for victims and perpetrators to present.

We have presented only two areas of forensic nursing practice in which we discuss cultural implications within both of those settings. However, the tenets that we put forward in both of these settings can be applied in other forensic settings. What is most important is that we recognize our own biases regarding any forensic population with whom we work and then commit to understanding the culture of the *other*. By doing so we can improve our own practice as well as provide more optimal care to all forensic patients.

## REFERENCES

Amar, A. F., Stockbridge, J., & Bess, R. (2008). Global voices on gender-based violence. *Journal of Forensic Nursing, 4*(4), 182–184.

American Nurses Association. (2009). *Scope and standards of clinical nursing practice*. Silver Spring, MD: American Nurses Publishing.

American Nurses Association. (2017). Forensic Nursing: Scope and Standards of Practice. In The American Nurses Association (Ed.). (2nd ed., pp. 171). Silver Spring, MD: American Nurses Association, International Association of Forensic Nurses.

Black, J. L. (2014). *Owlcation*. Retrieved from https://owlcation.com/social-sciences/psychological-Cultural-Differences-Sexual-Identity-Gender-Identity-and-Sexual-Orientation

Campinha-Bacote, J. (2002). The process of cultural competence in the delivery of healthcare services: A model of care. *Journal of Transcultural Nursing, 13*(3), 181–184; discussion 200–181. http://dx.doi.org/10.1177/10459602013003003

Campinha-Bacote, J. (2003). Cultural desire: the key to unlocking cultural competence. *Journal of Nursing Education, 42*(6), 239–240.

Donald, C., & Ehrenfeld, J. M. (2015). The opportunity for medical systems to reduce health disparities among lesbian, gay, bisexual, transgender and intersex patients. *Journal of Medical Systems, 39*(11). doi:10.1007/s10916-015-0355-7

Foucault, M. (1991). *Discipline and punish: The birth of a prison*. London: Penguin.

Gaventa, J. (2003). Power after Lukes: An overview of theories of power since Lukes and their application to development. Brighton: Participation Group, Institute of Development Studies. https:www.powercube.net/wp-content/uploads/2009/11/power_after_lukes.pdf

Giger, J. N., & Davidhizar, R. (2002). The Giger and Davidhizar Transcultural Assessment Model. *Journal of Transcultural Nursing, 13*(3), 185–188; discussion 200–181. http://dx.doi.org/10.1177/10459602013003004

Holmes, D. (2005). Governing the captives: Forensic psychiatric nursing in corrections. *Perspectives in Psychiatric Care, 41*(1), 3–13.

Holmes, D., & Federman, C. (2003). Killing for the state: the darkest side of American nursing. *Nursing Inquiry, 10*(1), 2–10.

Holmes, D., Perron, A., & Michaud, G. (2007). Nursing in corrections: lessons from France. *Journal of Forensic Nursing, 3*(3–4), 126–131.

Jacob, J. D., Holmes, D., & Buus, N. (2008). Humanism in forensic psychiatry: the use of the tidal nursing model. *Nursing Inquiry, 15*(3), 224–230. http://dx.doi.org/10.1111/j.1440-1800.2008.00420.x

Leininger, M. (2002). Culture care theory: A major contribution to advance transcultural nursing knowledge and practices. *Journal of Transcultural Nursing, 13*(3), 189–192; discussion 200–181. http://dx.doi.org/10.1177/10459602013003005

Leininger, M., & McFarland, M. R. (2002). *Transcultural nursing: Concepts, theories, research and practice* (3rd ed.). New York, NY: McGraw Hill.

Purnell, L. (2002). The Purnell Model for Cultural Competence. *Journal of Transcultural Nursing, 13*(3), 193–196; discussion 200–191. http://dx.doi.org/10.1177/10459602013003006

Stotzer, R. L. (2009). Violence against transgender people: A review of United States data. . *Aggression and Violent Behavior, 14*(3), 170–179. http://dx.doi.org/10.1016/j.avb.2009.01.006

World Professional Association for Transgender Health. (2018). *Standards of care for the health of transexual, transgender, and gender nonconforming people*. Retrieved from https://www.wpath.org/publications/soc

Zoucha, R. (2006). Considering culture in understanding interpersonal violence. *Journal of Forensic Nursing, 2*(4), 195–196.

# Index

NOTE: Page references followed by *f* and *t* denote figures and tables, respectively.